WHAT PEOPLE WITH DIABETES ARE SAYING ABOUT
28 DAYS TO DIABETES CONTROL!

A valuable and essential reference tool on how to best manage diabetes.

> —Lisa Yourman, mother of 13-year-old
> extreme athlete Sarah Yourman

Whether you are newly diagnosed or have lived with diabetes for 42 years, as I have, you will use this book long after your 28-day program is over. Keep it by your side to help you take good care of your diabetes.

> —Judith Jones Ambrosini, Healthy Living
> Writer, Diabetes Exercise & Sports
> Association board member, and author of
> "Judith's Cyber Kitchen" at diabetesnet.com

The key to managing diabetes is to learn as much about it as possible. Lance Porter's book is the perfect place to start.

> —Kris Freeman, Under-23 World Champion
> Cross Country Skier

An extremely helpful, straightforward book for all of us diagnosed with diabetes who wondered, "What do I do now?" Diabetes doesn't have to mean we give things up; we just have to learn how to be more organized, and Lance tells us how.

> —Midge Cross, member of the 2002 Ford
> Expedition to Everest

This book actually motivates you to make positive changes and remain positive even if you don't accomplish all your goals.

—Jamie Dillinger, RN, Diabetes Nurse
Specialist

An effective guide to help those of us with diabetes get better control quickly. I highly recommend this valuable resource.

—Will Cross, Arctic Explorer

This book is one small step to understanding diabetes control and one giant leap toward developing a proven strategy for a high-quality life free of diabetes complications.

—Bill King, Marathon Runner and DCCT
Study Participant

A long, healthy life is something you can get by following the plan in 28 Days to Diabetes Control! *A fantastic book. I wish it had been available years ago!*

—Ozzie Roberts, 85-year-old World Traveler

So much relevant and useful information for the newly diagnosed or veteran—at home or under the light of a headlamp in a tent at 20,000 feet!

—David Panofsky, Mountain Climber

28 DAYS TO

LOWER YOUR BLOOD SUGAR,
IMPROVE YOUR HEALTH,
AND REDUCE YOUR RISK OF
DIABETES COMPLICATIONS

DIABETES CONTROL!

LANCE PORTER

Editor-in-Chief of *Diabetes Positive!* magazine
Foreword by Michael Heile, M.D.

M. Evans and Company, Inc.
New York

M. Evans and Company, Inc.
216 East 49th Street
New York, NY 10017

Library of Congress Cataloging-in Publication Data

Porter, Lance.
   28 days to diabetes control! : lower your blood sugar, improve your
health, and reduce your risk of diabetes complications / Lance Porter ;
foreword by Michael Heile.
       p. cm.
   ISBN 1-59077-041-2 (paperback)
   1. Diabetes--Popular works. 2. Diabetes--Treatment--Popular works.
I. Title: Twenty-eight days to diabetes control!. II. Title.
   RC660.4.P677 2004
   616.4'6206--dc22
                                    2003022769

CONTENTS

PART TWO: 28 DAYS TO DIABETES CONTROL!

PART THREE: RESOURCES

FOREWORD

I was very honored when Lance Porter asked me to write this foreword for his book.

I first met Lance when he interviewed me for an article in *Diabetes Positive!* magazine. He contacted me because I was someone who knew diabetes both as a practicing physician and as a person with diabetes. I am a family practicioner in Cincinnati, Ohio, with a special interest in the care of people with diabetes (especially those who require insulin). And I have type 1 diabetes myself.

During that interview, Lance asked me questions not only about diabetes in general but also about the care of the diabetic patient. I was very impressed by his intense and genuine interest in understanding the dynamics of this disease—as well as its psychological impact on the patient. He had a degree of understanding you usually only see in someone with diabetes or in the loved one of a patient with diabetes. (Later, I learned that his father was diagnosed with type 2 diabetes years ago.) His questions and interest went much deeper than needed to write the story of my own personal success with diabetes. It was his intense interest and his tireless study that enabled him to write this phenomenal book.

When you read *28 Days to Diabetes Control!* you will see that Lance not only understands the treatment of diabetes, but also the art and empathy needed to empower those of us who have this complicated disease with the ability to control it. Beyond a shadow of a doubt, this book gets to the heart of common sense diabetes care that is critical to achieving control. It offers a very specific and practical approach to people with both types of diabetes.

28 Days to Diabetes Control! also offers important general health information for nondiabetics and people concerned about their potential to become diabetic. It is an *essential* guide for anyone who has a friend or family member with diabetes. I also recommend this to my fellow physicians and other health-care professionals who need to build more successful diabetes strategies and management plans for their patients.

I know from personal experience how hard diabetes is to control. I was diagnosed with juvenile-onset diabetes at the age of 21, just prior to graduation from college.

The standards of diabetes care then were very different than they are today. The insulin and dietary plan I was given was nearly impossible to follow. Even when it was followed perfectly, it was often unsuccessful. I thought my life was over. Through medical school, my sugars were horrendous on twice-daily injections. I was on a roller-coaster: my sugars were either 40 or 300. There was no such thing as a planned or predictable healthy meal while working 48-72 hour shifts at the hospital.

But the best advice my diabetes doctors offered was going back for dietary training.

Finally, after some persuasion, my primary care doctor allowed me to switch to multiple daily injections (often five or six) with insulin for meals, so that my life did not revolve around my insulin doses. This helped to some degree—but going into residency with diabetes was a nightmare. I remember running to code (resuscitate) a patient in the middle of the night at the hospital and bottoming out my blood sugars while giving chest compressions. Although it never happened, I feared it was inevitable that the coder (me) was going to "get coded" for low-sugar coma/seizures. As you can imagine, I was very concerned that my diabetes would affect my ability to be a dependable physician. I remember worrying every moment about what my blood sugar was and what it was going to do.

Before graduating residency, about seven years ago, I discovered the insulin pump. At that time, not many doctors knew much about the insulin pump—although it had been available for years. To me, it looked like the most natural way to administer insulin for tighter control and a better lifestyle. But again, my diabetes doctors were reluctant to approve a change (most likely out of lack of knowledge about this type of therapy).

After more persuasion, I convinced my residency professor to help me get on the pump. That was a momentous day! The roller-coaster of ups and downs and crazy feeling totally went away. I was able to get more predictable blood sugars for the first time. On that day everything calmed down and a sense of stability came over me. I got back the part of my life that poorly controlled diabetes had taken away.

During this period, researchers discovered that tight control of diabetes meant fewer long-term complications. Balancing your diet, exercise, and medications to control diabetes—as Lance shows you how to do in this book—does pay off!

Medical science has come light-years in the treatment of diabetes since I was first diagnosed. Today you don't have to learn how to control your diabetes through years of trial and error. You *can* take the bull by the horns and control this difficult disease. If you're newly diagnosed, *28 Days to Diabetes Control!* will get you off to an outstanding start. If you've been struggling with diabetes control for years, you will find the answers you've been searching for here. Enjoy your 28-day program and remember: control this disease or it will control you!

–Michael Heile, M.D.

Editor's note: In addition to practicing medicine and controlling his diabetes, Dr. Heile is a marathon runner and a gifted singer/songwriter who performs regularly in the Cincinnati area.

INTRODUCTION

YES, YOU CAN LIVE A LONG, HEALTHY, FANTASTIC LIFE WITH DIABETES!

According to the U.S. Department of Health and Human Services, there are 18.2 million people with diabetes in the United States. You are probably reading this book because you—or someone you love—just became part of that statistic.

You're probably not too happy about it. Learning that you have diabetes is not *good* news. But it's not as bad as you may think. It's not the end of the world, and it doesn't have to compromise your life. You can't *ignore* diabetes. But you don't have to be stopped by it. Read this book, discuss it with your doctor or diabetes educator, and then get with the program! Get your diabetes under control, and you can live out any dream you had before you were diagnosed.

The two absolutely essential things you must know about this disease are:

▶ One, that diabetes is *very serious*. Don't take it lightly! Diabetes can cause blindness, amputation, kidney failure, nerve damage, heart attack, stroke, and, ultimately, death.

▶ Two, that none of the devastating complications of diabetes is *inevitable*. Keeping your diabetes under control can help to prevent them. If you learn to maintain your blood sugar at normal or near-normal levels, you may *never* experience any of the complications of diabetes.

An important secondary benefit is that you will *feel* better. Keeping your diabetes under control will give you more energy, help you think more clearly, and improve your performance at school, at work, and at play.

The 28-day program in this book is designed to get you started on the right foot. It will help you understand how three key factors affect your blood sugar levels: food, exercise, and medication. And it gives you a simple, effective, easy-to-follow program that shows you how to *use* those three factors to keep your blood sugars at normal or near-normal levels.

HOW TO USE THIS BOOK

Diabetes is a complicated disease, and before you can control it, there are certain things you need to know.

The first step is to read Part One. Part One of this book provides you with the key information you must have to control diabetes. Although it is concise, it is comprehensive—everything you really need to know is there.

The second step is to *learn by doing*. That's what you'll do in Part Two of this book, which is the 28-day program itself. You can't learn how to control diabetes just by reading about it. Because everyone's diabetes is different, even your doctor can't tell you *exactly* what to do to bring your blood sugar down to normal or near-normal levels. You have to figure out for yourself how to balance your exercise, diet, and (if you use them) medications or insulin. The structured, practical 28-day program will help you work that out as efficiently as possible, with journal pages provided for each day, allowing you to record all the factors that affect your blood sugar levels. The instructions that come with each journal page explain how to analyze the information you're recording and make changes to get better results every day.

When you complete the 28-day program you will be the world's leading expert on *your own diabetes.* You will know precisely how the foods you eat and the exercise you do—along with your insulin or medications, if you use them—affect your blood sugar levels. You will have the knowledge and skills to control your diabetes and *keep* your diabetes under control for the rest of your life.

What should you do after that? Live your life! Do whatever you planned to do before you were diagnosed. Or make new plans, take new paths, dream new dreams—and make them come true. *You can do it!*

Let's get started.

PART ONE:

WHAT YOU MUST KNOW BEFORE YOU BEGIN YOUR PROGRAM

CHAPTER 1

WHAT IS DIABETES?

Diabetes is a chronic condition in which blood sugar (also called glucose) accumulates in your blood. The full name of the disease, *diabetes mellitus*, literally means "honey diabetes." Since the time of ancient Greece, people have noticed a sweet or honeyed smell in the urine of those affected by the disease.

There is no *cure* for diabetes. However, diabetes can be *controlled*. Controlling diabetes means keeping your blood sugar at levels that are the same as—or close to—those of a person who does not have diabetes.

There are two primary kinds of diabetes, and the *cause* of your elevated blood sugar depends on which kind of diabetes you have.

TYPE 1 DIABETES

Type 1 diabetes used to be called "juvenile diabetes," because it normally occurs in people under the age of 30. If you have type 1 diabetes, your pancreas no longer produces insulin, a vital hormone that helps your body turn sugar into energy. Without this essential hormone, the sugar in your system accumulates in your blood. Type 1 diabetes is considered to be an "auto-immune" disease. It occurs when the immune system mistakenly attacks the pancreas and destroys its ability to make insulin.

Although family history plays a role in the development of type 1 diabetes, 90 percent of the people who get it have no family history of the disease at all. No one knows for sure why it strikes some people and not others. People with type 1 diabetes have to take insulin to control their blood sugar.

TYPE 2 DIABETES

Type 2 diabetes used to be called "adult onset" because it normally occurs in people over the age of 30. Type 2 diabetes is more likely if you have a family history of diabetes. It is closely related to excess weight and a lack of physical activity. African-Americans, Latinos, Pacific Islanders, Asians, and Native Americans are all at high risk for type 2 diabetes.

Although type 2 diabetes normally strikes people over the age of 30, it is on the rise among children. Experts think this is directly related to a lack of physical activity and the increase in obesity among the young.

If you have type 2 diabetes, your pancreas still makes insulin. But it may not make enough, or your body may have become resistant to it. The first line of treatment for type 2 diabetes is exercise and weight loss—many people can control their blood sugar levels with exercise and diet alone. There are also oral medications that can be used to treat the disease. Type 2 diabetes tends to be progressive, and a substantial number of people with type 2 diabetes ultimately need to take insulin to control their blood sugar.

Of the two types of diabetes, type 2 is by far more common. Between 90 percent and 95 percent of all cases of diabetes in the United States are type 2, and the incidence of type 2 diabetes is increasing at an alarming rate, driven by our increasing weight and increasingly inactive, computer-focused lifestyles.

In a way, type 2 is the more dangerous of the two types of diabetes. Type 1 is impossible to ignore. If you have type 1 diabetes and you ignore it even for a few days, you wind up in the hospital. But type 2 often starts slowly. At first, your pancreas may still be making a fairly good amount of insulin, or you may only have mild insulin resistance, and your blood sugar levels may only be slightly elevated. If you ignore it, nothing catastrophic happens *immediately*. So some people with type 2 diabetes are less stringent about caring for their diabetes than people with type 1. But with any type of diabetes, ignorance is not bliss. Take care of it right from the start, or the results *will* be catastrophic in time.

GESTATIONAL DIABETES

In addition to type 1 and type 2 diabetes, there is a third kind of diabetes which is unique in that it is usually temporary: *gestational diabetes*. Gestational diabetes affects up to 4 percent of all pregnant women. Experts estimate that there are between 100,000 and 135,000 cases of gestational diabetes in the United States each year.

Risk factors for gestational diabetes include:

▶ The mother's age (older mothers are more likely to get gestational diabetes than younger mothers)

▶ Obesity

▶ Family history of type 2 diabetes

▶ Ethnic background: African-Americans, Hispanics, Native Americans, and Asians are at high risk

▶ Gestational diabetes in a previous pregnancy

▶ History of delivering a baby heavier than nine pounds at birth

The prevalence of gestational diabetes in certain high-risk groups can be as high as 14 percent.

Women are usually screened for gestational diabetes at the end of their second trimester of pregnancy, roughly 24–26 weeks after conception.

It is very important to take gestational diabetes seriously, because it has the potential to harm both the mother and baby. When you have gestational diabetes, your pancreas is working overtime to produce insulin, but the insulin does not bring your blood sugar down to normal levels. Insulin does not cross the placenta, but the extra sugar in your blood does. Since the baby is getting more energy than it needs to grow and develop, the extra energy is stored as fat. This can lead to a fat baby, which risks damage to the shoulders at birth. Additionally, the newborn may have very low blood sugar at birth and be at risk for breathing problems. Fat babies become children who are at risk for obesity and adults who are at risk for type 2 diabetes.

The treatment for gestational diabetes is exactly the same as for type 1 or type 2 diabetes: keeping your blood sugar at the same level as a mother who does not have diabetes, or as close to it as possible. In many cases, this can be accomplished by diet and exercise alone. In fact, nutrition and lifestyle management is the only treatment necessary for up to 75 percent of women with gestational diabetes. If that doesn't adequately control their blood sugar, insulin may be used as well.

Women who have gestational diabetes once are at high risk to have the same problem again in later pregnancies. They are also at higher risk of developing type 2 diabetes later in life. So experts strongly recommend that you take this experience as a warning, and do everything you can to return to a normal weight after pregnancy and make regular physical exercise part of your daily routine for the rest of your life.

In some cases, gestational diabetes turns out to not be pregnancy-related at all. Instead, it is possible that you had either type 1 or type 2 diabetes that just happened to be caught by the gestational diabetes screening that is routinely given to women around the 26th week of their pregnancies. In that case, of course, your diabetes will not go away when you deliver your baby. That's why it is essential that women with gestational diabetes be tested six weeks after delivery to make sure their blood sugar has returned to normal.

CHAPTER 2

DIABETES SYMPTOMS AND DIAGNOSIS

Diabetes is a tricky disease. Sometimes the symptoms are unmistakable. In other cases, a person can have diabetes for years and never show any signs of it.

SYMPTOMS

Some of the classic symptoms of diabetes include:

▸ Unusual thirst

▸ Having to urinate frequently

▸ Sudden or unexplained weight loss

▸ Unusual hunger

▸ Fatigue

▸ Mood swings and irritability

▸ Frequent skin, gum, or bladder infections

▸ Blurred vision

▸ Numbness or tingling in the extremities

▸ Cuts or bruises that are slow to heal

The symptoms of diabetes normally go away completely as soon as you get your blood sugar under control.

DIAGNOSIS

Diagnosing diabetes is a very simple procedure. Diabetes means "elevated blood sugar," and your doctor diagnoses it with a blood sugar test. The "gold standard" is a test of your blood sugar level after an eight-hour fast. The easiest time to do it is in the morning before you have anything to eat or drink. Normal people have fasting blood sugar levels below 100 mg/dL (milligrams per deciliter). A value between 100 and 125 mg/dL indicates that you have what is called "impaired fasting glucose," or pre-diabetes. A value of 126 mg/dL or higher indicates that you have diabetes. Your doctor may repeat the test just to make sure.

CHAPTER 3

FIVE ESSENTIAL FIRST STEPS

If you were just diagnosed with diabetes, your mind is probably spinning and your emotions are probably on a roller-coaster ride. But take heart! You're going to be just fine. Diabetes is *not* a death sentence. Now is the time to keep a cool head and put together a practical program to keep this disease in control. In addition to following the program outlined in this book, here are some other essential steps you need to follow to get your diabetes under control—and get on with your life.

ASSEMBLE A GOOD MEDICAL TEAM

Because diabetes can affect your health in a variety of ways, the best way to treat it is by assembling a health-care *team*. Ideally, your team should include:

Your primary physician. Everyone with diabetes needs to be in the care of a capable physician. *But it doesn't necessarily have to be the person who diagnosed your diabetes.* You're going to be seeing your doctor at least three or four times a year, and you'll be relying on this physician to recommend the other members of your health-care team. So find someone you like, trust, and are comfortable with. Don't settle for just anyone. Find a doctor who has *experience treating patients with diabetes* and is willing and able to take the time to listen to your concerns and answer your questions.

Make sure your doctor keeps up with the latest developments in diabetes treatment. Diabetes care is rapidly evolving, and unless your doctor keeps up with the latest advances, you may not get the quality of care you deserve and need. If your doctor doesn't take care of a lot of people with diabetes, you may be better off with an endocrinologist—a doctor who has advanced training in dealing with diabetes and other hormone-related diseases—or a diabetologist, a specialist who only takes care of people with diabetes.

It's your health that's at stake here. If your doctor doesn't help you get your blood sugar levels at near-normal levels in short order, do not be afraid to change doctors until you find one who will!

A certified diabetes educator. Ideally, in addition to your physician, you'll also want to see a certified diabetes educator. A diabetes educator will teach you the practical techniques of dealing with diabetes, including how to take your insulin or other medicine, how to measure your blood glucose levels, and much more. Your doctor may recommend an educator, or you can call the American Association of Diabetes Educators at 800-832-6874.

A registered dietitian. Eating the right diet is a critical part of diabetes therapy. Your certified diabetes educator can answer many of your questions about diet, but you may also want to see a registered dietitian. Again, your doctor may recommend one who works with people with diabetes. Or you can call the American Dietetic Association at 800-366-1655.

An ophthalmologist. Because diabetes can damage the eyes, you will definitely want an ophthalmologist (an eye doctor) on your health-care team.

Experts recommend that people with type 1 diabetes get a *dilated retinal examination* once a year, starting five years after the onset of diabetes. People with type 2 diabetes should have a yearly dilated retinal examination starting *immediately* after diagnosis—because type 2 diabetes is often not diagnosed until you have had the disease for many years. (Many people first learn they have diabetes when their ophthalmologist finds diabetic retinopathy during a routine eye exam.) Women with gestational diabetes are particularly at risk for diabetic retinopathy, and some experts recommend that they have their eyes examined every three months during their pregnancy.

Early detection is the key. Much can be done to prevent and treat diabetic eye disease. The sooner your ophthalmologist spots it, the better job he or she can do of stopping it.

A dentist. One of the complications of diabetes is dental problems, including cavities and gum disease. When diabetes is poorly controlled, the levels of sugar in your saliva are just as high as in your blood, and that causes tooth decay. High blood sugar levels also damage the blood vessels in your mouth, reducing the flow of oxygen and nutrients to the gum tissues and weakening their resistance to infection.

Your best defense against dental complications is good diabetes control. Keep your blood sugar levels at normal levels, and you're not likely to have any more dental problems than someone who does not have diabetes.

But it doesn't hurt to practice good dental hygiene! Brush your teeth twice a day, and floss to get at plaque between your teeth that the brush can't reach. Replace your brush often. See your dentist regularly. And have your teeth professionally cleaned at least every six months.

A podiatrist (foot doctor). If you have circulatory problems or nerve damage in your feet, you will also want to see a podiatrist. Even if you don't have problems, it's a good idea to visit the podiatrist every year to make sure everything is fine.

People with diabetes—especially if it is poorly controlled—often experience some degree of diabetic neuropathy, the impairment or damage of nerve function due to increased blood sugars. This can result in tingling, burning, or numbness in the hands or—even more frequently—the feet. It can also result in a decreased ability to feel pain, especially in the extremities.

The way to prevent neuropathy is to control your blood sugar levels. Good diabetes control has been proven to *dramatically* decrease your risk of neuropathy.

In any case, be sure to visually inspect your feet every day. Make sure you don't have a cut or blister you're not able to feel. It's important to take care of any kind of injury to the foot right away, because foot injuries in people with diabetes can be very hard to heal.

STEP TWO:

LEARN EVERYTHING YOU CAN ABOUT DIABETES

People with diabetes manage their own health. Your doctor and the rest of your health-care team will help, of course. But, day-to-day, *you* must administer your own treatment. Your medical team can *help* you get your diabetes under control. But only *you* can actually do it. It's generally accepted that 5 percent of diabetes care is up to your doctor, and 95 percent is up to you.

So read up! Do the research. Find out all you can about diabetes—so you can deal with it *effectively*. Reading this book is absolutely the best place to start.

Check out the diabetes magazines, too. Diabetes care is constantly changing. Important new products that can help you control your diabetes come on the market virtually every month. You would be wise to subscribe to at least one magazine to keep up with the latest advances. Good choices include *Diabetes Positive!*, *Diabetes Interview*, *Diabetes Self-Management*, and *Diabetes Forecast*.

It also helps to surf the Web. The American Diabetes Association has a Web site, as do many other organizations that can help you live well in spite of the challenge that diabetes represents. Almost all of the major manufacturers of diabetes medicines, supplies, equipment, and insulin also have their own sites, many of which are very helpful.

STEP THREE:

PREPARE

Prepare yourself, both physically and mentally, to deal with this new challenge. Gather the supplies you need, including your insulin or any other drugs your physician may have prescribed, and a blood glucose meter. Make a plan. Decide when you're going to exercise and what you're going to eat.

STEP FOUR:

MAINTAIN A POSITIVE ATTITUDE

Your long-term health depends on maintaining a positive attitude as much as anything else.

If you think you are depressed, tell your doctor right away. Depression is nothing to be ashamed of—people with diabetes suffer from depression at a rate two to four times higher than the general population. The key is to do something about it! Professional counseling, support groups, and antidepressant medicines can all help you get back on track. Exercise is also a highly effective antidepressant.

For fighting off everyday garden-variety blahs and generally keeping your chin up, positive thinking techniques—visualization, positive self-talk, affirmations, relaxation, and meditation—can be tremendously helpful. Now is the time to start learning about them.

STEP FIVE:

ACCEPT THE SITUATION, AND GET STARTED ON YOUR NEW LIFE

The people who do best with diabetes are those who, first of all, accept it. They take positive steps to deal with it. And then *they get on with their lives.* They feel they have a mission, a purpose, a reason for living. They feed their minds a steady diet of positive thoughts. They love, they work, they laugh, they play, they plan for the future and live their lives, just like anybody else.

Your diabetes and your health are completely under your control. Take good care of yourself and you'll live a long, happy, healthy life!

CHAPTER 4

NORMAL BLOOD SUGAR = LESS CHANCE OF COMPLICATIONS

Whatever type of diabetes you have, the most important single fact you can know is this: the closer you keep your blood sugar to normal levels, the less chance you will have of ever experiencing any of the complications of diabetes.

Even though that statement seems like common sense, and many people suspected as much for years, we didn't know *for a fact* how important close control of diabetes was until recently.

WHAT YOU MUST KNOW ABOUT THE DIABETES CONTROL AND COMPLICATIONS TRIAL (DCCT) AND THE UNITED KINGDOM PROSPECTIVE DIABETES STUDY (UKPDS)

The two studies that proved conclusively how important it is to keep your blood sugar close to normal were the Diabetes Control and Complications Trial and the United Kingdom Prospective Diabetes Study.

The Diabetes Control and Complications Trial (usually just called the DCCT), conducted from 1983 to 1993 by the National Institute of Diabetes and Digestive and Kidney Diseases, was, at the time, the most comprehensive diabetes study ever. It involved 1,441 volunteers with type 1 diabetes at 29 medical centers in the United States and Canada. This study compared the effects of two treatment regimens—*standard therapy* (typically, one or two shots of insulin a day) and *intensive control*—on the complications of diabetes. Participants in the intensive control arm of this study tested their blood sugar levels four or more times a day and took four daily insulin injections or used an insulin pump. They adjusted their insulin dose according to food intake and exercise, followed a diet and exercise plan, and met with their health-care team monthly.

The results: *Intensive control reduced the risk of eye disease by 76 percent. It reduced the risk of kidney disease by 50 percent. And it reduced the risk of nerve disease by 60 percent.*

Although the DCCT focused on people with type 1 diabetes, its findings were confirmed by an even larger study called the United Kingdom Prospective Diabetes Study (UKPDS), which compared conventional and intensive therapy in more than 5,000 newly diagnosed people with type 2 diabetes.

The UKPDS confirmed that reducing blood sugar levels dramatically reduces the risk of complications in people with type 2 diabetes. It also found that controlling blood pressure, among those with diabetes whose blood pressure is high, dramatically reduces the risk of diabetes complications—especially the risk of strokes and vision damage.

Make no mistake: keeping your diabetes under control greatly reduces your risk of all the major complications of diabetes, and can help you live a long, healthy, *fantastic* life.

CHAPTER 5

TESTING YOUR BLOOD SUGAR

It wasn't so long ago that the only way to check your blood sugar was to mix a few drops of urine with Benedict's Solution, which changes color in the presence of sugar when it is heated. The color the solution changed to gave you a very rough estimate of your blood sugar.

Even as recently as the 1970s, the standard way to check blood sugar was only slightly more sophisticated. Test strips were available that reacted with urine immediately, eliminating the need for mixing and heating a solution. But the result was essentially the same: the test strips turned color depending on the amount of sugar in your urine. By comparing the resulting color with a color chart, you got a rough idea of whether your blood sugar was low, normal, or high.

Today, blood glucose monitors give a digital readout of

blood sugar levels in a matter of seconds, with a single droplet of blood. More than any other single innovation in this disease, the invention and use of these awesome monitors make the tight control of diabetes possible. Make no mistake, the simplest blood glucose monitor on the market today is nothing less than a medical miracle.

CHOOSING A MONITOR

A blood glucose monitor is the one essential tool that every person with diabetes *must have* to keep their blood glucose levels under control. It's such an important tool that we review all the available monitors in *Diabetes Positive!* magazine every June and December. The pace of innovation in the development of new blood glucose monitors is fantastic, with six to eight new ones appearing every year.

When picking out a monitor, here are some key features to look for.

Alternate site testing. As recently as three or four years ago, all blood glucose monitors required you to prick your fingertip for the drop of blood the test requires. But now there are monitors that allow you to use "alternate sites"—that is, sites other than the fingertip—for your blood sample. The most common and most frequently used of these alternate sites is the forearm. Your forearm has fewer nerve endings than your fingers do. So forearm testing, for most people, is much less painful. Other alternate sites may include the palm, upper arm, thigh, or calf, but the forearm is the one most people use.

Because there are differences in the amount of muscle and fat found in different parts of your body, it may be possible to test in two different places at the same time and get two different results. This happens most often when your blood sugar levels are rapidly changing: after a meal, after an insulin dose, or after exercise. Changes in blood sugar tend to show up more quickly in a fingertip sample than a sample taken from the forearm. For that reason, experts recommend that you use the fingertip when you're testing less than two hours after a meal, after an insulin dose, after physical exercise, or at any other time you feel that your blood sugar may be rapidly changing. Testing on the forearm is fine when you're testing first thing in the morning, before a meal, or before exercise. "Alternate site" monitors give you that option.

Speed. Another factor you might want to consider is how long the monitor takes to compute a reading. The monitors on the market today take between five and 45 seconds to compute a reading. That may not seem like a wide range, but there's a big difference between waiting 45 seconds for your reading and waiting five seconds, especially when you're testing frequently. It's not hard to see why most people choose faster monitors.

Sample size. By and large, monitors that are approved for "alternate site" testing use much less blood than those that are approved for fingertip testing only. Although there are still monitors on the market that require a "full hanging drop" of blood, you'll probably be happier choosing one of the newer models that uses the "wicking" type test strip that requires only a tiny droplet of blood.

Meter memory. Whether a monitor records only the date, time, and results of a few dozen tests or it logs and presents months of diabetes information with onscreen charts, you'll need your blood sugar meter to have a good, easy-to-use memory. This function is especially important when you're trying to understand how your blood sugar is behaving over time.

Beyond those basic functions, you'll find monitors on the market with a dizzying array of features. Only you can decide which one is right for you!

HOW OFTEN TO TEST

According to the American Diabetes Association (ADA), most people with type 1 diabetes, and pregnant women taking insulin, should test three or more times a day. While there is no specific recommendation for people with type 2 diabetes, the ADA does recommend that you test as often as needed to reach your target blood sugar levels. Many health-care professionals encourage their patients with type 2 to test at least twice a day. It is also recommended that you record the results of every test, including the time the test was taken, and major factors that could have affected the results, especially information concerning insulin or medication, what you ate, and exercise.

Of course, there's nothing to keep you from testing *more* often than recommended. In fact, especially when you are newly diagnosed, frequent testing is the only way to know for a fact what's going on in your body. One of the most incredible people we ever profiled in *Diabetes Positive!* magazine is Ozzie Roberts, who is 85 years old, travels to the most remote regions of the world, and has never experienced *any* complications of diabetes. Even after 61 years with diabetes, Ozzie still tests *14 times a day!* As Ozzie says, he doesn't just want to know what his blood sugar *is*. He wants to know *what direction it is going in*, so he can head it off.

WHEN TO TEST

Excellent times to test your blood sugar include:

First thing in the morning, before you have anything to eat or drink. This test can tell you if you're staying at a safe blood sugar level overnight. If your levels are too low in the morning, you may have to reduce your insulin or medication, or have a bed-time snack.

Before lunch and dinner, to help you decide what and how much to eat, and also how much insulin or medication you should take.

Two hours after meals, to find out how what you ate has affected your blood sugar levels. You may find that certain foods cause an unacceptable spike in your blood sugar, for example, and you'll learn to avoid them.

Before exercise, to help avoid hypoglycemia (low blood sugar.) Exercise usually lowers your blood sugar level, so you don't want to exercise when your blood sugar is already low. Make sure your blood sugar is above 100 before you start exercising. Testing *after* exercise is also important, since the lowering effects of exercise sometimes don't kick in for hours.

When your insulin dosage or diabetes medication changes, to see how your body is reacting. More frequent testing is also recommended when you are ill, under stress, or making major changes in your daily routine.

THE SINGLE MOST IMPORTANT TIME TO TEST

Beyond doubt, the *single most important time* to test your blood sugar is just before you get behind the wheel of a car. When you're going for a drive, your short-term safety—and the safety of others on the road—is more important than your long-term blood sugar control. The Federal Aviation Administration requires pilots with diabetes to test their blood sugar before they fly, and to make sure it is at least 100. The same rule applies to driving—make sure your blood sugar is at least 100 before you get behind the wheel. If it is not, have a snack and test again before you turn the ignition key. If you're going for a long drive, be sure to take snacks with you, and test again every hour or so. One of the very first symptoms of low blood sugar is mental confusion, which can be fatal to you and to others when you are driving. So always test before you drive. No exceptions! Ever!

YOUR TARGET RANGE

What blood glucose level do you want to see when you test? Well, a normal blood sugar level *for someone without diabetes* is 70–110 mg/dL before a meal, and less than 120 two hours after a meal. Your doctor may set a slightly higher target range for you—typically from 90–120 mg/dL or 90–130 mg/dL before a meal, and less than 140 or 150 (some recommend 180) two hours after a meal, which is "near normal." To avoid the complications of diabetes, you don't want to let your blood sugar go too high. And to prevent problems with hypoglycemia (low blood sugar), you don't want it to go too low. Yes, it's a balancing act, but it's one you will master soon enough.

No matter how hard you try, you will not hit your target range 100 percent of the time. It can't be done. But keeping your *average* within range *is* possible. Even if you have the occasional bad day—and everybody does—your goal should be to keep your weekly averages in line with your doctor's recommendations.

If you test often enough and pay attention to what you eat, what you did, and what insulin or medication you took before testing, your blood glucose monitor will *teach you* exactly what you need to do to keep your blood sugar levels in a desirable range.

CHAPTER 6

UNDERSTANDING YOUR A1c

The blood glucose test you do at home tells you how much sugar is in your blood *at the moment it is tested*. There's another test available that tells you how much blood sugar has been in your bloodstream *on average* for the past three months. This test used to be called the Hemoglobin A1c or HbA1c test. Today it is simply called the A1c. A1c is the technical name for a component of hemoglobin that blood sugar binds to within your red blood cells. Once blood sugar binds with A1c it stays bound for the life of the cell, which is about three months. By measuring the amount of blood sugar bound to your A1c, laboratory technicians can get a very good reading of your average blood sugar levels for the past 90 days.

The DCCT and the UKPDS (see chapter 4) showed beyond a shadow of doubt that, for people with both type 1 and type 2 diabetes, the lower the A1c, the lower the risk of serious eye, kidney, and nerve disease. The studies also showed that any improvement in A1c levels can potentially reduce complications.

When calibrated to DCCT standards, an A1c reading of approximately 6.0 is considered to be the upper limit of the "normal" range. For many years, the American Diabetes Association has recommended that people with diabetes set themselves a goal of keeping their A1c below 7.0.

Recently, however, the American College of Endocrinology came out with a new set of recommendations. Their most important suggestion was that you set yourself a target of keeping your A1c below 6.5. Ask your doctor what target A1c is right for you.

Your A1c levels correlate very closely to your average blood glucose level. Knowing this relationship can help you decide the kind of targets you need to set for your home blood sugar tests to hit the A1c goal you're going for. The following table may help.

A1C	AVERAGE BLOOD GLUCOSE LEVEL		
4	NORMAL (NON-DIABETIC) LEVELS	60	MG/DL
5		90	MG/DL
6		120	MG/DL
7	ELEVATED LEVELS	150	MG/DL
8		180	MG/DL
9		210	MG/DL
10		240	MG/DL
11	SERIOUSLY ELEVATED LEVELS	270	MG/DL
12		300	MG/DL

The correlation between your average daily blood sugar reading and your A1c is why calculating the averages of your daily blood glucose readings is so important. If you're shooting for an A1c below 7, you need to keep your daily averages below 150 mg/dL. If you're shooting for an A1c of 6.5, you need to keep your daily averages below 135 mg/dL.

TESTING A1c AT HOME

In the past, the only way to check your A1c was at the doctor's office. Now, however, you can do it at home. A company called Metrika makes a disposable, pager-sized A1c monitor called the A1cNow that you can buy for $24.99 at any Walgreens drugstore at the time of this writing. The A1cNow gives you your A1c reading in just eight minutes, from a small drop of blood. No prescription is required.

KNOW YOUR A1c

A recent survey by the American Association of Diabetes Educators found that 75 percent of people with type 2 diabetes do not know their A1c number. That's shocking! What could be more important than knowing your A1c? It is the best available gauge of how well you're controlling your diabetes—and how much you are at risk for complications of the disease. If you haven't had your A1c tested in the past three months, run, don't walk, to your doctor's office or the nearest Walgreens to find out where you stand.

CHAPTER 7

WEIGHT CONTROL

The vast majority of people with type 2 diabetes are overweight. In fact, the fat in your body may be the *primary reason* you have diabetes. Fat is metabolically inactive and resistant to insulin. If you have the kind of diabetes primarily characterized by *insulin resistance*, your weight may be the cause of it. Weight loss, through diet and exercise, is one of the key goals of treatment for type 2 diabetes. Lose enough weight and you may be able to normalize your blood sugar levels without medication or insulin.

Losing weight isn't easy. If you've been overweight for many years, you may have convinced yourself that you *can't* lose weight. But you *can!* Here's the absolute truth: when you take in more calories than you burn up in the course of a day, you gain weight. But when you take in *fewer* calories than you burn up, you *lose* weight. This is a rule of nature, as certain as the rising and setting of the sun. It doesn't just work for *some* people. It doesn't just work for thin people. It works for *all* people.

There are two ways to make this law of nature work for you. One is to cut down on the calories you eat and drink. The other is to increase the amount of exercise you do to increase the number of calories you burn. Better still, do both at the same time.

STEPS TO CONTROL YOUR WEIGHT

To control your weight, the first step is to find out how many calories you're eating right now. To do this, you'll need to arm yourself with a book that gives the calorie counts of foods. There are several good ones available. *The Complete Book of Food Counts*, by Corinne T. Netzer (Dell), is one of the most comprehensive. For packaged foods, you can get the calorie count by checking the label. (Just be sure to notice that the calories given are *per serving*. Eat the whole package and you may be eating several servings!)

Then, start a food diary. It doesn't have to be anything fancy—an ordinary notebook or pad of paper will do. In this diary, write down what you eat and drink—every bite and every sip—and note how many calories you're getting. Total them up at the end of the day. On average, men need about 2,700 calories a day to maintain a healthy weight. Women need about 2,000. You may find that you're getting a lot more than that!

Don't set yourself up for failure by going on an extremely

low-calorie diet. For the first few days, it's best not to change the way you're eating at all. Just get in the habit of recording the calories you eat in your food diary.

After a few days, when you're comfortable keeping your food diary, start trying to reduce the number of calories you're getting gradually. Save 150 calories by drinking a bottle of water or a diet soda instead of a regular soda or fruit juice. Pass up your usual between-meals snack. Swear off french fries. Stop those midnight snacks. Make small changes and continue to keep your diary. Congratulate yourself on even modest reductions in the number of calories you're taking in. Even cutting a small number of calories makes a big difference over time. It takes 3,500 calories to make a pound of fat. Cut back 500 calories per day—or burn 500 more with exercise—and at the end of the week you *will* have lost a pound. Or—if you're still eating too much—at least you will have *avoided* gaining a pound!

Don't let your subconscious mind sabotage what you're doing. Remind yourself, over and over, how important it is to your diabetes control and your overall health for you to lose weight—and never doubt that you *can* do it. Tell yourself that you are a strong, self-disciplined person. Visualize the athlete inside you who is waiting to get out. Celebrate every bit of progress you make and rededicate yourself to making even more.

Above all, remember that if you are gaining weight, it is because you are eating more calories than you are burning up. Reverse that formula—burn more than you eat—and you absolutely, positively will lose weight.

CHAPTER 8

COUNTING CARBOHYDRATES

One of the most important skills anyone with diabetes can learn is "carbohydrate counting." Carbohydrates are foods that break down into sugars during digestion.

Why do we count carbohydrates and not protein or fat? Because carbohydrates have *by far* the greatest short-term impact on your blood sugar. Fat plays only a minor role in short-term blood sugar levels. Protein takes several hours to show up as blood sugar, so it also plays a very minor role in short-term blood sugar control. Carbohydrates are the key. For anyone with diabetes, counting carbohydrates is essential.

Carbohydrates can be found in:

▶ Grains—bread, pasta, cereal, and rice

▶ Fruits

▶ Vegetables

▶ Alcoholic beverages

▶ Cakes, cookies, and candies

▶ Milk and yogurt (but not cheese)

▶ Sugar, honey, corn syrup, and molasses

HOW TO COUNT CARBS

Carbohydrates are counted in *grams*. Grams are a unit of weight. Twenty-eight grams equal one ounce.

Some foods are almost entirely carbohydrate. Sugar and foods that are almost pure sugar—a lollipop or cotton candy—are easy to figure. Fifteen grams of table sugar is 15 grams of carbohydrate—simple as that.

But most foods are a mixture of nutrients. So how do you know how much of any given food is carbs? The easiest way is to read the label on the food package. The laws requiring that packaged foods be labeled for their nutritional content are a godsend for people with diabetes. An important note: as with calories, the carbs listed are not for the whole package, but just for one serving—and servings are often smaller than you would expect! Be sure to check the serving size. If you're eating two servings, double the carb count.

In addition, don't be confused if the package lists carbohydrates and sugars separately. The sugars are *included* in the carbohydrate number. Ignore the sugar listed on the package label. Sugars are included in the carb count.

For foods that are not packaged, like fresh fruits and vegetables, you'll need a book that lists the carb content of foods. One good choice is *Dr. Atkins' New Carbohydrate Gram Counter* (M. Evans).

CARBOHYDRATES AND INSULIN

If you take insulin, carbohydrate counting is essential to knowing how much insulin to take. You count the carbohydrates in a meal you are about to eat, and then adjust the amount of short-acting insulin you inject or the "bolus" on your insulin pump to "balance out" those carbohydrates as exactly as you can. When you do that, you're essentially doing what a healthy pancreas does automatically—releasing just the right amount of insulin to cover the carbohydrates you eat.

How much insulin you need to balance out a given amount of carbohydrate is determined by your *carbohydrate-to-insulin* ratio. Your diabetes health-care team can help you determine your own individual carbohydrate-to-insulin ratio—and experience will help you refine it. Checking your blood sugar regularly and keeping careful records of your carbohydrate intake, blood sugar levels, and insulin doses will soon show if the amount of insulin you're taking to cover your carbs is too much, too little—or just right.

If you have type 2 diabetes, counting and recording your carbohydrates is just as important for the same reason: because carbohydrates have the biggest effect on your blood sugars of all the foods you eat. Once you start counting carbs, it won't be long before you notice that eating certain foods causes your blood sugar to "spike," and that you can help keep your blood sugar in range by avoiding them. You will also discover foods you enjoy that you can eat plentifully without adversely affecting your blood sugar.

THE GLYCEMIC INDEX

All carbohydrates break down into sugar once you eat them. But they don't all break down into sugar *at the same rate*. Scientists refer to carbohydrates that break down into sugar very rapidly as having a "high glycemic index." Carbohydrates that break down into sugar more slowly have a "low glycemic index."

It won't come as any surprise to learn that a teaspoon of table sugar has a fairly high glycemic index. But you might be surprised to know that a slice of white bread breaks down into sugar in your body *just as fast* as pure table sugar. And a baked potato breaks down into sugar even *faster!* So do instant white rice, French bread, and most popular breakfast cereals.

On the other hand, some sweet fruits—highly recommended by dietitians because of their healthful vitamins and antioxidants—are relatively low on the glycemic index. For example, an apple breaks down into sugar only about half as fast as a slice of bread. So does a pear. So does a peach. And cherries are very low on the glycemic index—ten cherries break down into sugar in your body three times more slowly than a slice of bread.

Take time to learn something about the glycemic index. Try eating a food with a moderate or low glycemic index—like pasta—in place of a carbohydrate with a higher glycemic index, like bread. Then see what your blood sugar tests tell you. You may find that you can level out your blood sugars by replacing high glycemic index carbohydrates with those that are lower on the scale, rather than cutting out carbohydrates altogether.

CHAPTER 9

EXERCISE

Exercise has a *major* affect on your blood sugar level. Exercise acts like insulin: it burns up blood sugar. But that's just one reason why you must get *at least* 30 minutes of exercise—ideally, a combination of aerobic exercise and weight training—every day.

WHY IS EXERCISE SO IMPORTANT?

1) Exercise is essential for weight control. Extra good news: exercise increases your metabolic rate, and your metabolic rate tends to stay up even after you stop exercising. So

you go on burning more calories than usual for hours after you've finished your workout! An important note: even if you exercise and never lose a pound, you're still benefiting. Studies show that overweight people who exercise, even if they don't shed pounds, have half the death rate of sedentary skinny people.

2) Exercise improves insulin sensitivity in your body. People who exercise regularly can reduce the amount of insulin or oral medication they take. (In many cases, type 2 diabetes can be controlled by diet and exercise alone.)

3) Aerobic exercise reduces your risk of *dozens* of serious health problems, including gallstones, heart, and coronary artery disease—even cancer. A major study published in the September 10, 2003, *Journal of the American Medical Association* found that women aged 50 to 79 who walked briskly for 75 to 150 minutes per week had an 18 percent lower risk of breast cancer when compared with inactive women. Numerous studies show that people who exercise have a dramatically lower risk of colon cancer than those who do not. Other studies suggest that exercise helps protect you from cancers of the ovary, prostate, and lung.

4) Working out with weights helps you build lean muscle mass, which is metabolically active and sensitive to insulin. Fat is inactive and less sensitive to insulin. That's why athletes with diabetes generally require lower doses of insulin —they have more muscle and less fat. Weight training also builds your strength and can help protect you from osteoporosis by increasing your bone mineral density.

5) Exercise is a powerful antidepressant. Recent studies show

that exercise may be as effective as medication in fighting depression—and easier to stick with for the long run!

6) Exercise helps prevent insomnia. This has been shown by medical studies, but it's also common sense! If you sit around all day resting, you won't be tired enough to sleep through the night. Expend some energy, and you'll sleep better.

7) Exercise increases your overall sense of well-being. When you exercise, nerve cells in your brain release natural pain-killing chemicals called "endorphins." And endorphins are very good for you. Studies conducted over the last 20 years show that endorphins give you an increased sense of well being, decrease anxiety, increase your ability to cope with stress, and increase your tolerance for pain—and they strengthen your immune system!

8) Exercise improves your self-confidence and self-esteem. And it makes you look better!

GETTING STARTED

If you're already exercising, keep it up. You're absolutely doing the right thing. If not, be sure to get a physical and your doctor's approval before you start any exercise program, especially if you are overweight, over 40, or have been sedentary for a while. Then, find something that you think will be fun to do—and get moving!

What kind of exercise you do is up to you. Walking is the standard recommendation, because it requires no special equipment, and it can be done anywhere, anytime. But the right kind of exercise *for you* is whatever you like, enjoy, and will do on a consistent basis. Is there a sport you never tried before because you didn't have time? Let diabetes be your excuse to make time for it now! Exercise is meant to be fun. Find the kind of exercise that's fun for you, and your workout will become the highlight of your day.

Unless you can schedule another time in the day when you absolutely will exercise, then the best time to exercise is first thing in the morning. That way it can't be pre-empted by life's daily emergencies. It's already done!

AVOIDING HYPOGLYCEMIA

Exercise is incredibly good for you—but it is not entirely risk-free. Along with the pulled muscles and sprained ankles that everyone risks when they exercise, people with diabetes have one more hazard to worry about: hypoglycemia (low blood sugar). One of the key reasons to exercise is that it lowers your blood sugar. But that also means it increases your risk of hypoglycemia if you take insulin or oral diabetes medicine.

AVOIDING
EXERCISE-INDUCED
HYPOGLYCEMIA

There are two things you need to do to protect yourself from exercise-induced hypoglycemia.

First, knowing that exercise burns off blood sugar, reduce your dose of insulin or have a snack before you start your workout. Just as you adjust your dose of insulin to cover the carbohydrates in a meal you are about to eat, you need to adjust your pre-workout snack depending on how long or strenuous a workout you're planning. If you're going for a long hard run, obviously you'll need a more substantial snack than if you're just going for an easy 15-minute walk. Getting your snack just right may take a little bit of trial and error at first, but eventually you'll master it. As always, your best bet is to monitor your blood sugar frequently to make sure your levels aren't getting too high or too low. It makes sense to monitor your blood sugar right before you exercise. Most experts suggest that you not exercise if your blood sugar is under 100 or over 300. (That doesn't mean you should skip your exercise session. Just take steps to bring your blood sugar within that range, and then go out and do it!) And remember that hypoglycemia can strike several hours *after* your workout, so keep monitoring your blood sugar periodically.

Second, carry some form of sugar with you in case you feel the early warning signs of hypoglycemia coming on. This is a critically important precaution, whether you're exercising or not—an episode of hypoglycemia that hits when you're driving your car alone can be even more dangerous than one that happens while you're out walking.

Many athletes—with or without diabetes—carry a carbohydrate gel in a foil packet. There are several brands available at any sporting goods store. They're designed in such a way that you can actually eat their contents on the run. At the first signs of mild hypoglycemia (shaking, sweating, hunger, weakness, anxiousness), take some gel or any other source of carbohydrate or sugar.

Don't let diabetes stop you from exercising. Take reasonable precautions to protect yourself from hypoglycemia and you should be able to participate in just about any sport you choose.

WALK 10,000 STEPS
TO BETTER HEALTH

What's the latest "buzz" in the exercise world? Using a pedometer to count your steps. It's inexpensive (an electronic pedometer only costs about $25) and it's easy—you put the pedometer on in the morning and take it off just before you go to bed at night. Object of the game? To rack up 10,000 steps a day—the equivalent of about five miles—which many experts say will lead to better health. You get to count both the steps you take in the normal course of your day as well as any additional exercise you do to build up your totals.

Sedentary people average 2,000 to 3,000 steps a day. If you hit the recommended target of 10,000 steps, you're probably getting the 30 minutes of moderate activity public health guidelines recommend—and, of course, that's the whole point. The pedometer adds some pizzazz to the process, brings out the competitive spirit, and makes getting the exercise you need fun.

Here are some ideas on how to walk more steps during the course of the day:

1. Call that friend you were going to meet for coffee or lunch and suggest going for a walk together instead.

2. Use a cordless phone, and pace around while you're talking.

3. Take a "walk break" instead of a "coffee break."

4. If you have one of those cell phone plans with unlimited

minutes on nights and weekends, take your phone to the park (or some other place where you won't be in danger from traffic), and walk while you talk to family and friends.

5. Take the stairs instead of the elevator.

6. Instead of hunting for the closest possible parking space, look for the one farthest away.

7. Go down every aisle in the grocery store every time you shop—even if you only need a few things.

8. Make your dog the happiest pet on the block! Take him for a walk two or three times a day instead of just once.

9. Get a treadmill and walk while you watch TV, talk on the phone, or listen to music.

10. Just get up and go for a walk!

Keep in mind that 10,000 steps isn't cast in stone. If you're only getting 2,000 steps a day now, and you increase to 4,000 steps, that's a big improvement. On the other hand, if you're overweight and your goal is weight loss, 10,000 steps may not be enough to do it. You may have to do more. In a Japanese research project, people trying to lose weight were encouraged to do 12,000 to 15,000 steps a day.

DANCE THE POUNDS AWAY

One way to get your body moving and enjoy social interaction at the same time is to take up dancing. Dancing is an awesome low-impact aerobic exercise. There are literally hundreds of different dances—ballroom, swing, country, jazz, tap, ballet—and they all give you a great workout. It won't even cross your mind that you're exercising as you glide across the dance floor.

If you don't have a dance partner, don't let that stop you! Country line dancing and other group dances are perfect for people without partners. They're great exercise and a ton of fun.

If you don't know how to dance, it's not too late to learn! There are classes available in everything from belly-dancing to the Cotton-eyed Joe. It doesn't matter what kind you choose—they all get your body moving, burn off calories, and help control your blood sugar.

THE FASTER YOU GO, THE MORE YOU BURN

How many calories you burn with exercise depends not only on how long you work out, but also on how *intensely*. Here's a chart that shows roughly how many calories you burn in an hour with various levels of exercise intensity:

SLOW WALKING	2 MPH	216 calories per hour
FAST WALKING	4 MPH	408 calories per hour
JOGGING	5 MPH	762 colories per hour
RUNNING	8 MPH	930 calories per hour

Please note: these are rough estimates for a person who weighs 185 pounds. If you weigh less, you'll burn fewer calories. If you weigh more, you'll burn more.

As this chart shows, it pays to pick up the pace! As you get fitter and fitter, you'll be able to walk, jog, or run faster and faster. And the faster you go, the more calories you burn.

TOO OLD TO PUMP IRON? THINK AGAIN!

It may seem strange to you, but weight training actually gets more important to your well-being as you get older. Most people gain about ten pounds every ten years after the age of 40. But they also lose five pounds of lean muscle—so they're actually gaining 15 pounds of fat!

Dieting can help get rid of the fat—but it won't do anything to restore lost muscle. So weight training is essential if you want to stay strong and maintain your lean muscle mass as you get older. Weight training is tremendously beneficial even for the oldest of the old. Without exercise, people weaken rapidly in old age (by 30 percent from age 80 to 90). Their bones also lose mineral mass, increasing the risk of injury from even a minor fall. But research shows that even frail people in their eighties and nineties gain 40 percent to 80 percent in strength when put on a weight-lifting program. As a result, they typically spend less time in wheelchairs, walk faster and farther, and are less dependent on others to do things for them.

Of course, an 80 year old is not going to lift the enormous weights that a 20 year old can. But that's just fine! Studies show that resistance training with weights as light as a pound-and-a-half can boost strength and endurance in healthy elderly adults.

JOIN THE DIABETES EXERCISE AND SPORTS ASSOCIATION

As you continue to exercise longer and harder, you may find it helpful to join the Diabetes Exercise & Sports Association (DESA).

DESA was founded as the International Diabetic Athletes Association (IDAA) in 1985 by Paula Harper, a registered nurse with type 1 diabetes who was heavily involved in distance running and cycling. Even though she was a medical professional herself, she found it hard to find good information about exercise and diabetes management. After her fifth marathon in 1980, Paula had "I run on insulin" printed on the back of a T-shirt. She soon met other athletes with diabetes who wanted to share experiences, pass on information, and offer each other support.

In 2000, the board of the IDAA changed the name to Diabetes Exercise & Sports Association. Membership is open to everyone from "mall walkers" to Olympic athletes.

The primary benefit of joining DESA is the opportunity to share experiences with other athletes who have diabetes. It wasn't so long ago that people with diabetes were discouraged from participating in sports! And, even today, good information about the relationship between exercise and diabetes can be hard to come by. DESA is widely regarded as the best forum available today for athletes of all kinds to share and exchange their stories, tips, and information.

You can find out more at their Web site at: www.diabetes-exercise.org.

CHAPTER 10

INSULIN

In August 1921, a Canadian surgeon named Frederick Banting and his assistant, Charles Best, successfully extracted material from a dog's pancreas, which they called "insulin." First they used this new substance to lower high blood sugars in diabetic dogs. Just six weeks after that, they tried it for the first time on a human subject—Leonard Thompson, a 14-year-old boy dying of diabetes. It saved his life, and the modern era of diabetes management began. Within two years of its discovery, insulin was available from Eli Lilly and Company in large enough quantities to treat most severe diabetics.

To people with diabetes, the discovery of insulin was more than just revolutionary. It was a medical miracle! What once was a death sentence became a manageable disease, and people with diabetes could look forward to living long, healthy, fulfilling lives!

Over the years, insulins became better and better. The first crude insulin, made from beef pancreases, was purified and refined. Today we refer to it as "regular" insulin. Scientists added proteins, buffers, and zinc to make more stable, longer-acting insulins, including NPH (now also called "N"), Lente ("slow") and Ultralente insulin. Twenty years ago, medical science discovered ways to make synthetic human insulin from bacteria and yeast, and these "human" insulins have largely taken the place of the earlier insulins made from beef or pork. Eli Lilly's brand of human insulins is called Humulin. NovoNordisk's human insulins are called Novolin.

But even these synthetic "human" versions of the traditional insulins can cause problems. NPH and Lente peak—unpredictably—from roughly four to 12 hours after injection. As a result, morning doses may cause low blood sugar episodes (hypoglycemia) in the afternoon, and doses taken at dinnertime can cause dangerous low blood sugar episodes at night while you're sleeping.

Regular insulin is also difficult to use. It takes 30 to 60 minutes to start working, peaks from two-and-a-half to five hours later, and lingers in your system for up to eight hours. So, if you take it with meals, you're likely to have high blood sugars an hour or two after eating and low blood sugars three to six hours after eating.

To solve these problems, Eli Lilly and Company recently came up with a new, very fast-acting insulin called Humalog that makes it much easier to maintain good blood sugar control. NovoNordisk has a similar fast-acting insulin called NovoLog. Both these new insulins begin working almost immediately—within 10 or 15 minutes. They peak from one to three hours after injection. And they are out of your system in roughly four hours.

Humalog and NovoLog are perfect for taking just before—or even during—a meal. They go to work right away to help you metabolize the carbohydrates you eat. They do their job and then disappear. So they are much less likely to cause low blood sugar problems hours later.

Another very important new insulin called Lantus ("glargine") was recently introduced in the United States by a German company, Aventis Pharmaceuticals. Lantus is a very long-acting insulin that works for a full 24 hours and it is virtually "peakless." It is perfect for providing the baseline, or "basal," dose of insulin you need all day long. You take just one shot of Lantus a day to give you the low dose of insulin you need between meals and at night. Then you use Humalog or NovoLog with meals to give yourself the extra "bolus" dose of insulin you need to cover the carbohydrates you eat. A daily shot of Lantus, plus Humalog or NovoLog with each meal, can give you blood sugar control—and mealtime flexibility—similar to an insulin pump. Lantus has become the "basal," or long-acting, insulin of choice for most people who are dependent on insulin.

Although these new insulins are more expensive than the traditional ones, they help most people achieve lower A1c levels with less hypoglycemia. If you're not getting the kind of control over your diabetes you want, ask your doctor about these new products—or consider switching from multiple daily injections to an insulin pump.

WHAT YOU NEED TO KNOW ABOUT YOUR INSULIN

No matter what kind of insulin or combination of insulins you use, it is vital to know three things:

▶ When it starts to work

▸ When it peaks

▸ How long it lasts

Knowing these three key characteristics of your insulins can help you use them most effectively to control your blood sugar—and prevent hypoglycemia. The quick reference tables below and on the following pages lists all the most popular insulins and the characteristics of each.

ELI LILLY AND COMPANY

TYPE	STARTS TO WORK	PEAKS	LASTS
Humulin Regular	30–60 minutes	2–3 hours	4–6 hours
Humulin NPH	1–2 hours	4–10 hours	14–18 hours
Humulin Lente	1–3 hours	6–15 hours	16–20 hours
Humlin Ultralente	4–6 hours	Minimal peaking	24–36 hours
Humulin 70/30	15–30 minutes	2–3 hours and 8–12 hours	18–24 hours
Humalog	Less than 15 minutes	30–90 Minutes	Less than 5 hours
Humalog Mix 75/25	15–30 minutes	30–90 minutes and 1–6½ hours	12 hours

AVENTIS PHARMACEUTICALS
LANTUS INSULIN ACTIVITY

TYPE	STARTS TO WORK	PEAKS	LASTS
Lantus	1½ hours	Virtually no peak	24 hours

NOVO NORDISK
INSULIN ACTIVITY

TYPE	STARTS TO WORK	PEAKS	LASTS
Novolin Regular	30 minutes	2 ½–5 hours	8 hours
Novolin NPH	1 ½ hours	4–12 hours	24 hours
Novolin Lente	2 ½ hours	7–15 hours	22 hours
Novolin 70/30	30 minutes	2–12 hours	24 hours
Velosulin BR	30 minutes	1–3 hours	8 hours
NovoLog	10–20 minutes	40–50 hours	3–5 hours

CHAPTER 11

INSULIN DELIVERY SYSTEMS

People who are newly diagnosed with diabetes often ask, "Why can't I take my insulin in pill form?" The answer is that insulin is a protein, and if you took it as a pill it would be broken down during digestion before it could go to work. It works best when it is injected into the layer of fat that lies just below your skin.

If you control your diabetes with insulin, you can choose from three basic ways to get the insulin into your body.

1) **Needle and syringe.** The needle and syringe is still the most common of the three insulin delivery systems. Today's needles are much improved from years ago. They are sharper and finer, and some are coated with Teflon to make injections much less painful than they used to be.

Before you begin giving yourself insulin, be sure your diabetes educator shows you the correct technique. It's not rocket science, but you do need to know what you're doing! Recommended injection sites include the abdomen, outer upper arms, the thighs, the buttocks, and hip areas. Do not inject insulin in bony areas or near any of your joints—it needs to go into an area with a good fat layer below the skin.

Comprehensive information on anything to do with injections is available online at BDdiabetes.com. This site, put up by BD Healthcare, the world's leading manufacturer of syringes and needles, includes a narrated, animated demonstration on how to give yourself an injection. Before the demonstration begins, you get to pick whether you want to be shown how to draw and inject one insulin, or how to mix, draw, and inject two insulins. You also get to choose the syringe you use: a 1 cc syringe, a 1/2 cc syringe, a 3/10 cc syringe with whole-unit scale markings, or a 3/10 cc syringe with half-unit scale markings. The demo you see is customized to your choices.

One question people frequently ask is: "Can I inject through my clothes?" The answer: although nobody recommends it, almost everybody does it.

2) **Insulin pens.** An insulin pen is a compact, portable device that serves exactly the same function as a needle and syringe, but is handier and more convenient to use. There are a wide variety of pens available. Both Eli Lilly and NovoNordisk make disposable insulin pens that come preloaded with their insulins. BD Healthcare, Disetronic, and Owen Mumford make resusable insulin pens.

One of the great advantages of insulin pens is that they are less "medical looking" than a typical needle and syringe. Pull out a vial of insulin and a syringe in a crowded restaurant and everyone will wonder what the heck you're doing. An insulin pen is much less conspicuous. Many parents prefer to provide their children with an insulin pen for their lunchtime insulin dose at school.

One of the newest pens on the market is the InnoLet, from Novo Nordisk. The InnoLet is specifically designed to make accurate dosing easier, especially for people who may have problems with their eyesight. The large dosing dial, which looks almost exactly like a kitchen timer, has big numbers and clicks audibly at each dosing level. It's ugly, but it works. In a recent test, 84 percent of patients using InnoLet were able to accurately set and dispense an insulin dose intuitively without instruction, versus 41 percent using a conventional insulin pen and just 32 percent using a vial and syringe.

3) Insulin pump. An insulin pump is a computer-controlled device—about the size and shape of a pager—that painlessly and accurately delivers insulin all day long through a tiny tube inserted just under the skin. An insulin pump is the best and most intensive way that currently exists to control diabetes. In theory, it is possible to achieve control over your blood sugar with multiple daily injections that would be as tight as the control you achieve with a pump. But in the real world, it doesn't often work that way! In the real world, almost everybody gets *dramatically* better control with the pump—and a lot more freedom to go with it.

Here's why. Everybody, with or without diabetes, needs insulin for two reasons: a background amount of insulin for normal functions of the body without food, and a burst of insulin, on demand, when food is eaten. People without diabetes can count on their pancreas to produce just the right amount of insulin for both purposes. The pump is not automatic—you have to tell it what to do. But, with experience, you can program it to do exactly what a healthy pancreas does.

In multiple daily injection therapy, it is not always clear how much insulin is being used for background use and how much is being used for food. With the insulin pump, the two are clearly separate. The pump allows you to set a "basal" rate of delivery to cover your background needs. And then you can give yourself a "bolus," or a little extra, on demand, when you eat.

When you exercise, you can reduce the basal rate so your blood sugar doesn't go too low. When you're sick or have an infection, you can increase the basal rate so your blood sugar doesn't go too high. And you can increase or decrease your "bolus." You can give yourself a very small boost of insulin if you're just having an apple for a snack, or a larger one if you're sitting down to Thanksgiving dinner.

An insulin pump uses only short-acting insulin, so you don't have to eat according to a rigid schedule. You can skip a meal entirely if you want, because there's no long-acting or intermediate insulin in your body dictating that you must eat.

The pump is not entirely pain-free. Every two or three days you have to change the location of the "infusion set," and that feels about like an injection. But with multiple daily injections you have to take *12 shots* every three days! Compared to that, changing the infusion set is hardly worth mentioning.

Today's pumps are very easy to use. If you can get money out of an ATM, you can learn to use a pump. And they are very safe.

There's a misconception among many people with diabetes that you only "go on the pump" if your diabetes is really out of control. It's true that many people who absolutely cannot control their diabetes with injections are able to get control with the pump. But most people use the pump simply because they want to have the best control over their diabetes that they possibly can.

Another misconception is that the pump is strictly for people with type 1 diabetes. In fact, it's just as useful for type 2s who need insulin to control their diabetes.

Should you be using a pump yourself? It's certainly something you should at least consider. More than half of all doctors and certified diabetes educators who use insulin wear the pump. Most people who try the pump immediately become raving fans. Very few are willing to give it up once they've tried it.

CHAPTER 12

ORAL MEDICATIONS FOR TYPE 2 DIABETES

People with type 1 diabetes don't have a choice: they must take insulin, because their pancreas no longer makes it. Being dependent on external sources of insulin is part of the definition of type 1 diabetes.

People with type 2 diabetes may have some other choices. In type 2 diabetes, the pancreas still makes insulin. It just may not make enough, or your body may have become resistant to it.

The first line of defense against type 2 diabetes is diet and exercise. But if diet and exercise alone do not bring your blood sugar down to acceptable levels, your doctor may prescribe one or more oral medications. There are a tremendous number of different medications to choose from today, and new ones come out all the time.

Which drug—or combination of drugs—is right for you?

The truth is, not even your doctor knows for sure. Not all of the drugs work for everybody. And even if a drug works for you to begin with, it may not work as well—or at all—later on. So there's a little bit of trial and error involved. This 28-day program will absolutely show you whether your oral medications are working for you the way they should, and whether the dosage is appropriate.

An important note: even though you were diagnosed with type 2 diabetes rather than type 1, you still may need insulin to control your diabetes. Many people with type 2 diabetes do. Most people who manage their diabetes successfully with oral medications at first need insulin later on. If this is the case with you, don't fight it! You may not like the idea of giving yourself a shot. Nobody does. But after the first week or two, you won't give it a thought. The complications of diabetes are *extremely* serious! So if you must take insulin to control your type 2 diabetes, count yourself blessed that today's excellent insulins exist to keep you healthy.

CHAPTER 13

AVOIDING HYPOGLYCEMIA

One of the most dangerous side-effects of insulin—and also of some oral medications for type 2 diabetes—is *hypoglycemia*. "Hypoglycemia" simply means low blood sugar.

Treating diabetes with insulin is a constant juggling act. Sometimes you eat too much food and don't take enough insulin, and then you get *hyper*glycemia—high blood sugar. *Hypo*glycemia happens when you make the opposite mistake and take too much insulin without enough food. Hypoglycemia can also be brought on by exercise, because exercise, like insulin, burns up sugar. (see chapter 9.)

SYMPTOMS

The symptoms of mild hypoglycemia include nervousness, shakiness, grouchiness, sweating, dizziness, yawning, weakness, blurred vision, headache, and hunger. *Never ignore these symptoms!* Hypoglycemia is always a potential medical emergency, and you have to take care of it quickly. The cure is to eat or drink any kind of fast-acting carbohydrate: orange juice, a regular sugared soft drink (not sugar-free), candy, glucose tablets—anything you can get your hands on. The standard recommendation is to take 15 grams of carbohydrate. And then, if you don't feel better in 15 minutes, take another 15 grams of carbohydrate. Lifesaver candies—available all over the world—are as good a source of emergency sugar as any. One Lifesaver has about 2 grams of carbohydrate, so you'll need to gobble seven or eight pieces to get your 15 grams of carbohydrate. Never go *anywhere* without a roll of Lifesavers or some other source of instant sugar in your pocket or purse!

WHY YOU MUST ACT QUICKLY

Left untreated, hypoglycemia can get progressively worse, leaving you less and less able to help yourself. Without a quick dose of fast-acting sugar, your hypoglycemia may progress to what is called "moderate hypoglycemia"—

although those who have experienced it say there's nothing "moderate" about it! Symptoms of moderate hypoglycemia include confusion, poor coordination, inability to cooperate, and slurred speech. In the first stages of moderate hypoglycemia, you may still be able to save yourself by drinking some juice or eating some candy. But as it advances you may have to rely on someone else to squirt a tube of Insta-glucose or the equivalent between your gum and cheek. It's very important that your family and friends understand diabetes, know the symptoms of moderate hypoglycemia, and have some Insta-glucose gel on hand so they can do something about it. After the Insta-glucose takes effect, you should have a substantial snack, like some crackers with cheese.

SEVERE HYPOGLYCEMIA

The most serious kind of hypoglycemia is "severe hypoglycemia," which involves unconsciousness or seizures. If severe hypoglycemia strikes, you are powerless to help yourself. The treatment for severe hypoglycemia is a shot of glucagon or intravenous glucose. Just as you should never leave home without a roll of Lifesavers in your pocket, it is vital that you keep a glucagon emergency kit handy, wherever you may be. And make sure somebody there knows what to do with it!

Unfortunately, many people with diabetes are embarrassed to ask their family and friends to take the responsibility of learning to give a glucagon injection. And that can lead to disaster in an emergency situation. Somebody who has never given a shot in their life is not likely to be able to do it in an emergency! Experts recommend that you not only explain to a potential rescuer how to use the kit, but also let them practice by giving you one of your regular insulin shots. Again—obviously—as soon as the glucagon takes effect and the person wakes up, he or she should eat something as soon as possible.

Hypoglycemia is especially dangerous for those who live alone, as many older people do. For that reason, many doctors set a higher blood sugar "target range" for their older patients.

Whether you live alone or not, in the end it's up to you to protect yourself from hypoglycemia. Your best defense is to monitor your blood sugar frequently, carefully balance your insulin with your food intake, always keep some fast-acting sugar at hand, and act *immediately* when you feel the symptoms of hypoglycemia coming on.

WEAR YOUR MEDICAL I.D. BRACELET

In case of emergency, it's very important that the people who respond know you have diabetes. Here's just one scenario to illustrate how important this is: The symptoms of low blood sugar resemble those of drunkenness. If a police officer thinks you're drunk and throws you in jail to "sleep it off"—when what you really need is some fast-acting carbohydrate—it could lead to a life-threatening situation. So wear your medical I.D. bracelet. It could save your life.

One of the most popular bracelets is the one provided by a company called MedicAlert. A MedicAlert bracelet is engraved with a toll-free number as well as your own member-ship number. In case of emergency, the responder can call the toll-free number, 24-hours-a-day, and access your medical information. MedicAlert will also notify your family. Full information is available online at medicalert.org.

AlertAccess.com is another Web site that harnesses the power of the Internet to make your medical information and history available to health-care providers, worldwide, in case of an emergency.

When you subscribe to the service, you get an identification card and also a very important red sticker with an 800 number that wraps around the edge of your driver's license. In the event of an accident or any other medical emergency, the paramedic on the scene or the doctor in the emergency room can call the 800 number and then access your complete medical information—medical history, medications, insurance information, emergency contacts, or whatever else you want—via phone, fax, or over the Internet.

If you do not have either of these forms of identification, think about getting one in the near future. For more information, refer to Part 3 of this book.

CHAPTER 14

KETOACIDOSIS

Hypoglycemia is *low* blood sugar. Ketoacidosis is the opposite problem: it occurs when your blood sugar is *too high*.

Diabetic ketoacidosis is a very serious but treatable complication of diabetes that happens when there is not enough insulin in your body. It is not to be taken lightly: Before the discovery of insulin, it was fatal 100 percent of the time. With modern management methods, death occurs in about 2 percent of episodes. The good news: it's not a common occurrence. It happens, on average, twice in 100 patient years of diabetes, meaning that if you have diabetes for 50 years, you run the risk, on average, of having one episode of ketoacidosis during that time. It is most common in people under 19, and it is almost always affects those with type 1 diabetes. It is extremely rare for those with type 2.

In about 15 percent of cases, ketoacidosis is caused by newly diagnosed, previously unknown diabetes. In other words, someone who has just become diabetic has had their insulin levels fall so far before they are diagnosed that they wind up in the hospital with ketoacidosis. In another 25 percent of cases, ketoacidosis results from a missed insulin dose or doses. But the most frequent cause of ketoacidosis is an infection or illness. Any infection has the potential to make your blood sugar levels skyrocket, leading to the risk of ketoacidosis. Urinary tract infections are the biggest culprit.

The way to defend yourself from ketoacidosis is to keep tight control over your blood sugar levels, and test frequently. Whenever you feel sick, even from a common cold, it is very important to test your blood sugar more often than you usually do. Ketoacidosis normally develops slowly—unless you're vomiting. Any time vomiting continues for more than two hours, if you have type 1 diabetes, you should contact your doctor.

Ketoacidosis is characterized by high blood sugar levels (usually over 300 mg/dL), dehydration, and the presence of ketones (acids) in your blood. You can test for ketones using a urine strip. Many experts recommend that you check for ketones whenever your blood sugar is more than 240 mg/dL.

The first symptoms of ketoacidosis are:

▶ Extreme thirst

▶ Frequent urination

▶ High blood sugar levels

▶ High levels of ketones in your urine

As ketoacidosis progresses, you may experience:

▶ Constant fatigue

▶ Dry or flushed skin

▶ Nausea or vomiting

▶ Difficulty breathing

▶ A fruity odor on your breath

▶ Confusion

Ketoacidosis is very dangerous. If you have *any* of these symptoms, call your doctor or go to the nearest emergency room.

CHAPTER 15

DIABETES AND YOUR HEART

When most people think about diabetes complications, the thing that scares them most is blindness. And that fear is based in fact: diabetes is the number one cause of blindness in adults in America. But the most common—and deadliest—complication of diabetes is *heart disease*. Just having diabetes puts you at two to four times greater risk of cardiovascular disease or stroke. There are two keys to protecting yourself from heart disease.

The first is: *stop smoking*.

Cigarette smoke contains thousands of chemicals that hurt your body, including carbon monoxide, nicotine, and tar. Smoking irritates and damages the throat, lungs, heart, circulatory system, and digestive tract. Tobacco is linked to at least seven different kinds of cancer. And it is the leading cause of death from heart attacks and strokes—a risk you can't afford, because you are *already* at increased risk of cardiovascular disease!

Now here's the good news. It's easier to stop smoking now than it ever has been before.

In the past few years, a whole new class of nicotine-replacement products has been approved by the FDA to help smokers quit. Some of them are available over-the-counter, without a prescription, like Nicorette nicotine gum. Others, like Nicotrol nasal spray, require a doctor's prescription. Whether you choose to use a gum, a nasal spray, an inhaler, or a patch, the principle is the same. These products give you a dose of nicotine to replace the nicotine you're used to getting from cigarettes.

And they work! In clinical trials, each of these nicotine replacement therapies proved effective in helping people quit.

ZYBAN

And there's an even more effective aid. Two years ago, the FDA approved the first-ever pill designed to help you quit smoking. The brand name of the product is Zyban. The generic name is bupropion SR (sustained release). It's the exact same prescription drug that is found in Wellbutrin SR, a proven antidepressive.

To stop smoking using Zyban, you begin taking the drug a week before your quit date. Then you continue taking it for seven to 12 weeks after you stop smoking. In clinical trials, an impressive 49 percent of smokers who tried it were successful after a month. And because Zyban contains no nicotine, you can use it along with nicotine replacement therapy. People who took Zyban and used nicotine gum to curb momentary cravings were even more successful in quitting.

If you've tried to stop before and failed, take heart. Almost everyone who successfully quits smoking has tried unsuccessfully before. You can do it, too! Stopping smoking is never easy, but these new products make it easier than it has ever been before.

So set a date—and make it soon. Talk with your doctor. Choose the therapy you think will work for you. On your quit date, throw away all your cigarettes, lighters, and ashtrays. Join a support group. Plan alternate rituals—if you've always smoked after meals, for example, start taking a brisk five-or ten-minute walk instead.

And make it work! It's one of the most important things you can do for yourself.

GET YOUR CHOLESTEROL CHECKED

The second thing you should do to protect your heart, if you haven't done it recently, is get a complete cholesterol check-up (also called a "lipid panel.") The ordinary cholesterol screening, which evaluates total cholesterol and high-density lipoproteins (HDL—the "good" cholesterol), is not enough. You need to get the kind of test that requires a 12-hour fast and checks your total cholesterol, LDLs ("bad" cholesterol), HDLs, and triglycerides—another fatty substance in the blood shown to contribute to heart disease. The LDLs are what your doctor will be looking at, above all. These low-density lipoproteins damage your heart's coronary arteries by causing a build-up of calcified plaque inside them.

If the test results show that your LDL cholesterol is below 100 mg/dL, that's good. If it is greater than 100 mg/dL, the current guidelines recommend that your doctor start you on "therapeutic lifestyle changes"—meaning diet and exercise. Between 100 mg/dL and 130 mg/dL, adding drug therapy is considered optional. But if your LDL level is more than 130 mg/dL—and you have diabetes—adding drug therapy to lower your LDL cholesterol is recommended.

If your doctor decides to put you on cholesterol-lowering medications, he or she is likely to prescribe a category of drugs called "statins." After years of prescribing these drugs sparingly and analyzing the results, the experts now approve of them wholeheartedly and recommend prescribing them aggressively—especially for people with diabetes.

Statins really do save lives. In a five-year clinical study among people with high cholesterol and heart disease, those who took one of the most popular cholesterol-lowering drugs, Zocor, had 42 percent fewer deaths from heart disease.

AN ASPIRIN A DAY

You've probably heard that an aspirin a day—either an 81 mg "baby" aspirin or a standard 325 mg tablet—is frequently prescribed to people who have had heart attacks. Now guidelines suggest that an aspirin a day may be a good idea for some people who have *not* had a heart attack, but are at high risk because of other factors—including diabetes.

But aspirin therapy is not risk-free. Aspirin has rare but very dangerous side effects, including the possibility of gastrointestinal bleeding and hemorrhagic strokes (uncontrolled bleeding in the brain).

So the trick is to balance the benefit with the risk. The more risk factors you have for a heart attack, the more sense it makes to take aspirin. For people with little risk of a heart attack, there's no sense in taking chances with aspirin's side effects.

People with diabetes are two to four times as likely as people without to die from the complications of cardiovascular disease. So aspirin therapy is something you should at least discuss with your doctor.

CHAPTER 16

SEX

It would be great if you could leave diabetes behind when you close the bedroom door. But, unfortunately, you can't. Diabetes can intrude on your sexual life in small ways and in large ways. The small ways include such things as having to remember that sex is exercise, and as such has an effect on your blood sugar. It may not seem romantic, but it's wise to check your blood sugar before sex just as you do before exercise. If your blood sugar level is below 100, you would be wise to have a snack to bring it up. Otherwise, you run the risk of becoming hypoglycemic.

Another nuisance is what to do with your insulin pump during sex. Actually, this is an easy one. Almost all pumps have a "quick connect" feature that allows you to take them off when you shower, swim, or have sex. Taking the pump off for a short time rarely causes any problems, as long as you remember to put it back on again. Even if your infusion set pulls completely out in a fit of passion, it rarely causes a disaster. Just choose another insertion point and replace it when you're done.

Diabetes intrudes on your sex life in a more serious way when it causes sexual dysfunction. In one study of men with type 2 diabetes, 34 percent reported frequent erectile problems, and another 24 percent reported occasional problems. Diabetes can cause these problems in two ways: first, as a result of damage to the blood vessels, restricting the flow of blood required to create an erection; and second, as a result of damage to the nerves, resulting in a lessening of sensation.

Furthermore, some medications taken for type 2 diabetes and related problems like high blood pressure or high cholesterol can be the cause of sexual dysfunction. Drinking too much and smoking can also cause the problem.

Although male sexual problems related to diabetes get most of the coverage in the press, women frequently have diabetes-related sexual dysfunction, too. Women with diabetes sometimes have problems with vaginal lubrication, and they may experience a lessening of sexual response due to nerve damage.

The first line of defense against diabetes-related sexual dysfunction, as with all diabetes complications, is to maintain tight control over your blood sugar levels. Stopping smoking, getting regular exercise, and losing weight may also help.

If problems persist despite your best efforts, be sure to talk to your doctor. In years past, sexual dysfunction was a taboo topic. But no more! The huge success of Viagra—which has been specifically proven to work on men with erectile dysfunction caused by type 2 diabetes—has focused the attention of medical researchers on this problem. Now there is a second pharmaceutical product on the market, called Levitra, which was also tested specifically on men with diabetes. And there are other very effective therapies that your doctor may suggest.

So, whether you are a man or a woman, don't hesitate to bring up the subject with your doctor. Don't suffer in silence just because it makes you uncomfortable to bring the subject up! And don't wait for your doctor to take the lead. Speak up! Be matter-of-fact. There are treatments available for both men and women that may help you enjoy a more satisfying sex life.

CHAPTER 17

TRAVELING WITH DIABETES

If you're planning a trip by air in the near future, you need to be aware of how airline security rules put in place by the FAA after September 11, 2001, may affect you. As of this writing, you are only allowed to take one carry-on bag on board, along with a pocketbook or briefcase. Items that you may *not* carry on board a plane: knives; any other cutting instruments, such as straight razors, box cutters, metal scissors, ice picks, metal nail files, or corkscrews; baseball and softball bats; golf clubs; pool cues; ski poles; and hockey sticks. Umbrellas and walking canes are allowed on the plane with you, as well as syringes, *with proof of medical need.*

Here are some tips for traveling with diabetes under the current airline restrictions:

1. To satisfy the requirement of "proof of medical need," get a letter from your doctor, on office letterhead, stating that you are being treated for diabetes mellitus and that you must have your medications and the means to deliver them—along with your testing equipment, supplies, emergency glucose, and other food—in your possession at all times. If you're carrying insulin, be sure to keep it in its original box with the original label, even if some has already been used out of the vial. The same for oral medications: keeping them in the prescription bottle you got from the pharmacy can save explanations.

2. Always carry your diabetes prescriptions—and prescriptions for any other medications you require—with you. This also helps to establish medical need when your bags are searched, and could be essential if you need refills while you are out-of-town.

3. Pack all your medications, including your insulin and glucose tablets and substantial snacks, in your carry-on bag—*never in your checked baggage.* Pack with the assumption that your checked baggage will be lost, your flight will take three times longer than scheduled, and that *nothing* will be available to eat on the plane. (The airlines have eliminated food service on most flights, as a cost-cutting measure.)

4. Call your airline in advance and get the *exact measurements* they allow for carry-on bags. And don't push your luck. The last thing you want is to have the airline refuse your carry-on because it is too large.

5. Bring a government-issued photo ID, and get to the airport at least an hour before your departure for domestic flights, earlier for international.

Ozzie Roberts, who travels all over the world, says that the one word of explanation for your diabetes supplies that is understood all over is "medical." Don't hesitate to use it!

One of the keys to living a positive life with diabetes is: don't let it keep you from doing what you enjoy. If you've always loved traveling—or you've always dreamed of traveling but put it off—pack your bags. With a little planning and preparation, there's nowhere you can't go.

CHAPTER 18

PREVENTING DIABETES

It may seem strange to have a chapter in a book written for people who already have diabetes on how to prevent it. But there's a good reason to include it. Family history is a factor in type 2 diabetes. So your brothers and sisters and your children are at risk for type 2 diabetes if you have it. If your husband or wife has shared your diet and lifestyle for many years, he or she may be at risk also. You are in a position to let people you love know they are at risk—and help them diminish that risk.

The exception to what I just said is type 1 diabetes. No one is certain what triggers it in the first place, so unfortunately there's no way to stop it.

Type 2 *can* be prevented. On August 8, 2001, the results of a landmark study called the Diabetes Prevention Program (DPP) were released by the National Institute of

Diabetes and Digestive and Kidney Diseases.

Participants in the study were people at high risk for developing type 2 diabetes. The DPP participants were overweight and had impaired glucose tolerance—their blood glucose levels were higher than normal, but they were not yet diabetic.

Two different approaches were tested to see if they could keep these at-risk people from developing diabetes. One group tried diet and exercise. The other group was given Glucophage (metformin).

Both approaches worked. The diet and exercise group reduced their risk of developing diabetes by a whopping 58 percent! The Glucophage group also reduced their risk of developing diabetes, by 31 percent.

What did the people in the diet and exercise group have to do to get such great results? Did they have to starve themselves until they were as skinny as supermodels? Not at all! On average, this group did 30 minutes of physical activity per day—mostly walking. They lowered the amount of fat in their diet and lost just 5 to 7 percent of their body weight—typically about 15 pounds.

This study is particularly encouraging because it proved that diet and exercise work for everybody—African-Americans, Latinos, Native Americans, Asian-Americans, and Pacific Islanders, as well as Caucasians. All these groups were included in the trial, and all were successful.

It was also encouraging to see that the diet and exercise approach worked *better* among adults older than 60 than any other age group. This is very important, because American adults over 60 have the highest rate—20 percent—of type 2 diabetes.

So don't let the people you love put themselves at risk for a disease they can avoid. The same things that are recommended above all for people with diabetes—weight control and exercise—have been proven to effectively prevent it.

PART TWO:

28 DAYS TO DIABETES CONTROL!

USING THE
28-DAY PROGRAM
TO CONTROL
YOUR DIABETES

Now we get down to business!

Having read the first part of this book, you've learned the basics about diabetes. Now you're ready for step two: learning to control *your* diabetes.

The key to mastering your diabetes in the next 28 days is to complete the journal pages in this section. The journal includes spaces for every factor that affects blood sugar levels. Filling out these pages will take all the mystery out of why your blood sugar is sometimes high, and sometimes low. In the course of this program you will learn *exactly* how food, exercise, and (if you use them) medication or insulin raise or lower the levels of sugar in your blood. Keeping this journal, and analyzing it, will teach you everything you need to know to get your diabetes under control—and keep it under control for the rest of your life.

HOW THE JOURNAL WORKS

There are four categories of information on the journal pages.

1) Food. Because food has a huge impact on your blood sugar levels as well as your weight, for the next 28 days you are going to record everything you eat and drink—every bite of food and every sip of beverage. There are spaces on the journal pages to write down what you have for breakfast, lunch, and dinner, as well as your snacks.

In addition, you're going to count and record the *calories* and the *carbs* in each meal. If you need a refresher on counting calories, please refer back to chapter 7. If you need a reminder on how to count carbs, please refer to chapter 8.

2) Exercise. Daily exercise is vital both for your diabetes control and for your general health. For the next 28 days you're going to be exercising every day and making a note of it. There are two blanks for exercise in case you choose to do two exercise sessions in a day—an aerobic exercise and a weight-lifting routine, for example.

Be sure to enter *when* you exercised under "Time of day," so you can relate that to the times of your blood sugar tests and see how exercise affects your blood sugars. Under "Type of exercise," indicate what you did: walking, for example. Under "duration," write the number of minutes you worked out. Under "intensity," indicate how hard you exercised: easy, average, or hard.

3) Medications or insulin. If you take oral medications or insulin to help control your diabetes, obviously it is important to make a note of them. There are six blanks in the journal pages to let you record when, what, and how much you took through the day.

4) Blood sugar tests. It is your blood sugar test that makes everything else make sense. There's no way to exaggerate how important frequent blood sugar testing is. If diabetes is the question, blood sugar tests are the answer! It is your blood sugar tests that will tell you *everything*.

There are eight blanks in the journal pages for blood sugar tests. For the first seven days, you should test eight times a day, no matter what type of diabetes you have. For the last 21 days, testing four times a day should be sufficient. If you have been in the habit of testing only once or twice a day, that may seem like an awful lot. But keep in mind that I'm not asking you to test eight times a day for the rest of your life. Only for the next seven days. There is no substitute.

Here is when you should test during the first week of your program:

1. First thing in the morning, before you have anything to eat

2. Two hours after breakfast

3. Just before lunch

4. Two hours after lunch

5. Before exercise

6. Just before dinner

7. Two hours after dinner

8. Before going to bed

There's nothing to stop you from continuing to test eight times a day throughout the program if you're comfortable with it, and the journal pages include eight blanks for test results all the way to the end. But it is not absolutely necessary. For the last 21 days, testing four times a day should be enough. A good strategy is to stick with the recommended schedule, but skip every other test. One day, test on the even numbers shown, and test on the odd numbers the following day. That way you're covering all eight test times every two days.

Be sure to total up your blood sugar tests at the end of each day and divide by the number of tests you did to get your daily average.

The journal pages also include a place to record your body weight, because weight loss is a key goal of therapy for the vast majority of people with diabetes. Weigh yourself at the same time every day. I recommend doing it in the morning right after you get up, before you have anything to eat or drink.

Here is a sample journal page, filled out.

DAY 1

Sept. 1

BREAKFAST

	CALORIES	CARBS
Toast with Butter	200	18
2 Fried Eggs	150	1
1 cup O.J.	120	31
1 cup 2% Milk	130	13
BREAKFAST TOTALS:	600	63

LUNCH

	CALORIES	CARBS
Grilled Chicken	390	0
Green Salad	17	3
Italian dressing	120	3
LUNCH TOTALS:	527	6

DINNER

	CALORIES	CARBS
6 ounces Salmon	351	0
1 cup zucchini	28	7
1 cup rice	340	74
Dinner roll	110	18
DINNER TOTALS:	829	99

SNACKS

	CALORIES	CARBS
Orange	65	16
Cup of yogurt	130	15
SNACKS TOTALS:	195	31
DAILY TOTALS:	2,151	199

EXERCISE

TIME OF DAY	TYPE OF EXERCISE	DURATION	INTENSITY
4:00 p.m.	Walk	20 min.	Medium

MEDICATION OR INSULIN TAKEN

TIME OF DAY	TYPE	AMOUNT
8 a.m.	glucophage	500 mg
Noon	glucophage	500 mg
8 p.m.	glucophage	500 mg

BLOOD SUGAR TESTS

TIME OF DAY	READING	TIME OF DAY	READING
7 a.m.	98	8 p.m.	114
11 a.m.	120	9:30	108
Noon	118		
2 p.m.	132		
4 p.m.	115		
6 p.m.	99		

TODAY'S AVERAGE BLOOD SUGAR READING: 113

BODY WEIGHT: 220

Once you have Day One of your journal completed, you'll be in a position to make changes that will help you to get better control the following day. With eight daily blood sugar tests to guide you, the effects of your diet, your exercise, and your medications or insulin will be obvious. Every day, you'll look back at what happened before. Identify problem areas. Decide what to change, make the change, and see what happens. It won't take long before the cause and effect of blood sugar control becomes second nature to you. You'll see what makes your blood sugar go up, and what brings it down. Step-by-step and day-by-day, analyzing your journal pages will teach you exactly what you need to know to control your diabetes.

An important note: this 28 day program will *not* work unless you are on a medical regimen that makes it possible for you to control your blood sugars. Earlier, I said that your diabetes care is 5 percent up to your doctor, and 95 percent up to you. And that's absolutely true. But the 5 percent the doctor does is very important! You can't write your own prescriptions. If you're not on the right medicine, or you're not taking the right insulins, you may not be able to get control over your blood sugar levels no matter how hard you try.

You're going to know soon enough. Follow this program faithfully for just four or five days, and take a look at your daily blood sugar averages. Make sure you're taking your medicine or insulin *just the way your doctor ordered*. If you're 20 or 30 mg/dL higher than you want to be on your blood sugar daily averages, that's all right. You can easily bring that down by increasing your exercise program, by dropping some carbohydrates from your diet, or by slightly increasing your dosage of insulin or medication. That's what this program is all about—learning to balance your food, exercise, and medication so that your average daily blood sugars fall right where you want them.

But if your blood sugars are *way* out of line—if they are *twice* as high as you want them to be—you need to get with your doctor as soon as possible. Take this book with you to show that you're serious about bringing your diabetes under control. Show your doctor your first few journal pages. It could be that the medicine you're taking is not working for you. You may need to switch medicines, change your dosage, add another medicine, or start taking insulin. If you're taking insulin already, your insulin-to-carbohydrate ratio may be way off. Or you may need to take different kinds of insulin, switch from one or two shots a day to multiple injections, or try an insulin pump.

Doctors aren't psychic—they don't know what's going on with your diabetes unless you tell them. Lots of patients have high blood sugars because they don't follow doctors' orders. But that's not the case with you! You're taking your medicine or insulin, getting daily exercise, and you're recording all the factors that affect your blood sugar. You're serious enough about controlling your diabetes to test your blood sugar eight times a day. You deserve to be on a medical regimen that *works!*

If you're doing everything your doctor told you to do, and your first few days' blood sugars are not even in the ballpark, raise the red flag right away! Get on a medical regimen that gives you a chance for success.

DAY 1

Your goal on Day 1 is simple: just fill out Day 1 in the journal. If you've never counted calories or carbs before, that will be challenge enough. Your first day counting calories and carbs is the hardest, because you have to look *everything* up. Believe me, it gets much easier. If you're like most people, there are certain things you eat almost every day. When you're filling out your journal for Day 2, there will be a lot of things you can just pick up from your journal entries on Day 1. By the end of your first week, you'll only have to look things up occasionally. You'll have most of your favorites memorized.

Please take this process seriously, and do it right. Make sure you *measure* what you eat and drink. That means you're going to have to get out a measuring cup to find out how many cups are in the glass of juice you drink every morning.

Remember, you only have to do this today. Tomorrow when you fill that same glass, you'll already know how much it holds.

Don't try to cut back on what you eat or drink today. That can come later. The goal for today is simply to *record* what you eat. Be sure to total up the number of calories and carbs for each meal, and for the day.

Of course I want you to fill out the *whole* journal, not just the food diary. I want you to get some exercise and record what you did. Under "Medications or insulin taken" be sure to note when, what, and how much you took through the day. Do your eight blood sugar tests, and average them at the end of the day.

You can do this! Take a deep breath, roll up your sleeves, and go to work.

DAY 1

_____

BREAKFAST

	CALORIES	CARBS
_____	_____	_____
_____	_____	_____
_____	_____	_____
_____	_____	_____
_____	_____	_____
BREAKFAST TOTALS:	_____	_____

LUNCH

	CALORIES	CARBS
_____	_____	_____
_____	_____	_____
_____	_____	_____
_____	_____	_____
_____	_____	_____
LUNCH TOTALS:	_____	_____

DINNER

	CALORIES	CARBS
_____	_____	_____
_____	_____	_____
_____	_____	_____
_____	_____	_____
_____	_____	_____
DINNER TOTALS:	_____	_____

SNACKS

	CALORIES	CARBS
_____	_____	_____
_____	_____	_____
_____	_____	_____
_____	_____	_____
SNACKS TOTALS:	_____	_____
DAILY TOTALS:	_____	_____

EXERCISE

TIME OF DAY	TYPE OF EXERCISE	DURATION	INTENSITY

MEDICATION OR INSULIN TAKEN

TIME OF DAY	TYPE	AMOUNT

BLOOD SUGAR TESTS

TIME OF DAY	READING	TIME OF DAY	READING

TODAY'S AVERAGE BLOOD SUGAR READING: _____

BODY WEIGHT: _____

DAY 2

Welcome to Day 2. Here's where the fun begins! You now have something you've never had before: a complete record of everything you did yesterday that could affect your blood sugar levels—along with blood sugar tests that show the results. You have what a scientist would call *data*. Yes, it's only one day. But it's a start!

Early in the day, sit down and look at the data you entered yesterday. Start out with your blood sugar tests. You know what your target range is. How often did you hit it? What was your daily average? Was it below 150, which would put you within the ADA's suggested target of keeping your A1c below 7? Or if you're shooting for the more aggressive target of 6.5 that the American College of Endocrinology suggests, was it below 135?

If not, what can you do to bring it down? You might start with your highest reading of the day. How can you bring that one reading down? Have fewer carbs in the previous meal? Get some exercise before that reading? Pick one thing to adjust to bring down your highest reading from yesterday and do that one thing today.

This is the process you'll be using for the next 27 days: *analyze and adapt*. Analyze what happened yesterday. And adapt your behavior to get a better result today. Now that you have a record of what you ate, what you did, what medicine or insulin you took, and what the results were on your blood sugar tests, you're in a position to analyze what's going on, make simple changes, record the results, and analyze again.

If you had a huge bowl of spaghetti for dinner and your bedtime and morning sugars were sky-high, you don't need an expert to tell you that a huge bowl of pasta is not a good dinner for someone with diabetes! It's just too many carbohydrates. Maybe a dinner of chicken or fish with a salad and green vegetables might be better—with a single piece of bread or a small portion of spaghetti on the side. Or maybe you just need to adjust the insulin you took to cover that meal.

If weight control is one of the goals you want to accomplish on this program, today is the day to start cutting just a few calories out of your diet. Remember, on average, men need about 2,700 calories a day. Women need about 2,000. What was your total yesterday?

One of the easiest places to start is with the calories you *drink*. For example, a 12-ounce can of Coke contains 150 calories. Some people go through a six-pack a day. That's 900 calories! Orange juice is certainly a healthy drink, full of vitamin C. But an eight-ounce glass of orange juice has 120 calories. Alcoholic beverages are packed full of calories, too. A regular 12-ounce beer has around 150 calories, and a light beer has

100 to 120. A four-ounce glass of wine is 100 calories. So you can wind up getting too many calories in the beverages you consume—even if you're disciplined about what you eat.

Sweet drinks are packed with carbohydrates, too. The calories in most sweet beverages are pure carbs. If you want to cut some of the carbs out of your diet to level out your blood sugars, drinks are a painless place to start. Many people enjoy the diet version of their favorite soft drink just as much as the high-calorie kind. Another option is good, old-fashioned, water! Pick up a cold, refreshing bottle of water instead of a 12-ounce can of Coke, and you've saved 150 calories and 40 grams of carbohydrate. Or try the new flavored waters that have minimal calories and carbs.

DAY 2

_____

BREAKFAST

	CALORIES	CARBS
BREAKFAST TOTALS:		

LUNCH

	CALORIES	CARBS
_____	_____	_____
_____	_____	_____
_____	_____	_____
_____	_____	_____
_____	_____	_____
LUNCH TOTALS:	_____	_____

DINNER

	CALORIES	CARBS
_____	_____	_____
_____	_____	_____
_____	_____	_____
_____	_____	_____
DINNER TOTALS:	_____	_____

SNACKS

	CALORIES	CARBS
_____	_____	_____
_____	_____	_____
_____	_____	_____
_____	_____	_____
SNACKS TOTALS:	_____	_____
DAILY TOTALS:	_____	_____

Day 2

EXERCISE

TIME OF DAY	TYPE OF EXERCISE	DURATION	INTENSITY

MEDICATION OR INSULIN TAKEN

TIME OF DAY	TYPE	AMOUNT

BLOOD SUGAR TESTS

TIME OF DAY	READING	TIME OF DAY	READING

TODAY'S AVERAGE BLOOD SUGAR READING: _____

BODY WEIGHT: _____

DAY 3

It's Day 3, and now you have two days' records to look back over.

The first thing you need to look at is the one thing you changed yesterday to bring down your highest blood sugar from Day 1. Did it work? If so, great! If not, try to figure out why it didn't.

Now, for the first time, you have enough written history of all the factors that affect your blood sugars to start to look for *patterns*. Analyzing patterns and adapting your behavior is something you will do throughout this program. Of course, looking for patterns will be more productive when you have several days worth of information to analyze. But at least you can start.

Are you having high blood sugars consistently at the same time of day? After a certain meal? Take a look at what you've been eating at that meal. How do the carbs compare to the other meals of the day? What can you change to bring those "pattern highs" down?

DAY 3

_____

BREAKFAST

	CALORIES	CARBS
_____	_____	_____
_____	_____	_____
_____	_____	_____
_____	_____	_____
_____	_____	_____
BREAKFAST TOTALS:	_____	_____

LUNCH

	CALORIES	CARBS
_____	_____	_____
_____	_____	_____
_____	_____	_____
_____	_____	_____
_____	_____	_____
LUNCH TOTALS:	_____	_____

DINNER

	CALORIES	CARBS
_____	_____	_____
_____	_____	_____
_____	_____	_____
_____	_____	_____
_____	_____	_____
DINNER TOTALS:	_____	_____

SNACKS

	CALORIES	CARBS
_____	_____	_____
_____	_____	_____
_____	_____	_____
_____	_____	_____
SNACKS TOTALS:	_____	_____
DAILY TOTALS:	_____	_____

Day 3

EXERCISE

TIME OF DAY	TYPE OF EXERCISE	DURATION	INTENSITY

MEDICATION OR INSULIN TAKEN

TIME OF DAY	TYPE	AMOUNT

BLOOD SUGAR TESTS

TIME OF DAY	READING	TIME OF DAY	READING

TODAY'S AVERAGE BLOOD SUGAR READING: _____

BODY WEIGHT: _____

DAY 4

Day 4. Now we're getting somewhere!

It would be great if there were a one-size-fits-all way to control diabetes. But there isn't. Every single person with diabetes is unique. What works for you might not work for your neighbor. A food that drives your blood sugars way up may not have the same effect on someone else. You have to figure out your *own* way to control your diabetes.

And you're well on you're way to doing it! With every day that goes by, you have more data, more information, more recorded history that you can go over, analyze, and learn from.

So look back on what happened in your first three days. Analyze and adapt. Decide what you're going to change today to get your blood sugars under better control. Above all: keep exercising, keep testing, and keep filling out your journal!

DAY 4

_____

BREAKFAST

	CALORIES	CARBS
BREAKFAST TOTALS:		

LUNCH

	CALORIES	CARBS
_____	_____	_____
_____	_____	_____
_____	_____	_____
_____	_____	_____
_____	_____	_____
LUNCH TOTALS:	_____	_____

DINNER

	CALORIES	CARBS
_____	_____	_____
_____	_____	_____
_____	_____	_____
_____	_____	_____
_____	_____	_____
DINNER TOTALS:	_____	_____

SNACKS

	CALORIES	CARBS
_____	_____	_____
_____	_____	_____
_____	_____	_____
_____	_____	_____
SNACKS TOTALS:	_____	_____
DAILY TOTALS:	_____	_____

Day 4

EXERCISE

TIME OF DAY   TYPE OF EXERCISE   DURATION   INTENSITY

_____

_____

MEDICATION OR INSULIN TAKEN

TIME OF DAY	TYPE	AMOUNT

BLOOD SUGAR TESTS

TIME OF DAY   READING   TIME OF DAY   READING

_____   _____

_____   _____

_____

_____

_____

_____

TODAY'S AVERAGE BLOOD SUGAR READING: _____

BODY WEIGHT: _____

DAY 5

It's Day 5—and keeping your journal should be getting a little easier. You're starting to get the hang of counting calories and carbohydrates. You've found that there are certain foods you eat almost every day, and you know their calories and carbs by heart.

How's the exercise program going? Many people with diabetes diagnosed in their 40s, 50s, and 60s have been inactive for years. And it's hard to change habits of long standing. So if you're having a hard time getting your exercise program started, you're not alone.

But don't give up! This is one area you *have* to change. The human body must have exercise to remain healthy. Years ago, doctors routinely recommended "bed rest" for a variety of ailments. Now doctors realize that bed rest is the *worst* thing you can do. Today, people who have quadruple bypass surgery are encouraged to get up and walk the hospital halls within a couple of days of surgery. Why? It's either get moving—or die. That's how important exercise is.

If you have been excusing yourself from exercise because of a bad knee, arthritis, or a weak back, stop! It's time to adopt a new attitude. There is a "work-around" for everything. Exercise is so important that doctors and physical therapists have devised ways for *everyone* to get in a good workout. If you have arthritis or a bad knee or a weak back, you can still exercise. One option is water aerobics, where you work out in a swimming pool. The water supports most of your body weight, making it possible for almost anybody to exercise. There are also exercise programs that can be done while you're seated in a chair. People whose hands are too arthritic to grip even a light weight can exercise by strapping weights around their wrists with velcro. All these programs are available if you look for them.

So if you've been putting off the exercise part of this program, today is the day to get with it. No excuses. Find something you can do and get moving!

DAY 5

BREAKFAST

	CALORIES	CARBS
BREAKFAST TOTALS:		

LUNCH

	CALORIES	CARBS
_____	_____	_____
_____	_____	_____
_____	_____	_____
_____	_____	_____
_____	_____	_____
LUNCH TOTALS:	_____	_____

DINNER

	CALORIES	CARBS
_____	_____	_____
_____	_____	_____
_____	_____	_____
_____	_____	_____
_____	_____	_____
DINNER TOTALS:	_____	_____

SNACKS

	CALORIES	CARBS
_____	_____	_____
_____	_____	_____
_____	_____	_____
_____	_____	_____
SNACKS TOTALS:	_____	_____
DAILY TOTALS:	_____	_____

Day 5

EXERCISE

TIME OF DAY   TYPE OF EXERCISE   DURATION   INTENSITY

_____

_____

MEDICATION OR INSULIN TAKEN

TIME OF DAY	TYPE	AMOUNT

BLOOD SUGAR TESTS

TIME OF DAY	READING	TIME OF DAY	READING

TODAY'S AVERAGE BLOOD SUGAR READING: _____

BODY WEIGHT: _____

DAY 6

Day 6: You're doing great!

This program isn't easy—I know it. I'm asking you to do a lot of new things all at once. I'm asking you to get in the habit of counting both the carbohydrates you eat and the calories you consume each day. I'm asking you to test your blood sugar *eight times a day*. (Although that's only for two more days!) I'm asking you to keep this daily journal, which you may never have done before. I'm asking you to get exercise every day, which may be new to you. And I'm asking you to go back over your journal pages every day, actively looking for changes you can make in your diet, exercise, and medications or insulin to bring your blood sugar readings down as close as possible to normal levels.

That's not just a lot—that's an *awful* lot. If you've done it all every day so far, you should stop and congratulate yourself.

You've done something exceptional, and you've shown awesome self-discipline. You're fantastic! You're a star! You're a champion—keep it up!

If you haven't done everything perfectly, but you've done *most* of it—frankly, that's fantastic, too. Congratulations! Even if you've missed a couple days' exercise, or haven't always tested eight times a day, as long as you're filling out most of your journal sheets, you've got more data on how to control your diabetes *already* than most people ever compile in their lifetime! But don't settle for less than your best. Your goal is to fill in every blank, and I want you to hang in there and fill out as much as you possibly can. Don't start over and promise you'll do it perfectly next time. Just keep going. Keep testing, keep exercising, and keep filling out your journal to the best of your ability.

The more you do, of course, the more you'll learn and the better control you'll achieve. But if you do *most* of what I ask, you'll still learn a *lot*. So don't beat yourself up if you missed a test, or even missed a day. Instead, look for the positive. Look for the tests you did, and see what they tell you. Congratulate yourself on every bit of exercise you recorded, and build on your successes. Even if you aren't perfect, you are precious and irreplaceable. This program is important, and you're worth the effort. I know it's hard, but I also know you're strong. You can do it!

DAY 6

_____

BREAKFAST

	CALORIES	CARBS
BREAKFAST TOTALS:		

LUNCH

	CALORIES	CARBS
_____	_____	_____
_____	_____	_____
_____	_____	_____
_____	_____	_____
_____	_____	_____
LUNCH TOTALS:	_____	_____

DINNER

	CALORIES	CARBS
_____	_____	_____
_____	_____	_____
_____	_____	_____
_____	_____	_____
DINNER TOTALS:	_____	_____

SNACKS

	CALORIES	CARBS
_____	_____	_____
_____	_____	_____
_____	_____	_____
_____	_____	_____
SNACKS TOTALS:	_____	_____
DAILY TOTALS:	_____	_____

Day 6

EXERCISE

TIME OF DAY   TYPE OF EXERCISE   DURATION   INTENSITY

_____

_____

MEDICATION OR INSULIN TAKEN

TIME OF DAY	TYPE	AMOUNT

BLOOD SUGAR TESTS

TIME OF DAY   READING   TIME OF DAY   READING

_____   _____

_____   _____

_____

_____

_____

TODAY'S AVERAGE BLOOD SUGAR READING: _____

BODY WEIGHT: _____

DAY 7

Congratulations! You've made it to an important milestone. Day 7 is the end of your first full week on this program. This is also the last day you need to test your blood sugar eight times.

You'll notice that there's an extra journal page today. Don't panic—it's for your first set of weekly averages. It's very simple. All you need to do is add up your daily total calories this evening and divide by seven. Add up your daily total carbs and divide by seven. And add up each day's average blood sugar level and divide by seven to get your average blood sugar reading for the week.

You're doing great! Keep up the good work.

DAY 7

_____

BREAKFAST

	CALORIES	CARBS
BREAKFAST TOTALS:		

LUNCH

	CALORIES	CARBS
_____	_____	_____
_____	_____	_____
_____	_____	_____
_____	_____	_____
_____	_____	_____
LUNCH TOTALS:	_____	_____

DINNER

	CALORIES	CARBS
_____	_____	_____
_____	_____	_____
_____	_____	_____
_____	_____	_____
_____	_____	_____
DINNER TOTALS:	_____	_____

SNACKS

	CALORIES	CARBS
_____	_____	_____
_____	_____	_____
_____	_____	_____
_____	_____	_____
SNACKS TOTALS:	_____	_____
DAILY TOTALS:	_____	_____

Day 7

EXERCISE

TIME OF DAY	TYPE OF EXERCISE	DURATION	INTENSITY

MEDICATION OR INSULIN TAKEN

TIME OF DAY	TYPE	AMOUNT

BLOOD SUGAR TESTS

TIME OF DAY	READING	TIME OF DAY	READING

TODAY'S AVERAGE BLOOD SUGAR READING: _____

BODY WEIGHT: _____

WEEK 1 AVERAGES

AVERAGE DAILY
BLOOD SUGAR READING

_____

AVERAGE DAILY
TOTAL CALORIES

_____

AVERAGE DAILY
TOTAL CARBOHYDRATES

_____

TOTAL MINUTES OF EXERCISE

_____

AVERAGE BODY WEIGHT

_____

DAY 8

Take a little time this morning to sit down and look at the data you accumulated during this first seven days of this program. You've accomplished a lot! You know more about how your body reacts to food, exercise, and your insulin or medication than most people with diabetes. Hopefully you've made adjustments that are bringing 80 percent to 90 percent of your blood sugar readings within your target range. Don't even *try* to get to 100 percent. It can't be done. Even people who do a fantastic job of controlling their diabetes get the occasional reading that is out of range. And everybody has a bad day from time to time, when nothing seems to go right. Take those exceptions in stride. They won't hurt you. The key is to keep your *averages* in line—particularly your weekly averages.

If the vast majority of your tests do not fall within your target range, don't be afraid to get professional advice. Talk to your doctor or your certified diabetes educator. By all means, show them your first week's records. Because of their experience in dealing with hundreds of patients with diabetes, they may be able to spot things you didn't notice. The data you've collected will be *tremendously* helpful to them.

Look back at your first full week and analyze it. With a full week behind you, certain patterns are sure to stand out. As you've been doing all along, decide what you should do to correct anything that looks like a problem. Make the change, keep on testing, and see what happens. It's an on-going science experiment, and you are the one who will benefit from the results.

Starting today, you no longer need to test eight times a day, although eight spaces are still provided for test results in case you want to continue. But at this point, four times a day should be enough.

Now set your goal for the coming week. If your weekly average was a little bit higher than you were shooting for, make up your mind to get it within your target range this week. If you were within your target range but just barely, try to get right in the middle this time. If you were right on the bull's-eye, congratulations! Keep it there!

DAY 8

BREAKFAST

	CALORIES	CARBS
BREAKFAST TOTALS:		

LUNCH

	CALORIES	CARBS
_____	_____	_____
_____	_____	_____
_____	_____	_____
_____	_____	_____
_____	_____	_____
LUNCH TOTALS:	_____	_____

DINNER

	CALORIES	CARBS
_____	_____	_____
_____	_____	_____
_____	_____	_____
_____	_____	_____
_____	_____	_____
DINNER TOTALS:	_____	_____

SNACKS

	CALORIES	CARBS
_____	_____	_____
_____	_____	_____
_____	_____	_____
_____	_____	_____
SNACKS TOTALS:	_____	_____
DAILY TOTALS:	_____	_____

Day 8

EXERCISE

TIME OF DAY   TYPE OF EXERCISE   DURATION   INTENSITY

_____

_____

MEDICATION OR INSULIN TAKEN

TIME OF DAY	TYPE	AMOUNT

BLOOD SUGAR TESTS

TIME OF DAY   READING   TIME OF DAY   READING

_____   _____

_____   _____

_____

_____

_____

_____

TODAY'S AVERAGE BLOOD SUGAR READING: _____

BODY WEIGHT: _____

DAY 9

Now that you're starting to get your blood sugars under control, it's time to focus on something else that is critically important to managing your diabetes: your weight.

Losing weight is important for so many reasons that it would take an entire book to list them. In terms of your diabetes, it is important because losing weight lowers your insulin resistance. If you have type 2 diabetes, your body's natural insulin works better the less you weigh. If you have type 1, the insulin you inject works better the less you weight. Losing weight also tends to lower your cholesterol levels and blood pressure. It reduces your risk of heart attack or stroke. And it reduces your risk of cancer.

So how is it going so far? Many people find that when they start counting calories and keeping a detailed food diary, their weight automatically starts going down. It makes sense, doesn't it? If you know a sugary soft drink is going to add 150 calories to your daily calorie count, you may go for a bottle of water instead. All it takes is a few smart decisions like that in the course of the day to make a difference. Exercise also aids in weight loss, so it wouldn't be surprising if you've lost two or three pounds already.

Please do *not* go on a strict diet at this point—or any kind of a diet at all. Why? Because a "diet" is something people go on for a while, then go off. And they almost always gain all the weight they lost back when they go off of it.

So don't starve yourself. Don't go on a very low calorie diet. But *do* keep your food diary every day with scrupulous honesty. Be *aware* of what and how much you're eating, and try to make better choices during the day. Try to make the kinds of changes you can live with for the rest of your life.

Remember, it takes about 2,000 calories for the average woman to maintain a healthy weight, and about 2,700 for the average man. If you've been eating a lot more than that, just getting down to normal is an accomplishment. Congratulate yourself! If you want to lose weight steadily, a reasonable goal might be to cut 500 calories out of your total each day. For a woman, that might make your daily target 1,500 calories a day. For a man it might be 2,200 calories. That's not a starvation diet by any means, but it should enable you to lose a pound a week. Or a couple of pounds, if you're exercising hard. The beauty of counting calories is that *what* you eat is up to you. You know the target you're aiming for. Within that limit, your food choices are unlimited.

If you're looking for a food to cut out of your diet completely, here's a suggestion: potato chips. Look at the nutrition label on a typical bag of chips and you'll see that a serving contains 150 calories, 10 grams of fat, and 15 grams of carbohydrate.

That's bad enough, but the real problem is that a serving is only one ounce—about 20 chips. There are *12 servings* in the standard 12-ounce bag you buy at the grocery store. Open a bag of chips when you sit down to watch TV, and it's all too easy to finish off the bag in a couple of hours. That's 1,800 calories, 120 grams of fat, and 180 grams of carbohydrate! Wash it down with a couple cans of Coke and you've just taken in more calories, more fat, and more carbohydrates than you need *all day!*

Can't bring yourself to give up potato chips completely? Here are a couple of suggestions:

▶ If you know that you have the willpower, count out a single serving of chips and eat them from a bowl, not the bag. When the bag is sitting next to you on the couch, it's just too easy to keep reaching in there for more.

▶ If you don't think you can limit yourself to a single serving that way, buy your chips in individual snack-size bags. Yes, they're more expensive that way, but it may be worth it if they keep you from eating too many.

▶ Have a healthy substitute instead! If you really like salty, crunchy snacks, liberally season a handful of baby carrots and munch on them instead.

DAY 9

BREAKFAST

	CALORIES	CARBS
BREAKFAST TOTALS:		

LUNCH

	CALORIES	CARBS
_____	_____	_____
_____	_____	_____
_____	_____	_____
_____	_____	_____
_____	_____	_____
LUNCH TOTALS:	_____	_____

DINNER

	CALORIES	CARBS
_____	_____	_____
_____	_____	_____
_____	_____	_____
_____	_____	_____
_____	_____	_____
DINNER TOTALS:	_____	_____

SNACKS

	CALORIES	CARBS
_____	_____	_____
_____	_____	_____
_____	_____	_____
_____	_____	_____
SNACKS TOTALS:	_____	_____
DAILY TOTALS:	_____	_____

Day 9

EXERCISE

TIME OF DAY	TYPE OF EXERCISE	DURATION	INTENSITY

MEDICATION OR INSULIN TAKEN

TIME OF DAY	TYPE	AMOUNT

BLOOD SUGAR TESTS

TIME OF DAY	READING	TIME OF DAY	READING

TODAY'S AVERAGE BLOOD SUGAR READING: _____

BODY WEIGHT: _____

DAY 10

Welcome to Day Ten! Congratulations. You're doing great!

This is a great day to increase the amount of exercise you're getting. If you were totally sedentary when you began this program, you may still be working your way up to 30 minutes of exercise a day. Good for you! Keep going! The human body is incredibly responsive, and many people who can't walk a mile when they first try find they can walk two or three miles within a matter of weeks.

If you're already doing 30 minutes a day, that's awesome—but remember, 30 minutes a day is the recommended *minimum*. For optimal health, experts recommend an hour of exercise a day.

There are two ways to increase your exercise time: one is just to do more of whatever it is you're doing already. The other is to add a second exercise period of an entirely different kind.

(That's why there are two blanks in your journal for exercise.) Athletes call this "cross training."

If you've been walking for 30 minutes a day so far, you might want to add a session of light weight-lifting and calisthenics—push-ups, crunches, and so on—later in the day. The ideal exercise program includes aerobic exercise (like walking, jogging, or running) to strengthen your heart and lungs, and resistance training to strengthen your muscles—especially the muscles of your upper body, which don't get much of a workout from walking.

Exercise doesn't have to be drudgery. Trying to keep a hula hoop going is a fantastic, fun workout. Is there a sport you never tried before because you didn't have time? Let diabetes be your excuse to *make* time for it now! Always wanted to learn judo, or take a class in yoga? Always wondered what Tai Chi is all about? Or Tae Bo? What's stopping you?

Exercise is *meant* to be fun. Find the kind of exercise that's fun for you, and your workout will become the highlight of your day.

DAY 10

_____

BREAKFAST

	CALORIES	CARBS
BREAKFAST TOTALS:		

LUNCH

	CALORIES	CARBS
_____	_____	_____
_____	_____	_____
_____	_____	_____
_____	_____	_____
_____	_____	_____
LUNCH TOTALS:	_____	_____

DINNER

	CALORIES	CARBS
_____	_____	_____
_____	_____	_____
_____	_____	_____
_____	_____	_____
_____	_____	_____
DINNER TOTALS:	_____	_____

SNACKS

	CALORIES	CARBS
_____	_____	_____
_____	_____	_____
_____	_____	_____
_____	_____	_____
SNACKS TOTALS:	_____	_____
DAILY TOTALS:	_____	_____

Day 10

EXERCISE

TIME OF DAY	TYPE OF EXERCISE	DURATION	INTENSITY

MEDICATION OR INSULIN TAKEN

TIME OF DAY	TYPE	AMOUNT

BLOOD SUGAR TESTS

TIME OF DAY	READING	TIME OF DAY	READING

TODAY'S AVERAGE BLOOD SUGAR READING: _____

BODY WEIGHT: _____

DAY 11

Today I want you to make a special effort to focus on spotting *patterns* in your journal.

At this point you have ten days of really good data to look at. If you've got a highlighter pen handy, use it. Go over the past ten days and highlight the single highest and the single lowest blood sugar reading for each day. Is there a pattern? Are most of your highs falling after a specific meal, for example?

If so, take a look at what you normally eat at that meal. Is there something that you're eating or drinking at that meal that's causing the high readings? If you eat three or four different foods at that meal, try eliminating or replacing one of those foods one day, another the next, and so on. Test two hours after the first bite of the meal, and you'll soon find the problem food. Something you really like? Don't worry! In many cases, you don't have to *eliminate* the food from your diet—just eat a smaller quantity of it.

Conduct little experiments like this. Count on your blood glucose monitor to tell you what's going on. Analyze and adapt: these are the keys to diabetes control.

DAY 11

——————

BREAKFAST

	CALORIES	CARBS
BREAKFAST TOTALS:		

LUNCH

	CALORIES	CARBS
LUNCH TOTALS:		

DINNER

	CALORIES	CARBS
DINNER TOTALS:		

SNACKS

	CALORIES	CARBS
SNACKS TOTALS:		
DAILY TOTALS:		

Day 11

EXERCISE

TIME OF DAY   TYPE OF EXERCISE   DURATION   INTENSITY

_____

_____

MEDICATION OR INSULIN TAKEN

TIME OF DAY	TYPE	AMOUNT

BLOOD SUGAR TESTS

TIME OF DAY   READING   TIME OF DAY   READING

_____   _____

_____   _____

_____

_____

_____

_____

TODAY'S AVERAGE BLOOD SUGAR READING: _____

BODY WEIGHT: _____

DAY 12

Going into your twelfth day, I hope you're beginning to realize this program is not *that* hard to do. Counting carbs and calories only takes a few minutes when you get the hang of it and learn the numbers for most of your favorite foods. Exercising, once you get over the initial shock, is fun and feels good! I don't know if anybody thinks testing their blood sugar is actually *fun*, but after all the testing you've done so far, it should be no big deal.

By now, controlling your diabetes should be much less confusing. You're beginning to see the *cause and effect* from the entries on each of your journal pages. You know what it means to "master" your diabetes: to balance your food, exercise, medication, and insulin to control your blood sugar. You're well on your way!

DAY 12

_____

BREAKFAST

	CALORIES	CARBS
BREAKFAST TOTALS:		

LUNCH

	CALORIES	CARBS
_____	_____	_____
_____	_____	_____
_____	_____	_____
_____	_____	_____
_____	_____	_____
LUNCH TOTALS:	_____	_____

DINNER

	CALORIES	CARBS
_____	_____	_____
_____	_____	_____
_____	_____	_____
_____	_____	_____
_____	_____	_____
DINNER TOTALS:	_____	_____

SNACKS

	CALORIES	CARBS
_____	_____	_____
_____	_____	_____
_____	_____	_____
_____	_____	_____
SNACKS TOTALS:	_____	_____
DAILY TOTALS:	_____	_____

EXERCISE

TIME OF DAY	TYPE OF EXERCISE	DURATION	INTENSITY

MEDICATION OR INSULIN TAKEN

TIME OF DAY	TYPE	AMOUNT

BLOOD SUGAR TESTS

TIME OF DAY	READING	TIME OF DAY	READING

TODAY'S AVERAGE BLOOD SUGAR READING: _____

BODY WEIGHT: _____

DAY 13

It's lucky day 13! You now have a dozen days behind you.

Sometime today, take a moment for a little celebration. Look back at your first couple of days and remember how hard it was to look up everything you ate, to measure everything, to get this whole program started. Think about how *little* you knew about diabetes control then—and how much you know now.

Your knowledge of diabetes and diabetes control has come a long way. Your blood sugar readings should be falling in line much more consistently. It's very likely that your weight is dropping, too.

So take a moment to pat yourself on the back. You're doing great!

DAY 13

_____

BREAKFAST

	CALORIES	CARBS
_____	_____	_____
_____	_____	_____
_____	_____	_____
_____	_____	_____
_____	_____	_____
BREAKFAST TOTALS:	_____	_____

LUNCH

	CALORIES	CARBS
_____	_____	_____
_____	_____	_____
_____	_____	_____
_____	_____	_____
_____	_____	_____
LUNCH TOTALS:	_____	_____

DINNER

	CALORIES	CARBS
_____	_____	_____
_____	_____	_____
_____	_____	_____
_____	_____	_____
_____	_____	_____
DINNER TOTALS:	_____	_____

SNACKS

	CALORIES	CARBS
_____	_____	_____
_____	_____	_____
_____	_____	_____
_____	_____	_____
SNACKS TOTALS:	_____	_____
DAILY TOTALS:	_____	_____

EXERCISE

TIME OF DAY	TYPE OF EXERCISE	DURATION	INTENSITY

MEDICATION OR INSULIN TAKEN

TIME OF DAY	TYPE	AMOUNT

BLOOD SUGAR TESTS

TIME OF DAY	READING	TIME OF DAY	READING

TODAY'S AVERAGE BLOOD SUGAR READING: _____

BODY WEIGHT: _____

DAY 14

Congratulations! You've made it to the end of the second week of your program. You're halfway home. This evening, do your weekly averages and compare them to your averages for Week 1. Take a moment to celebrate every improvement and positive change you've made since you started this program!

By this evening you should have fourteen days of exercise behind you. You are well on your way to establishing daily exercise as a habit that will last for the rest of your life. Nothing could be more important!

Your blood sugar levels should by now be falling fairly consistently in your target range. Notice that you're feeling better, have more energy, are having fewer mood swings, and you're thinking more clearly? Those are the benefits of good blood sugar control—along with a *dramatic* reduction in your risk of the complications of diabetes.

If things aren't going that well, don't quit. Everyone progresses at a different rate, and tomorrow is another day. The benefits of this program are *long-term*. So don't worry if you have a couple of blank pages in your journal, if you haven't done every single blood test, or if you've missed a couple of days of exercise. Go at it again tomorrow, and give it your best. One solid week of recording everything you eat, testing regularly, getting your exercise, and analyzing the results will prove to you how much better you can feel—and will teach you more about controlling your diabetes than you can learn any other way.

Now is the time to set your goals for next week. Congratulate yourself on what you've done so far. Renew your commitment to get your diabetes under control. Onward!

DAY 14

BREAKFAST

	CALORIES	CARBS
BREAKFAST TOTALS:		

LUNCH

	CALORIES	CARBS
_____	_____	_____
_____	_____	_____
_____	_____	_____
_____	_____	_____
_____	_____	_____
LUNCH TOTALS:	_____	_____

DINNER

	CALORIES	CARBS
_____	_____	_____
_____	_____	_____
_____	_____	_____
_____	_____	_____
_____	_____	_____
DINNER TOTALS:	_____	_____

SNACKS

	CALORIES	CARBS
_____	_____	_____
_____	_____	_____
_____	_____	_____
_____	_____	_____
SNACKS TOTALS:	_____	_____
DAILY TOTALS:	_____	_____

Day 14

EXERCISE

TIME OF DAY   TYPE OF EXERCISE   DURATION   INTENSITY

_____

_____

MEDICATION OR INSULIN TAKEN

TIME OF DAY	TYPE	AMOUNT

BLOOD SUGAR TESTS

TIME OF DAY   READING   TIME OF DAY   READING

_____   _____

_____   _____

_____

_____

_____

TODAY'S AVERAGE BLOOD SUGAR READING: _____

BODY WEIGHT: _____

WEEK 2 AVERAGES

AVERAGE DAILY
BLOOD SUGAR READING

_____

AVERAGE DAILY
TOTAL CALORIES

_____

AVERAGE DAILY
TOTAL CARBOHYDRATES

_____

TOTAL MINUTES OF EXERCISE

_____

AVERAGE BODY WEIGHT

_____

DAY 15

By this stage of the program you should be saying to yourself: "I can do this!"

And you're right—you can! Remember back when you were first diagnosed and gaining control over your diabetes seemed overwhelming? Now your diabetes routines are starting to be integrated into your lifestyle. The time is near when you'll find that diabetes control only takes a few minutes out of your day. You may spend more time in the shower than you spend on tasks related to controlling your blood sugar.

So let yourself think ahead. What were your goals and dreams before you were diagnosed? Time to dust them off and really think about what you want to do. Assuming that you keep your blood sugar under control, diabetes does *not* need to limit you. Decide what you want. And then *do it*.

DAY 15

———————

BREAKFAST

	CALORIES	CARBS
BREAKFAST TOTALS:		

LUNCH

	CALORIES	CARBS
_____	_____	_____
_____	_____	_____
_____	_____	_____
_____	_____	_____
_____	_____	_____
LUNCH TOTALS:	_____	_____

DINNER

	CALORIES	CARBS
_____	_____	_____
_____	_____	_____
_____	_____	_____
_____	_____	_____
_____	_____	_____
DINNER TOTALS:	_____	_____

SNACKS

	CALORIES	CARBS
_____	_____	_____
_____	_____	_____
_____	_____	_____
_____	_____	_____
SNACKS TOTALS:	_____	_____
DAILY TOTALS:	_____	_____

Day 15

EXERCISE

TIME OF DAY	TYPE OF EXERCISE	DURATION	INTENSITY

MEDICATION OR INSULIN TAKEN

TIME OF DAY	TYPE	AMOUNT

BLOOD SUGAR TESTS

TIME OF DAY	READING	TIME OF DAY	READING

TODAY'S AVERAGE BLOOD SUGAR READING: _____

BODY WEIGHT: _____

DAY 16

If one of your goals is to lose weight, this is the perfect day to see how you're doing. You're far enough into the program now that you should have lost a couple of pounds—maybe even more.

If you haven't, stop and analyze why. Look at the entries on your journal sheets for exercise and total daily calories. Remember, when you burn more calories than you consume, you lose weight. When you consume more than you burn, you gain.

I recently did an interview with my friend Will Cross, who illustrated this simple fact very dramatically. Will just got back from a two-month trek to the South Pole. During the trek, Will ate a whopping 5,000 calories a day—sometimes more. And 50 percent of it was fat! (The reason for so much fat was because fat is very calorie dense, and he was trying to pack in as many calories as possible. He actually melted a pound of butter in his coffee every morning.)

Did he gain weight? No—he *lost* 30 pounds. Because he was walking for ten hours a day in sub-freezing cold, pulling a 150-pound sled, he was burning more calories than he could possibly consume.

If you're not losing weight, it's because you're *not* burning more calories than you consume. Your options are to burn more (increase your exercise), or consume less (eat fewer total daily calories.) Or do a little of both—increase your exercise and decrease your calories at the same time.

DAY 16

———————

BREAKFAST

	CALORIES	CARBS
BREAKFAST TOTALS:		

LUNCH

	CALORIES	CARBS
_____	_____	_____
_____	_____	_____
_____	_____	_____
_____	_____	_____
_____	_____	_____
LUNCH TOTALS:	_____	_____

DINNER

	CALORIES	CARBS
_____	_____	_____
_____	_____	_____
_____	_____	_____
_____	_____	_____
_____	_____	_____
DINNER TOTALS:	_____	_____

SNACKS

	CALORIES	CARBS
_____	_____	_____
_____	_____	_____
_____	_____	_____
_____	_____	_____
SNACKS TOTALS:	_____	_____
DAILY TOTALS:	_____	_____

EXERCISE

TIME OF DAY	TYPE OF EXERCISE	DURATION	INTENSITY

MEDICATION OR INSULIN TAKEN

TIME OF DAY	TYPE	AMOUNT

BLOOD SUGAR TESTS

TIME OF DAY	READING	TIME OF DAY	READING

TODAY'S AVERAGE BLOOD SUGAR READING: _____

BODY WEIGHT: _____

DAY 17

One goal of this 28-day program is to get you in the habit of getting *at least* 30 minutes of exercise every single day.

If you're doing your 30 minutes, congratulations! If not, don't beat yourself up about it—but don't give up on it either. Exercise is *tremendously* important for your diabetes control as well as your overall physical and psychological well-being.

If you've found something you like to do but you're missing more days than you hit, really consider doing it first thing in the morning. In the rush of the day, it's too easy for something "more important" to come up. When it's already done, it can't be pre-empted.

If you haven't found a kind of exercise you like to do, put some real effort into thinking of something. I would be very sorry if you finished this program without getting into the habit of getting exercise, consistently, for at least 30 minutes a day.

Throughout this book I've told you that your blood sugar is controlled by what you eat, how much you exercise, and by the medicine or insulin you take. And that's true. But there are "wild cards" that make it almost impossible to keep blood sugar in the target range 100 percent of the time. These wild cards include stress, illness, and hormones. Sometimes in the morning you may have a "rebound high," which is actually your body's emergency response to a low that occurred during the night. Furthermore, you will occasionally have an out-of-range reading that just can't be explained by *anything*. Just understand that these things are a normal part of life.

You can't let an occasional unexpected result throw you off track. Keep on doing the right things to keep your blood sugar as close to normal as you can. Your control will never be *perfect*—but it will be close enough to let you live a long, rewarding life, free of diabetes complications.

DAY 17

BREAKFAST

	CALORIES	CARBS
BREAKFAST TOTALS:		

LUNCH

	CALORIES	CARBS
_____	_____	_____
_____	_____	_____
_____	_____	_____
_____	_____	_____
_____	_____	_____
LUNCH TOTALS:	_____	_____

DINNER

	CALORIES	CARBS
_____	_____	_____
_____	_____	_____
_____	_____	_____
_____	_____	_____
_____	_____	_____
DINNER TOTALS:	_____	_____

SNACKS

	CALORIES	CARBS
_____	_____	_____
_____	_____	_____
_____	_____	_____
_____	_____	_____
SNACKS TOTALS:	_____	_____
DAILY TOTALS:	_____	_____

Day 17

EXERCISE

TIME OF DAY   TYPE OF EXERCISE   DURATION   INTENSITY

_____

_____

MEDICATION OR INSULIN TAKEN

TIME OF DAY	TYPE	AMOUNT

BLOOD SUGAR TESTS

TIME OF DAY   READING   TIME OF DAY   READING

_____   _____

_____   _____

_____

_____

_____

_____

TODAY'S AVERAGE BLOOD SUGAR READING: _____

BODY WEIGHT: _____

DAY 18

It's Day 18, and I want you to try something a little different today. Leaf through your completed journal pages without looking for anything in particular. You've got a lot to look at now—so just glance through the pages. Appreciate how much you've done and how much you've learned.

As you page through your journal, something may jump out at you that you never noticed before—something that may explain why one day was so much better than all the others, for example. If it does, great! You've noticed something new that may help you as you strive to achieve better control.

If nothing jumps off the page, that's okay, too. Just enjoy the satisfaction of looking back at your completed pages, and take pride in what you've accomplished in this short period of time.

DAY 18

BREAKFAST

	CALORIES	CARBS
_____	_____	_____
_____	_____	_____
_____	_____	_____
_____	_____	_____
_____	_____	_____
BREAKFAST TOTALS:	_____	_____

LUNCH

	CALORIES	CARBS
_____	_____	_____
_____	_____	_____
_____	_____	_____
_____	_____	_____
_____	_____	_____
LUNCH TOTALS:	_____	_____

DINNER

	CALORIES	CARBS
_____	_____	_____
_____	_____	_____
_____	_____	_____
_____	_____	_____
_____	_____	_____
DINNER TOTALS:	_____	_____

SNACKS

	CALORIES	CARBS
_____	_____	_____
_____	_____	_____
_____	_____	_____
_____	_____	_____
SNACKS TOTALS:	_____	_____
DAILY TOTALS:	_____	_____

Day 18

EXERCISE

TIME OF DAY	TYPE OF EXERCISE	DURATION	INTENSITY

MEDICATION OR INSULIN TAKEN

TIME OF DAY	TYPE	AMOUNT

BLOOD SUGAR TESTS

TIME OF DAY	READING	TIME OF DAY	READING

TODAY'S AVERAGE BLOOD SUGAR READING: _____

BODY WEIGHT: _____

DAY 19

It's Day 19. Congratulations! You're doing a fantastic job.

Today, think about increasing your exercise program just a little. The human body is incredibly responsive. If you started exercising regularly on Day 1, your body has almost certainly adapted to the exercise and accepted it as part of your daily routine. So now is a good time to go a little faster, a little farther, or a little longer. You know that half-an-hour of exercise a day is the *minimum* for good health. Long-term, your goal should be to do an hour. Please, don't jump from 30 minutes to 60 minutes all at once. Take it gradually. If you've been walking for 30 minutes every day for the last eighteen days, you should be able to go to 40 or possibly even 45 minutes without too much trouble. Stay at that level for another three or four weeks. Then, when 45 minutes no longer feels like a challenge, increase to an hour.

Here's another suggestion. You've started exercising regularly—and that's fantastic. By the end of this 28-day program, your regular daily exercise will be such a part of your routine that you wouldn't even *think* about giving it up. Ever. But to ensure that, pick a goal to help keep you motivated. Go on the Web or visit your local running-shoe store and find a 5K (3.1 mile) run/walk scheduled in your area three or four months from now. Sign up for it. Be there.

Even if you were totally sedentary when you started this program, you can almost certainly be ready to walk a 5K in three or four months if you train for it seriously. Close your eyes and picture yourself striding (maybe even jogging or running!) across the finish line, proudly picking up your T-shirt. Having a specific goal makes all the difference in staying motivated, and training for a 5K race rather than just going out for your daily walk is a super goal. Wake up the athlete inside you. Call on your own competitive spirit. Even if you don't win the race, go out there and show 'em what you can do—and have fun while you're ensuring your health.

DAY 19

BREAKFAST

	CALORIES	CARBS
BREAKFAST TOTALS:		

LUNCH

	CALORIES	CARBS
_____	_____	_____
_____	_____	_____
_____	_____	_____
_____	_____	_____
_____	_____	_____
LUNCH TOTALS:	_____	_____

DINNER

	CALORIES	CARBS
_____	_____	_____
_____	_____	_____
_____	_____	_____
_____	_____	_____
_____	_____	_____
DINNER TOTALS:	_____	_____

SNACKS

	CALORIES	CARBS
_____	_____	_____
_____	_____	_____
_____	_____	_____
_____	_____	_____
SNACKS TOTALS:	_____	_____
DAILY TOTALS:	_____	_____

Day 19

EXERCISE

TIME OF DAY	TYPE OF EXERCISE	DURATION	INTENSITY

MEDICATION OR INSULIN TAKEN

TIME OF DAY	TYPE	AMOUNT

BLOOD SUGAR TESTS

TIME OF DAY	READING	TIME OF DAY	READING

TODAY'S AVERAGE BLOOD SUGAR READING: _____

BODY WEIGHT: _____

DAY 20

It's Day 20, and you've gone from simply learning about controlling your blood sugar levels to mastering it.

Now it's time for a little advanced-placement exercise. Today, before each of your four (or more) blood sugar tests, try *predicting* the result. Think about it. You've been testing regularly for the past 19 days. You've diligently analyzed all the factors that affect your blood sugar: diet, exercise, and medication or insulin. So before you do your first blood test in the morning, think back to what you ate last night, how much exercise you did yesterday, and make your prediction. Then go ahead and test and see how you close you are.

If you're within 20 or 30 points of what you expected, that's right on the money. Within 40 or 50 points is darned close. I'm willing to bet your predictions are in the ballpark more often that not.

Being able to predict your blood sugar is a *big step*. Remember when you did your first blood sugar test and had *no idea* what the result would be—and probably very little idea of what the number meant anyway? You've come a long way. Now you know exactly what that number means, what it should be, and what factors determine it. Learning to make a reasonable prediction of your blood sugar level means you're well on your way to achieving diabetes control.

DAY 20

———————

BREAKFAST

	CALORIES	CARBS
BREAKFAST TOTALS:		

LUNCH

	CALORIES	CARBS
LUNCH TOTALS:		

DINNER

	CALORIES	CARBS
DINNER TOTALS:		

SNACKS

	CALORIES	CARBS
SNACKS TOTALS:		
DAILY TOTALS:		

EXERCISE

TIME OF DAY	TYPE OF EXERCISE	DURATION	INTENSITY

MEDICATION OR INSULIN TAKEN

TIME OF DAY	TYPE	AMOUNT

BLOOD SUGAR TESTS

TIME OF DAY	READING	TIME OF DAY	READING

TODAY'S AVERAGE BLOOD SUGAR READING: _____

BODY WEIGHT: _____

DAY 21

Congratulations!

This is the last day of the third week of your program. A major milestone! You're three-quarters of the way through. Just one more week to go.

The reason for the length of this program is that 28 days is the amount of time it takes to make a new habit *permanent*. Exercise every day for 28 days, and you're not likely to stop suddenly on day 29. Keep your blood sugars under tight control for 28 days, and you're not likely to let them go when this program is done. Get in the habit of counting every calorie you eat, and you'll do it subconsciously even when this program is finished and you're no longer writing down every bite of food you eat and every beverage you consume during the course of the day.

You have made positive changes and integrated healthy habits into your lifestyle. These changes will make you healthier for the rest of your life, and keep your risk of diabetes complications to the absolute minimum. Keep it up for one more week, and these positive changes will become *permanent*.

DAY 21

_____

BREAKFAST

	CALORIES	CARBS
_____		
_____		
_____		
_____		
_____		
BREAKFAST TOTALS:		

LUNCH

	CALORIES	CARBS
LUNCH TOTALS:		

DINNER

	CALORIES	CARBS
DINNER TOTALS:		

SNACKS

	CALORIES	CARBS
SNACKS TOTALS:		
DAILY TOTALS:		

Day 21

EXERCISE

TIME OF DAY   TYPE OF EXERCISE   DURATION   INTENSITY

_____

_____

MEDICATION OR INSULIN TAKEN

TIME OF DAY	TYPE	AMOUNT

BLOOD SUGAR TESTS

TIME OF DAY   READING   TIME OF DAY   READING

_____   _____

_____   _____

_____

_____

_____

_____

TODAY'S AVERAGE BLOOD SUGAR READING: _____

BODY WEIGHT: _____

WEEK 3 AVERAGES

AVERAGE DAILY
BLOOD SUGAR READING

_____

AVERAGE DAILY
TOTAL CALORIES

_____

AVERAGE DAILY
TOTAL CARBOHYDRATES

_____

TOTAL MINUTES OF EXERCISE

_____

AVERAGE BODY WEIGHT

_____

DAY 22

You're in the home stretch.

This is a week for fine-tuning and for improving any area where you haven't made as much progress as you'd like. Look back at your journal pages for the first three weeks and your first three weekly averages. Make a note of how you've done, and set your goals for this week.

If you haven't been as faithful to the program as you'd like, you still have this week to finish strong. I know I sound like a broken record, but I'm going to say it again: if you record everything you eat, your exercise, your medications, and the results of four tests a day for one solid week, you'll gain insights into controlling your diabetes that will benefit you for a lifetime.

If you've had trouble sticking with this program, don't be afraid to ask for help. Your friends and family can help you manage your diabetes if you let them. Teach them what you know about diabetes. If you're going to diabetes education classes, take family members along. Let them read this book. Just knowing that people close to you understand this disease and what you are going through to control it is very encouraging.

Family members need to understand the changes you're making in your diet and lifestyle to level out your blood sugars and control your weight. Explain this program to them, and let them help you analyze your data. They may see something you haven't noticed!

DAY 22

_____

BREAKFAST

	CALORIES	CARBS
BREAKFAST TOTALS:		

LUNCH

	CALORIES	CARBS
LUNCH TOTALS:		

DINNER

	CALORIES	CARBS
DINNER TOTALS:		

SNACKS

	CALORIES	CARBS
SNACKS TOTALS:		
DAILY TOTALS:		

Day 22

EXERCISE

TIME OF DAY   TYPE OF EXERCISE   DURATION   INTENSITY

_____

_____

MEDICATION OR INSULIN TAKEN

TIME OF DAY	TYPE	AMOUNT

BLOOD SUGAR TESTS

TIME OF DAY   READING   TIME OF DAY   READING

_____   _____

_____   _____

_____

_____

_____

TODAY'S AVERAGE BLOOD SUGAR READING: _____

BODY WEIGHT: _____

DAY 23

The end is in sight!

This is the day to pick up the phone and make an appointment with your diabetes doctor—whether you've made great strides in your diabetes control or not. Try to get an appointment within a week or two of finishing this program.

If you've made good progress and your blood sugar readings are starting to fall within range consistently, your doctor needs to know. You may be able to reduce the amount of medication or insulin you take. In any case, it's important to check in with your physician when anything about your diabetes changes—even when the change is for the better.

If you are disappointed with your results so far, then it's doubly important to see your doctor. If you're doing everything right to the best of your ability, then the problem may be with your medical regimen. You may do better with different oral medications or a different insulin regimen. Take your journal with you to your appointment—your doctor will be absolutely overjoyed to have so much information to work with. Doctors aren't psychic. They can't gaze into your eyes and figure out what's wrong. But with 28 days of detailed data to look at, your doctor doesn't need a crystal ball.

DAY 23

_____

BREAKFAST

	CALORIES	CARBS
BREAKFAST TOTALS:		

LUNCH

	CALORIES	CARBS
_____	_____	_____
_____	_____	_____
_____	_____	_____
_____	_____	_____
_____	_____	_____
LUNCH TOTALS:	_____	_____

DINNER

	CALORIES	CARBS
_____	_____	_____
_____	_____	_____
_____	_____	_____
_____	_____	_____
_____	_____	_____
DINNER TOTALS:	_____	_____

SNACKS

	CALORIES	CARBS
_____	_____	_____
_____	_____	_____
_____	_____	_____
_____	_____	_____
SNACKS TOTALS:	_____	_____
DAILY TOTALS:	_____	_____

Day 23

EXERCISE

TIME OF DAY	TYPE OF EXERCISE	DURATION	INTENSITY

MEDICATION OR INSULIN TAKEN

TIME OF DAY	TYPE	AMOUNT

BLOOD SUGAR TESTS

TIME OF DAY	READING	TIME OF DAY	READING

TODAY'S AVERAGE BLOOD SUGAR READING: _____

BODY WEIGHT: _____

DAY 24

Day 24—*charging* down the home stretch!

My sincere hope is that by now this is starting to seem like the *easiest thing in the world*. Controlling your diabetes doesn't have to consume you. It is destined to be just a small part of your life. The rest is a blank canvas, just as it was before you were diagnosed. You can make it into any kind of masterpiece you want.

Today I want you to concentrate on making this process intrude on your real life *as little as possible*. Don't get me wrong; I want you to fill out your journal page, get your exercise, and do your tests. I want you to count and record your carbs and your calories, just like always.

But you're an *expert* at all that by now. A blood sugar test, which may have taken you five minutes full of apprehension when you started this program, now probably takes you 30 seconds or less, including packing and unpacking your monitor. Counting the carbs in a meal? At first you had to measure, look things up, use all your fingers and toes to make the calculations. But now? You could teach a class on carbohydrate counting! You know the carb content of dozens of foods by heart. Bask in your success. It's well deserved.

So, for today, concentrate on efficiency. Control your diabetes—but in the least possible amount of time. Focus on the things that matter in your life. If family or friends have been helping you through this program, take the time to thank them. If you've been neglecting your dog or your house or your job while you worked on controlling your diabetes, now is a good time to start catching up. From this day on, diabetes will only be a small part of your life.

DAY 24

_____

BREAKFAST

	CALORIES	CARBS
BREAKFAST TOTALS:		

LUNCH

	CALORIES	CARBS
_____	_____	_____
_____	_____	_____
_____	_____	_____
_____	_____	_____
_____	_____	_____
LUNCH TOTALS:	_____	_____

DINNER

	CALORIES	CARBS
_____	_____	_____
_____	_____	_____
_____	_____	_____
_____	_____	_____
_____	_____	_____
DINNER TOTALS:	_____	_____

SNACKS

	CALORIES	CARBS
_____	_____	_____
_____	_____	_____
_____	_____	_____
_____	_____	_____
SNACKS TOTALS:	_____	_____
DAILY TOTALS:	_____	_____

Day 24

EXERCISE

TIME OF DAY   TYPE OF EXERCISE   DURATION   INTENSITY

_____

_____

MEDICATION OR INSULIN TAKEN

TIME OF DAY	TYPE	AMOUNT

BLOOD SUGAR TESTS

TIME OF DAY   READING   TIME OF DAY   READING

_____   _____

_____   _____

_____

_____

_____

_____

TODAY'S AVERAGE BLOOD SUGAR READING: _____
BODY WEIGHT: _____

DAY 25

It's Day 25. You have shown *fantastic* self-discipline and commitment to make it this far, and you should be proud of yourself.

Please make this the day you really commit yourself to continuing with this program after the 28 days are done. I'll warn you—already your subconscious mind is thinking, "Whew! Only three more days after today, and then we can *relax!*"

Don't let it take charge. Look in the mirror and say to yourself, "I like the path I'm on. Every day I am going farther and farther down the road to good health. And I'm going to keep right on going down that road when this program is done."

DAY 25

_____

BREAKFAST

	CALORIES	CARBS
BREAKFAST TOTALS:		

LUNCH

	CALORIES	CARBS
_____	_____	_____
_____	_____	_____
_____	_____	_____
_____	_____	_____
_____	_____	_____
LUNCH TOTALS:	_____	_____

DINNER

	CALORIES	CARBS
_____	_____	_____
_____	_____	_____
_____	_____	_____
_____	_____	_____
_____	_____	_____
DINNER TOTALS:	_____	_____

SNACKS

	CALORIES	CARBS
_____	_____	_____
_____	_____	_____
_____	_____	_____
_____	_____	_____
SNACKS TOTALS:	_____	_____
DAILY TOTALS:	_____	_____

Day 25

EXERCISE

TIME OF DAY   TYPE OF EXERCISE   DURATION   INTENSITY

_____

_____

MEDICATION OR INSULIN TAKEN

TIME OF DAY	TYPE	AMOUNT

BLOOD SUGAR TESTS

TIME OF DAY   READING   TIME OF DAY   READING

_____   _____

_____   _____

_____

_____

_____

TODAY'S AVERAGE BLOOD SUGAR READING: _____

BODY WEIGHT: _____

DAY 26

This is a perfect day to go back through your journal pages and look for patterns again.

You now have 25 days worth of high-quality data to look at. So get out your highlighter and go over every page since you did it last, marking the highs and lows for each day.

With just two days left in the program, is it too late to make adjustments? No! You'll be making adjustments to keep your diabetes in control for the rest of your life. With the knowledge and skills you have now, you'll be able to spot potential problems early, make adjustments quickly, and never let your diabetes get out of control.

DAY 26

_____

BREAKFAST

	CALORIES	CARBS
BREAKFAST TOTALS:		

LUNCH

	CALORIES	CARBS
_____	_____	_____
_____	_____	_____
_____	_____	_____
_____	_____	_____
_____	_____	_____
LUNCH TOTALS:	_____	_____

DINNER

	CALORIES	CARBS
_____	_____	_____
_____	_____	_____
_____	_____	_____
_____	_____	_____
_____	_____	_____
DINNER TOTALS:	_____	_____

SNACKS

	CALORIES	CARBS
_____	_____	_____
_____	_____	_____
_____	_____	_____
_____	_____	_____
SNACKS TOTALS:	_____	_____
DAILY TOTALS:	_____	_____

EXERCISE

TIME OF DAY	TYPE OF EXERCISE	DURATION	INTENSITY

MEDICATION OR INSULIN TAKEN

TIME OF DAY	TYPE	AMOUNT

BLOOD SUGAR TESTS

TIME OF DAY	READING	TIME OF DAY	READING

TODAY'S AVERAGE BLOOD SUGAR READING: _____

BODY WEIGHT: _____

DAY 27

It's the second-to-last day of your program, and you've done a fantastic job! I can't begin to say how proud I am of what you've done.

What I want you to think about today is *balance*. Diabetes control is all about balance. You balance out the carbs you eat with exercise, medication, and/or insulin to keep your blood sugar where you need it to be. You balance out the calories you consume with the amount of exercise you do to normalize your weight.

Life is about balance, too. For people with diabetes, the key is striking the right balance between managing the disease and living their lives. Yes, you *have* to control your diabetes. But you *don't* have to let your diabetes control you. This program has taught you the skills you need to live a life in balance, with your diabetes in control and the confidence to take on any challenge that life presents you.

Never let your diabetes hold you back from doing what you want to do. You may not want to compete in the Olympic Games, walk to the South Pole, or fly a small plane around the world. But you *could.* People with diabetes have done all those things—and more. Here is a short list of extraordinarily accomplished people with diabetes to prove it. The next time you're feeling down, open to this page and let these people inspire you.

Gary Hall, Jr. Already an Olympic champion swimmer with two gold and two silver medals in the summer games in Atlanta, Gary was training for the 2000 Games in Sydney when he was diagnosed with type 1 diabetes. He was told twice in one day by doctors that he would never swim again at the world-class level. But he proved them wrong by winning two more golds, a silver, and a bronze in Sydney. He's currently training for the 2004 Games in Athens, Greece, where he plans to win some more.

Nicole Johnson. Miss America, 1999.

Douglas Cairns. On February 19, 2003—after five months, 63 flights, 26,306 nautical miles, and stops in 22 countries— Douglas completed the first-ever flight around the world in a small plane by a pilot with diabetes. Until 1996, people with insulin-dependent diabetes could not get a pilot's license. But now, recognizing the advances that have been made in diabetes management, the U.S. Federal Aviation Administration will issue a private pilot's license to a person with diabetes. Douglas did the portions of the trip over the United States solo, including the longest single leg, from Hawaii to San Francisco, which is considered a domestic U.S. flight. In countries where people with diabetes are not allowed to fly by themselves, he was accompanied by a "safety pilot" to make the flight legal, although Douglas did all the flying himself.

Kris Freeman. Kris recently won the 30K cross-country classic in the Under-23 World Championships, and is considered a medal favorite in cross-country skiing events at the upcoming Winter Olympics in 2006.

Doug Burns and Kim Seeley. Champion bodybuilders.

Alison Scheel and Stephen Manley. Ironman-length triathletes.

Bill King and Dr. Michael Heile. Marathon runners.

Michael Hunter. Competitive aerobatic pilot.

Will Cross. One of the great adventurers of all time. Will has walked to both the North and South Poles. Next stop? Everest!

John Dennis. Sailed single-handedly over 11,000 miles from New York to England, and England to South Africa.

David Panofsky. Led a climbing expedition to 22,834-foot Cerro Aconcagua in Argentina that put seven insulin-dependent climbers on the summit of the highest mountain in the western hemisphere.

Diabetes didn't stop these people—and it won't stop you from doing *anything you want to do.*

DAY 27

_____

BREAKFAST

	CALORIES	CARBS
BREAKFAST TOTALS:		

LUNCH

	CALORIES	CARBS
_____	_____	_____
_____	_____	_____
_____	_____	_____
_____	_____	_____
_____	_____	_____
LUNCH TOTALS:	_____	_____

DINNER

	CALORIES	CARBS
_____	_____	_____
_____	_____	_____
_____	_____	_____
_____	_____	_____
_____	_____	_____
DINNER TOTALS:	_____	_____

SNACKS

	CALORIES	CARBS
_____	_____	_____
_____	_____	_____
_____	_____	_____
_____	_____	_____
SNACKS TOTALS:	_____	_____
DAILY TOTALS:	_____	_____

Day 27

EXERCISE

TIME OF DAY   TYPE OF EXERCISE   DURATION   INTENSITY

_____

_____

MEDICATION OR INSULIN TAKEN

TIME OF DAY   TYPE   AMOUNT

BLOOD SUGAR TESTS

TIME OF DAY   READING   TIME OF DAY   READING

_____   _____

_____   _____

_____

_____

_____

_____

TODAY'S AVERAGE BLOOD SUGAR READING: _____
BODY WEIGHT: _____

DAY 28

Well, my friend, here it is: Day 28. The final day of the program—and the first day of the rest of your new and improved life with diabetes. CONGRATULATIONS!

The skills you've learned in the past 28 days are yours to use for the rest of your life. If your blood sugars ever again get off track, you know what to do. Record what you eat, your exercise, and—if you use them—your medications or insulin. Analyze and adapt. You have the skills. You are *in control*.

So finish out the day in style! Fill out the last day's journal in your best handwriting. Do your totals for the week. Take time to compare your blood sugars from Week One with Week Four. Compare how fit you are to your physical condition a month ago. Compare your weight from Day One to today. Contrast what you know about managing diabetes now to what you knew 28 days ago.

Congratulate yourself on your accomplishments and celebrate your success! You were faced with a problem, and you confronted it head-on. You got this book, you followed the program, and now you have the problem *under control*. You are a champion!

Don't stop doing the things you've been doing for the past four weeks. Keep exercising on a daily basis. Test your blood sugar regularly. Balance your food, exercise, and insulin or medication to keep your blood sugars in your target range. Count your calories and keep your weight trending downward until you hit your goal.

I wish you the very best!

DAY 28

_____

BREAKFAST

	CALORIES	CARBS
_____	_____	_____
_____	_____	_____
_____	_____	_____
_____	_____	_____
_____	_____	_____
BREAKFAST TOTALS:	_____	_____

LUNCH

	CALORIES	CARBS
_____	_____	_____
_____	_____	_____
_____	_____	_____
_____	_____	_____
_____	_____	_____
LUNCH TOTALS:	_____	_____

DINNER

	CALORIES	CARBS
_____	_____	_____
_____	_____	_____
_____	_____	_____
_____	_____	_____
_____	_____	_____
DINNER TOTALS:	_____	_____

SNACKS

	CALORIES	CARBS
_____	_____	_____
_____	_____	_____
_____	_____	_____
_____	_____	_____
SNACKS TOTALS:	_____	_____
DAILY TOTALS:	_____	_____

Day 28

EXERCISE

TIME OF DAY   TYPE OF EXERCISE   DURATION   INTENSITY

_____

_____

MEDICATION OR INSULIN TAKEN

TIME OF DAY	TYPE	AMOUNT

BLOOD SUGAR TESTS

TIME OF DAY   READING   TIME OF DAY   READING

_____   _____

_____   _____

_____

_____

_____

_____

TODAY'S AVERAGE BLOOD SUGAR READING: _____

BODY WEIGHT: _____

WEEK 4 AVERAGES

AVERAGE DAILY
BLOOD SUGAR READING

_____

AVERAGE DAILY
TOTAL CALORIES

_____

AVERAGE DAILY
TOTAL CARBOHYDRATES

_____

TOTAL MINUTES OF EXERCISE

_____

AVERAGE BODY WEIGHT

_____

PART THREE:
RESOURCES

HELPFUL

ORGANIZATIONS

American Diabetes Association
Attn: National Call Center
1701 N. Beauregard St.
Alexandria, VA 22311
1-800-DIABETES (800-342-2383)
www.diabetes.org
Questions: askada@diabetes.org

American Heart Association
National Center
7272 Greenville Avenue
Dallas, TX 75231
1-800-AHA-USA-1 (800-242-8721)
www.americanheart.org

American Stroke Association
National Center
7272 Greenville Avenue

Dallas, TX 75231
1-888-4-STROKE (888-478-7653)
www.strokeassociation.org

American Dietetic Association
120 S. Riverside Plaza, Suite 2000
Chicago, IL 60606-6995
1-800-877-1600
Nutritional information line: 1-800-366-1655
Find a registered dietition: Extension 5000
findrd@eatright.org
www.eatright.org

American Association of Diabetes Educators
100 W. Monroe Street, Suite 400
Chicago, IL 60603
1-800-338-3633
Questions: aade@aadenet.org
www.aadenet.org

Diabetes Exercise and Sports Association (DESA)
8001 Montcastle Drive
Nashville, TN 37221
1-800-898-4322
Questions: desa@diabetes-exercise.org
www.diabetes-exercise.org

Juvenile Diabetes Research Foundation International
120 Wall Street
New York, NY 10005-4001
1-800-533-CURE (1-800-533-2873)
Questions: info@jdrf.org
www.jdrf.org

Joslin Diabetes Center
One Joslin Place
Boston, MA 02215
1-617-732-2400
www.joslin.harvard.edu

MedicAlert Foundation International
2323 Colorado Avenue
Turlock, CA 95382
1-888-633-4298
Questions: customer_service@medicalert.org
www.medicalert.org

Alert Access, LLC
5000 SW 75 Avenue, Suite 203
Miami, FL 33155
Customer Service: 1-877-462-5378
1-305-666-5240
Questions: info@alertaccess.com
www.alertaccess.com

National Institute of Diabetes and Digestive and Kidney Diseases (NIDDK)

National Diabetes Information Clearinghouse
1 Information Way
Bethesda, MD 20892-3560
1-800-860-8747
1-301-654-3327
E-mail: ndic@info.niddk.nih.gov
www.diabetes.niddk.nih.gov

Centers for Disease Control and Prevention (CDC)
1600 Clifton Road
Atlanta, GA 30333
1-800-311-3435
1-404-639-3534
www.cdc.gov

MAGAZINES

Diabetes Forecast
American Diabetes Association
1701 N. Beauregard Street
Alexandria, VA 22311
1-800-342-2383

Bill Outlaw, Director, Membership/Subscription Services
1-800-806-7801 (Diabetes Forecast Customer Service)
www.diabetes.org
1 YR (12 issues): $28.00
2 YR (24 issues): $52.00

Diabetes Self-Management

R.A. Rapaport Publishing, Inc.
150 West 22nd Street
New York, NY 10011
1-212-989-0200
James Moorehead, Circulation Director
1-800-234-0923 (Subscription Services)
1 YR (6 issues): $18.00
www.diabetesselfmanagement.com

Diabetes Interview

King's Publishing, Inc.
6 School Street., Suite 160
Fairfax, CA 94930-1650
1-415-258-2828
Jennifer Armor, Circulation Director
1-800-488-8468 (Subscription services)
Web site: www.diabetesworld.com
1 YR (12 issues): $19.95
2 YR (24 issues): $33.95

Diabetes Positive!

Positive Health Publications, Inc.
13010 Morris Road., 6th Floor
Alpharetta, GA 30004
Alyson Muse, Circulation Director
1-770-576-2036
1 YR (12 issues): $14.95
2 YR (24 issues): $24.95

WEB SITES

www.pubmed.org

The National Library of Medicine's database of medical journals. Some of the journals and articles are marked as easier to read, and some are also available in Spanish.

www.webmd.com

WebMD is a general health-care Web site that includes a lot of helpful information for people with type 1 or type 2 diabetes.

www.2aida.org

AIDA is a free diabetic software simulator of glucose insulin action and dose and diet adjustment. Forty case scenarios can be simulated.

www.diabetes123.com

Comprehensive information for the treatment and management of both type 1 and 2 diabetes.

www.childrenwithdiabetes.com

This site was founded by the father of a child with type 1 diabetes. An excellent support site for children with diabetes and their families.

www.diabetesmonitor.com

Focuses on the self-care of diabetes. You can participate in chat rooms and online discussions.

www.mendoza.com

A directory of diabetes care. Includes articles on diabetes management as well as listings and information about diabetes supplies and medications.

www.healthtalk.com

HealthTalk Interactive helps people with diabetes share their experiences through radio-format audio webcasts. Program archives and transcripts are available.

www.diabetic.com

Diabetic.com offers an online library, recipes, a Certified Diabetes Educator locator, and a superstore of diabetes products, including low-carb foods and over-the-counter medications.

Praise for *Betrayed*

"Pop culture's current crop of female lawyers owes a great deal to the attorneys at Rosato & Associates. . . . The deliciously dramatic and slightly over-the-top *Betrayed* reaffirms that after more than twenty novels, the Edgar Award–winning Scottoline is still able to create surprising, suspenseful plots with likable, daring heroines at the center." —*The Washington Post*

"Compelling." —*Publishers Weekly*

"*Betrayed* is populated with the kind of smart, funny women you love to watch working crime scenes." —*All You* magazine

"Scottoline writes terrific legal fiction with warm, smart characters and lots of humor and heart. Her legion of fans will be happy with this one, and it should find her new readers as well." —*Booklist*

"The most successful melding to date of Rosato & DiNunzio's cases and Scottoline's family-centered standalones." —*Kirkus Reviews*

"This is an author who knows what she wants to say and knows how to say it entertainingly." —*The Huffington Post*

"Takes the reader on a fast-paced thrill ride." —*RT Book Reviews*

"Action-packed." —*Record-Courier*

"A fast-moving thriller full of twists and turns." —*Bitter Lawyer*

Also by Lisa Scottoline

Fiction
Keep Quiet
Accused
Don't Go
Come Home
Save Me
Think Twice
Look Again
Lady Killer
Daddy's Girl
Dirty Blonde
Devil's Corner
Killer Smile
Dead Ringer
Courting Trouble
The Vendetta Defense
Moment of Truth
Mistaken Identity
Rough Justice
Legal Tender
Running from the Law
Final Appeal
Everywhere That Mary Went

Nonfiction (with Francesca Serritella)
Have a Nice Guilt Trip
Meet Me at Emotional Baggage Claim
Best Friends, Occasional Enemies
My Nest Isn't Empty, It Just Has More Closet Space
Why My Third Husband Will Be a Dog

BETRAYED

A Rosato & DiNunzio Novel

Lisa Scottoline

ST. MARTIN'S GRIFFIN ✖ NEW YORK

BETRAYED. Copyright © 2014 by Smart Blonde, LLC. All rights reserved. Printed in the United States of America. For information, address St. Martin's Press, 175 Fifth Avenue, New York, N.Y. 10010.

www.stmartins.com

The Library of Congress has cataloged the hardcover edition as follows:

Scottoline, Lisa.
    Betrayed : a Rosato & Associates novel / Lisa Scottoline. — First edition.
        p. cm. — (Rosato & associates ; 2)
    ISBN 978-1-250-02770-2 (hardcover)
    ISBN 978-1-250-02768-9 (e-book)
    1. Rosato & Associates (Imaginary organization)—Fiction. I. Title.
    PS3569.C725B48 2014b
    813'.54—dc23   2014025233

ISBN 978-1-250-07436-2 (trade paperback)

St. Martin's Griffin books may be purchased for educational, business, or promotional use. For information on bulk purchases, please contact the Macmillan Corporate and Premium Sales Department at 1-800-221-7945, extension 5442, or write to specialmarkets@macmillan.com.

First St. Martin's Griffin Edition: September 2015

10 9 8 7 6 5 4 3 2 1

With love and thanks to Laura Leonard and Nan Daley,
my partners in crime fiction

Everything we hear is an opinion, not a fact.
Everything we see is a perspective, not the truth.
—Marcus Aurelius

BETRAYED

Chapter One

Judy Carrier eyed her reflection in the shiny elevator doors, wondering when mirrors stopped being her friend. Her cropped yellow-blonde hair stuck out like demented sunrays, and her pink-and-blue Oilily sweater and jeans clashed with her bright red clogs. Worst of all was her expression, easy to read on a face as flat as an artist's palette, with troubled blue eyes set wide over a small nose and thin lips pressed unhappily together.

Judy tried to shake off her bad mood when the elevator halted and the doors slid open with a *ping*. ROSATO & DINUNZIO, LLC, read the shiny brass plaque, and she crossed the reception area, empty of clients on a Saturday morning. The office was quiet, but Judy knew she wouldn't be the only one in, because lawyers regarded weekends as a chance to work uninterrupted, which was their version of relaxing.

She heard her cell phone ringing and slid it from her pocket because she'd been playing phone tag with a client, Linda Adler. She checked the screen, but it read "Mom calling," with a faceless blue shadow. Judy had never bothered to put in a profile picture for her mother because the shadow seemed oddly perfect. Judy had grown up a Navy brat, but her family never developed the us-against-the-world closeness of a typical military family. The Carriers moved, skied, and hiked together, but their activities were a sort of parallel play for adults, and now they scattered all over the globe and emailed each other photos of themselves moving, skiing, and hiking. Judy clicked IGNORE and returned the phone to her pocket.

She rounded the corner to the hallway and brightened at the sight of her best friend, Mary DiNunzio, who turned when she spotted Judy and came hustling down the hall toward her, grinning from ear to ear. Mary had recently made partner, becoming Judy's boss, but neither of them knew how that would play out over time. Judy avoided thinking about it, and in any event, Mary made the most adorable boss ever in her tortoiseshell glasses, navy sweater, jeans, and loafers, with her little legs churning and her light brown ponytail bouncing.

"Judy, I was waiting for you! I have great news!" Mary reached her, light brown eyes warm with anticipation.

"Hi, cutie, tell me." Judy entered her office, and Mary followed her excitedly inside.

"Actually, I have great news and even greater news. Which do you want first?"

"The great news. We'll start slow." Judy slid her woven purse from her shoulder, tossed it onto the credenza, and went around to her chair. She sat down behind a desk cluttered with a laptop, case correspondence, a Magic 8 ball, ripped Splenda packets, and an empty can of Diet Coke. Law books, case reporters, notes, and files stuffed her bookshelves. She was going for creative clutter, but lately worried she was entering hoarder territory.

"First, I have breaking wedding news." Mary leaned back against the credenza, flushed with happiness. "You remember I told you about that high-end salon, J'taime?"

"Yes." Judy was going to be maid of honor at Mary's wedding, though she'd never been in a bridal party before. She was studying by watching bride shows on cable, but none of them told her that being maid of honor was like being executor of a vast and complicated estate, without the fee.

"They had a cancellation, so I got an appointment next Friday night! How great is that? Can you come?"

"Of course." Judy had already been to two bridal shops and seen Mary try on a zillion wedding dresses, but they all looked the same to her, like vanilla soft-serve without the cone.

"They have Vera Wang and all the big names."

"Cool!" Judy kept her smile in place, but wondered why she felt so negative, the Debbie Downer of bridesmaids. She wasn't jealous that Mary was getting married, but she wished she had what Mary had, which wasn't the same thing. It was more that Mary was moving forward, already a partner and soon a wife, while Judy got left behind, stuck. Judy didn't know how to get herself to the next level or what she was doing wrong. She'd always been on top, earned the best grades at school and succeeded at work. But now she sensed she was blowing her lead, at life.

"You don't mind going to a third shop, do you? My mother will be there."

"Great!" Judy answered, meaning it, since she was closer to Mary's mother than her own. The DiNunzios were warm and loving South Philly Italians, so they'd practically adopted her, whereupon she'd permanently gained ten pounds.

"The only problem is that I put a deposit on the veil at David's Bridal, and I can't know if it will go with the dresses at J'taime. But if I lose the money, so what?"

"Right, it wasn't that expensive," Judy said, though she'd forgotten how much the veil cost. The answer was, probably, a fortune. She'd learned that everything associated with weddings cost the same—a fortune.

"Okay, now to the even greater news."

"More wedding updates?" Judy braced herself to hear the latest drama with the DJ, the menu, the reception hall, the church, the invitations, or Mary's future mother-in-law, Elvira Rotunno, whom they called El Virus.

"No, this is about work." Mary cleared her throat, brimming with renewed enthusiasm. "Bennie told me to tell you, since she's in trial prep, that she just got a major piece of business and she's assigning it to you! Girl, you'll be a partner in no time!"

"Really?" Judy said, but she felt caught up short. She and Mary never referred to the fact that Judy was still an associate, tacitly saving her face, as if she didn't know her own employment status. "Great, what kind of case is it?"

"It's not one case, it's *seventy-five*." Mary beamed. "Bennie got them in as referral business from Singer Crenheim in Manhattan. The big league!"

"Why are there so many cases?" Judy didn't get it. "What are they about?"

"That's the only bummer." Mary paused. "They're asbestos cases, defense side, representing a company called Bendaflex."

"Oh no." Judy groaned in dismay. "Nobody likes asbestos cases, even asbestos firms."

"Judy, these cases will generate *millions* in fees."

"But they'll take two or three years to try." Judy was trying to process the information, which struck her as lawyer hell.

"They won't take that long because you don't have to try the whole case, just the damages phase. The liability was already decided."

"Even worse," Judy said, aghast. Mass tort trials like asbestos were often bifurcated, which meant that the question of liability was separated from the question of damages. Evidently, their new client Bendaflex had lost on liability, so there were a slew of individual damage cases that had to be tried. Literally the cases were damage control. "How did Bennie get these, anyway?"

"The cases were consolidated in the Southern District of New York, then remanded back to the various states for damages trials. She got all of the Pennsylvania cases, and most of them came out of the Navy Yard."

"For real?" Judy didn't think it could get worse. "My father was a lieutenant commander in the Navy, remember? He used to tell me about how there was asbestos all over those ships, in every shipyard in the country. Anything hot was insulated with asbestos, mainly pipes. Grinders would grind the old asbestos off, and pipe fitters blew the new asbestos on." Judy remembered her father's anger, and guilt, when he'd told her the stories, even though nobody knew that asbestos was deadly back then. "These poor guys, they'd be standing in the hull of a ship, sweating their butts off in a *snowglobe* of asbestos. No masks, no ventilation, no nothing. They're all dead now of mesothelioma. Johns Manville declared bankruptcy, and other companies, like Bendaflex, are fighting not to pay what they owe, decades later. And I'm supposed to help? Is this why I became a lawyer?"

Mary's smile faded. "I hear you, but we're lucky to get that much business in this economy."

"It's not worth it. The cases don't even present a legal question, only how much damages each plaintiff is owed, and since we represent Bendaflex, the answer has to be, as little as possible." Judy flashed-forward, disgusted. "I'll have to argue down the value of a man's life, probably in front of his widow and his children."

Mary sighed.

"My argument will have to be that the plaintiff, who's dead, wasn't going to earn that much, because, after all, he wasn't good enough to earn a promotion. And as far as pain and suffering, don't pay him for that because he died within a year, so he didn't suffer that long. Too bad he was only forty-three."

Mary frowned, sympathetic. "You don't have to try the cases yourself, just supervise them. With the money that comes in, you can hire whoever you need."

"Still." Judy fought a rising tension in her chest. "You wouldn't want to do it, would you?"

"I couldn't even if I wanted to." Mary shook her head, her tone turning defensive. "The cases came to Bennie, and she assigned them to you. I can't countermand her, as her partner."

Judy felt a twinge that Mary was taking Bennie's side, but she should have known it would happen, someday. Mary and Bennie were the sole partners of this all-woman firm, and nobody in her right mind opposed Bennie Rosato. Bennie was a world-class trial lawyer who'd grown the firm to national prominence and she hadn't reached the top by being a creampuff. On the contrary, the woman owned a coffee mug that read I CAN SMELL FEAR.

Suddenly, there was a commotion outside Judy's office, and they turned their attention to the door. Judy's boyfriend, Frank Lucia, materialized in the threshold, flashing the easy, confident grin that was one of the reasons she'd fallen in love with him. He'd been out of town last night, and she still got a thrill out of seeing him, especially looking so handsome in his puffy black jacket, tie-and-work-shirt combo, and jeans.

"Frank, what a surprise!" Judy said, brightening.

"I had to stay over in Baltimore and I missed my girl, so I thought I'd take her out to breakfast!" Frank burst into the office, threw open his big arms, and bounded around the desk, gathering Judy up and hugging her. "How you doing, babe?"

"Okay." Judy felt a warm rush of love, breathing in his familiar smells of aftershave and mortar dust. Frank was a smart, straight-up Italian hunk who owned a successful specialty masonry company, and they'd lived together for the past few years.

"Let's go eat, I'm starved." Frank raked big fingers through his thick, wavy hair, the same espresso-brown as his large, bright eyes.

Mary beamed. "What a guy! Frank, you have to teach Anthony to surprise me sometimes. He's not exactly spontaneous."

"Ha! Ditch him at the altar, Mare. I'll hook you up with one of my boys!"

Mary grinned. "How's your hand? Did you get the cast off?"

"It's all good, I only have this thing now." Frank showed his left hand, and a black cloth brace peeked from his sleeve. He grabbed Judy's arm. "Babe, let's get out of here."

"Okay." Judy let Frank pull her up, but her gaze fell on her desk clock, which read 10:15, and she remembered something. "Wait, how are you in town this early? Did you drop off the dog at the vet's? You said you would."

"Ruh-roh." Frank's grin turned sheepish. "Don't worry about it."

"What do you mean?" Judy stopped. "She had to get flea-dipped. Did you take her or not?"

"I forgot." Frank shrugged. "Sorry."

"Oh, honestly." Judy felt disappointed, but not completely surprised. She had been trying to figure out whether Frank was marriage material, and she was starting to worry she had an answer. "I just washed the sheets, the comforter, and the towels I put on top of the couch and chairs."

"It's not the end of the world." Frank glanced at Mary, and Judy knew that he hated to fight, especially in front of anyone. "We'll get her dipped tomorrow."

"They're closed on Sunday."

"No worries, we'll do it on Monday."

"That's too late." Judy had explained this to him ten times, but she couldn't seem to make him hear her. "Remember, we have to treat the house and the dog simultaneously? There can't be any delay."

"Okay, we'll treat them both, then. What's the big deal?"

"But you didn't drop her off, so that means that I have to wash everything all over again on Sunday night, if we want to drop her off on Monday."

"Would you rather me go home and try to take the dog in now, instead of taking you to breakfast?"

"Honestly, yes. The dog has to get dipped, and I have to work. I would really appreciate that."

"Okay, fine." Frank rolled his eyes and waved a cranky goodbye. "We'll do it your way. See you later. Bye, Mary."

Judy and Mary held each other's gaze for a moment then Judy shrugged. "What am I supposed to do? That was the right decision, wasn't it? Things have to get done but he wants to play all the time."

"I think he was trying to do a nice thing, but I totally get where you are coming from."

Suddenly Judy's phone started ringing, and she slipped it from her pocket in case it was Linda Adler. But it was her aunt Barb calling, and the phone screen came to life with a candid photo of her adored aunt, her mother's younger sister. "Excuse me, let me get this, it's Aunt Barb."

"Tell her I said hi," Mary said, because everybody loved Aunt Barb. She lived about an hour away, in Kennett Square, Pennsylvania, and they'd all been out to her house for beer and barbecue. Last year, Judy's uncle Steve, Barb's husband, had passed, and the whole office had gone to his funeral.

"Aunt Barb, hi, how are you?" Judy answered the call, realizing that she hadn't seen her aunt in a few months, though they talked on the phone all the time.

"Hello, honey," her aunt said, and Judy knew immediately that something was wrong. Her aunt sounded grave, when she was usually so warm and happy.

"What's the matter?"

"Am I catching you at a bad time?"

"No, why? What's the matter, Aunt Barb?"

"Didn't your mom call you?"

"Yes, but I was busy." Judy's mind raced. She regretted ignoring that call from her mother. "What's going on? Is Mom okay?"

"Yes, your mom's fine. In fact, she's here at the house with me."

"What?" Judy asked, surprised. Her parents lived in Santa Barbara, and her mother rarely visited her or Aunt Barb, and never unannounced.

"We'd love it if you could come out today, too, if you're not busy."

Judy's mouth went dry. Something was up. "Sure, okay, but why? What's the matter?"

"We'll talk about it when you come, sweetie."

"Tell me." Judy swallowed hard. "Please."

Aunt Barb hesitated. "Are you sitting down?"

Chapter Two

An hour later, Judy reached Kennett Square, a small town in semi-rural Chester County, and she pulled onto the gravel driveway in front of her aunt's small brick house, cut the ignition, and checked her reflection in the rearview mirror. Her eyes were still wet from crying, but her skin wasn't as mottled as it had been when she'd first heard the horrifying news.

I have breast cancer, her aunt had said, and Judy hadn't heard anything else. She sniffled, reached for a crumpled Dunkin' Donuts napkin, and wiped her eyes one last time. She pulled her key out of the ignition, got her purse, jumped out of the car, and hurried down the driveway past the garage. The sun was high in a cloudless sky, and the October air unseasonably warm, the lovely weather incongruous given the heartbreaking news. Judy couldn't imagine losing her aunt. Her aunt was too young to die.

She broke into a jog as soon as she saw her aunt, who looked so different from the last time she had seen her, only five months ago. Barbara Elizabeth Moyer was a tall, strong woman and had always been on the huggably beamy side, but no longer. Her fisherman's sweater and jeans drooped on a much thinner frame, and her long, thick silvery hair had vanished, replaced by a red bandanna knotted at her nape, over a newly bald head. She was only in her early fifties, but her face had acquired the gauntness of an older person, emphasizing the prominence of her cheekbones and her large, deep-set blue eyes. She sat alone at her wrought-iron table with a glass top, surrounded by the fading reds, pinks, and yellows of her beloved roses, now past their season.

"Aunt Barb!" Judy called out, tears returning to her eyes. She threw open her arms just as her aunt stood up and gave her a hug.

"Honey, don't worry, everything's going to be all right."

"No it's not!" Judy blurted out, burying her head in her aunt's bony shoulder, knowing that she was saying the exact wrong thing at the exact wrong time.

"Yes, it will, you'll see." Her aunt clucked softly, patting her back. "Don't worry."

"What happened?" Judy sobbed. "When did this . . . happen?"

"About nine months ago. Don't cry, really, sweetie." Aunt Barb gave her a final pat on the back. "I'm going to be well again, you'll see."

"You will be, I *know* you will be," Judy said, her words slightly blubby, but her tears subsiding. She let her aunt go and wiped her cheeks with her hand. "So, I mean, can you explain? How did I not know? I mean, what's going on? And where's Mom?"

"In the kitchen. Here, sit down and I'll catch you up." Aunt Barb pressed Judy into the wrought-iron chair opposite her, her eyes glinting in the bright sun. "So . . . I found a lump in my left breast, a puckering, kind of. Turns out, it was stage II breast cancer."

"Oh my." Judy swallowed hard, trying not to cry again. Stage II sounded terrifying, though she wasn't about to ask what was the highest stage. She would look it up later online.

"We thought we could get it with chemo, and it melted the tumor considerably, but they still found abnormal cells in my left breast, in my ducts." Aunt Barb paused but didn't tear up, strong and in control. "My cancer isn't encapsulated, which means it's not contained in one tumor, but throughout the tissue."

Judy tried to stay calm. She knew she was about to become familiar with terms like *encapsulated,* which she would look up later, too. She noticed for the first time that her aunt no longer had eyebrows and that her fair skin had a grayish tinge.

"The good news is it's not in my lymph nodes, including my sentinel node, so my prognosis is good. Everybody's cancer is different, that's what I'm learning. My doctor expects the mastectomy will do the trick, and I might not even need radiation."

Judy knew radiation was a cancer treatment, but it horrified her to think about irradiating a human being, especially one she loved so much.

"The mastectomy is scheduled for Monday."

"*This* Monday? In, like, two days?"

"Yes, but don't let it scare you. It doesn't scare me. Frankly, after seeing what your uncle went through with blood cancer, I feel lucky to have a surgical solution." Aunt Barb paused, her forehead etched with grief that was still fresh. "So I try to look on the bright side. I have to lose my breasts, but what I really care about is my life. And after all, every plant needs pruning, so that it can thrive as a whole. I'm just getting pruned, that's all."

"There you go," Judy said, pained. "You're a rose, Aunt Barb."

"Exactly." Aunt Barb smiled. "Besides, I know a lot of women who have had mastectomies, so there's no mystery. It should last about a few hours, and they'll discharge me on Wednesday, with a few drains."

Judy hid her fear. She didn't know a person could have a drain. Showers should have drains, not people.

"A lot of people have reconstruction, implants, or have expanders put in, but I decided not to." Aunt Barb set her mouth, a Cupid's bow, albeit determined. "I don't want to put myself through that. I hate the idea of more surgeries, or longer recovery, or spending more money. I mean, what's the point? I'm already so flat, and I can deal with padded bras."

"I see that," Judy said, meaning it. She couldn't imagine a more personal decision, and she didn't know what she would do, but she knew it was so like her aunt. "Why didn't you tell me, or Mom?"

"I didn't want you to worry." Aunt Barb frowned with regret. "That's why I canceled dinner on you, last month. Sorry."

"But on the phone, you never said anything." Judy talked to her aunt at least twice a week, checking in.

"I hid it."

Judy tried to think back in time, bewildered, as if understanding the chronology would lend her any comfort. "But I saw you on my birthday. You looked fine. You looked great."

"I was just starting chemo, and I didn't tell you then because I didn't want you to associate your birthday with news like that."

"Oh no." Judy almost burst into new tears, at the memory. They had celebrated in this very backyard, sharing a double-cheese pizza and a few cold Miller Lites among the lovely roses, in full bloom. Her aunt was an expert rosarian, and her heirloom Gallica rosebushes drooped now with the last of their massive crimson blooms, shaped more like a peony to the untrained eye.

"Right before I saw you, I had my first treatment. I hadn't lost my hair yet, that happened on day seventeen, just when they said it would. Chemo was awful, I felt tired and foggy. Chemo brain, they call it. It made my nails weird, dried my skin, and obviously, I'm prematurely bald. I'm going for a Pirate Queen look." Aunt Barb patted her bandanna. "Not bad, huh?"

"Very Gilbert and Sullivan." Judy managed a smile, because they both loved G&S operettas.

"My friend gained weight during chemo, but I lost twenty-five pounds. So there's the good news." Aunt Barb chuckled ruefully. Then she sighed, tilting her face to the sun. "Anyway, enough. It's a beautiful day, you're here, and we're in the presence of Reine Victoria."

"You mean the rose you were trying to grow? You did it?"

"Yep, go take a whiff. There's still one or two blooms left, in the middle, the pink." Aunt Barb gestured to the rosebushes on her right. "Reine Victoria is a Bourbon rose, one of the most fragrant. It can smell like pears."

Judy got up, crossed to the bushes, and smelled a rose with pinkish blooms. Its perfume filled her nostrils with a fruity sweetness. "Wow, that's so cool. Aromatherapy."

"Also, its thorns aren't that bad. I hate thorns. Who needs attitude from a flower?"

Judy heard her phone ringing in her back pocket, reached for it, and saw that the screen read Linda Adler, the client she'd been trying to reach. "Oh, damn."

"Feel free to get that, honey," Aunt Barb called to her.

"Nah, I'll get it later." Judy let the call go to voicemail because her conversation with Linda would have been a long one, and her aunt deserved her undivided attention. Judy went back to the table and sat down.

"So how's work, honey?"

"I'm not going to complain, in the circumstances."

Aunt Barb touched her hand. "No, please don't act differently around me. Tell me. I'm sick of talking about lymph nodes."

"Okay, well, I have a cool sex-discrimination case for this

woman who just called me, but I also just got dumped with seventy-five new cases, all damages trials." Judy didn't add that her goal in the damages cases would be to diminish the value of a lost human life, a heartbreaking thought right now.

Suddenly Aunt Barb turned to face the house, where Judy's mother was coming out the back door, carrying a floral-patterned tray. Judy didn't call to her because it was too far away, but she was struck, as always, by her mother's beauty, even in her late fifties. Delia Van Huyck Carrier had round blue eyes, now slightly hooded, and a squarish face and high cheekbones that bespoke her paternal Dutch heritage. She kept in trim shape and had great style, even in her standard airplane outfit: an oversized gray sweater, black leggings, and black ballet flats. She crossed the lawn toward them, her lips pursed and her head tilted slightly down, showing the top of her head with its loose, lemony blonde topknot.

"Hi, Mom!" Judy stood up, went to her mother, and gave her an awkward hug, around the tray, a pitcher of iced tea, glasses, napkins, and a platter of chocolate chip cookies.

"Hello, honey." Judy's mother set the tray on the tabletop, and the glasses clinked. "You might want to wipe your nose."

"Oops, sorry. How are you?" Judy plucked a napkin from the tray and blew her nose, sensing that her mother seemed oddly cooler than usual. Aunt Barb stiffened as soon as her mother came over, and Judy realized that the two sisters had been fighting, which wasn't atypical, though she would have guessed there was an exception for breast cancer.

"I'm good." Her mother's Delft-blue eyes narrowed in the sunlight, which caught the golden strands of her fine, smooth hair. "Dad says hi. How are you, all right?"

Of course not, Judy wanted to say, but that wasn't the right answer. "I guess so, but I'm worried about Aunt Barb. You didn't know about this, did you?"

"No, she kept it from us. I took the red-eye as soon as I found out. Sit down, please."

Judy sat down. *Taking the red-eye* was code for *showing concern,* even though her mother seemed completely pissed off. "Mom, is something bothering you?"

"No, I'm just determined to get my kid sister through her operation. I'm staying for the duration."

"You make it sound like a war."

"It is a war," her mother shot back, meeting her eye. "And we're going to win."

"Delia, it's not a war, to me." Aunt Barb shook her head, frowning. "We work on visualization in group, and I don't see it as a war, or 'my battle with cancer,' like the obits say. My cancer is part of me, and I have to work on it to heal myself, the same as my faults or my dark side."

"You don't have a dark side, Aunt Barb," Judy said, her throat thick.

"Nonsense, dear," her mother interjected. "We all have a dark side."

Judy recoiled. "Mom, what gives? Play nice."

Aunt Barb cocked her kerchiefed head. "Your mother and I had words, and now we're at an impasse, agreeing to disagree."

"About what?"

"Speak of the devil," her mother hissed, turning toward the house, as the back door opened.

Chapter Three

Judy looked over, and a middle-aged Hispanic woman with fluffy black hair in a pixie cut came out of the house. She was cute, roundish, and only about five feet tall, but gave the impression of being strong and sturdy as she crossed the lawn on short legs. She had on a faded Eagles T-shirt and jeans and carried a brown tote bag on her shoulder.

Aunt Barb motioned her over. "Iris, come meet my niece!"

Judy turned to her aunt, pleasantly surprised. "So that's the Iris I've heard so much about? Your gardening buddy?"

"Yes." Aunt Barb gestured to Judy when Iris reached the table. "Iris, this is Judy, and Judy, Iris Juarez."

"Hi, Iris, it's great to finally meet you!" Judy extended a hand, and Iris shook it, her grip strong and her nails manicured red, with tiny rhinestones on the tip.

"Please to meet you, too," Iris said, with a thick Spanish accent. She smiled easily, but almost shyly. Her smallish eyes were a rich, earthy brown with deep crow's-feet, and her skin had a dark brownish hue. Thin gold crucifixes dangled from her ears.

Aunt Barb gestured to a chair. "Iris, sit down, please. Join us a second. You have time before work, don't you?"

"Yes." Iris pulled out the remaining wrought-iron chair and sat down, perched on the edge. She placed a silver cell phone, one of the older models, on the table.

Aunt Barb picked up an empty glass. "Would you like some iced tea?"

"No." Iris shook her head, and Judy noticed her mother and aunt exchange chilly glances. Granted, Iris wasn't what Judy had expected, but she seemed like a perfectly nice woman.

Judy asked her, "Iris, where are you from?"

"Kennett Square."

"No, I mean, before that. You're from Mexico originally, right?"

"Yes. Guerrero."

"Where is that?" Judy had been to Mexico, but her Spanish wasn't as good as her Latin, which was excellent, if useless.

"Down." Iris waved her hand toward the ground.

Judy got the gist. "Oh, south. Do you have family there?"

"No, no." Iris winced, and Judy sensed she'd said the wrong thing.

Her aunt interjected, "Iris's husband died six years ago, as did her sons. In a car accident."

"Oh no, I'm so sorry." Judy swallowed hard, and her mother reached silently for the iced tea and poured herself a glass.

Her aunt forced a smile. "Judy, Iris grew corn, back in Mexico. She kept the farm going, all by herself, one of the few women in the village. She can grow anything, anywhere. She's a master in this garden, I tell you, a *master.* I've taken classes from horticulturalists who don't have her touch." Aunt Barb nodded toward the rosebushes. "She should get the credit for Reine Victoria, not me."

"Really?" Judy said, happy to have the subject changed.

Iris was already shaking her head. "No, Barb show me."

"Iris, that's not true." Aunt Barb turned to Judy, newly animated, and Judy could tell that her aunt wanted her to get to know Iris, especially since Judy's mother was giving the woman the silent treatment.

Judy smiled at Iris. "So what brought you here? Why did you leave Mexico?"

"I need work. The police, they take my farm."

"Why did they do that?"

"I don't know." Iris frowned, shaking her head. Her soft shoulders slumped. "The police, not good. I hab no choice, I go."

Aunt Barb interjected, "Iris is the strongest woman I know. She inspires me every day, especially now." Aunt Barb faced Iris, touching her arm. "Iris, tell Judy what you went through to get here. It was impossible, truly."

"Oh no." Iris waved her off again, shyly. "Is too long a story."

"No, tell me." Judy smiled. "How did you get here from Mexico?"

"I run," Iris answered.

Judy thought she misunderstood. "You ran? Like, running, in a race?"

"Yes." Iris pumped her arms, as if she were running.

"For how long?"

"Three night."

"For how long, each night?"

"All." Iris chuckled, showing a glimpse of a gold tooth in front.

"You ran *all* night, for three nights?" Judy asked, incredulous. The woman had to be fifty-five years old, and she hardly had an athletic build.

"In dessert," Iris added, and Judy understood that she meant desert.

"What desert?"

"Sonora." Iris looked at Aunt Barb. "Sonora, is call?"

"Yes, the Sonoran desert in Arizona." Aunt Barb turned to Judy. "She ran all night for three nights, from seven o'clock at night until seven the next morning. The desert is cold at night. There were ten other people, only two were women, none as old as she was. During the day, they hid inside bushes, despite snakes, rats, and a hundred-and-twenty-degree temperatures, in July."

"Really?" Judy asked, aghast. Meanwhile, she realized why her mother was so angry. Iris must have entered the country illegally, and her mother didn't approve. Judy didn't like the idea either, but she felt rapt by Iris's story. She asked her, "Iris, why the Sonoran desert? How did you get there?"

"I go bus to Peidras Negros. A man, a *coyote,* I pay him one thousand to go United Stays."

"A thousand dollars to take you to the United States?" Judy was getting the hang of her accent.

"Yes. Today, is *four thousand.*" Iris's dark eyes widened at the sum.

"When did you come?"

"Four."

"Four years ago?"

"I have water, beans, tuna, food with cans, on back." Iris gestured to her back, indicating a backpack. "Is so hot, we no have water lef'. We see farm with pig, many pig. We are happy, so happy. We drink from water. We fill bottle."

"You drank the water for the pigs? From *a trough?*" Judy's stomach turned over.

"*Pera* we see, in sun, water so dirty." Iris wrinkled her flattish nose in disgust and pantomimed holding up a bottle of water to the sun. "In water, is germ. I am sick, so sick."

"Oh no."

"I have my teacher. I use my teacher."

"Your teacher?" Judy didn't understand. "Like your leader? Was there a leader?"

"No. Teacher." Iris pulled on her T-shirt and picked up a glass, and put her shirt over the top. "I put water on teacher." Judy understood. "You used your T-shirt to strain the water?"

"Yes. Yes."

"Where were you going?"

"Phoenix. We go, we see wire." Iris pointed up. "We go under to Phoenix."

"You followed overhead cables to Phoenix, like those big towers?"

"Yes. A lady, she die." Iris winced again. "No water, she die. We go, go, go. We no stop."

"That's horrible," Judy said, meaning it. "You must have been so afraid."

"Yes. Sad. Worry. Nervous," Iris added, pronouncing it like nairbus.

"How did you get here, to Pennsylvania?"

"A man, in car, he take us. Five day. Chicago, Las Vegas, Florida, North Carolina." Iris mangled the phrase North Carolina, but Judy got the idea.

"Why did you come?"

"A man say work is here, in Pennsylvania." Iris pronounced it Pennsylvania, with a short a.

"What do you do here?" Judy asked, but suddenly Iris's cell phone on the table rang.

" 'Scuse." Iris picked it up and checked it, but her expression changed dramatically. She didn't answer the phone, pressing her lips together tightly, and her forehead wrinkled with concern.

Aunt Barb asked, "Iris, is something the matter? You can take that call if you want to?"

"No, no," Iris answered, but she was obviously worried and

the phone went silent. She jumped to her feet and hoisted her tote bag to her shoulder. "Barb, I go work now."

Aunt Barb blinked. "But you don't have to be there until three thirty. It's only two, isn't it?"

"I go, Barb." Iris forced a jittery smile and waved at the table, backing away. "Bye, nice meetin' you."

"You, too!" Judy gave her a wave, wondering what was bothering her.

"Good-bye!" Aunt Barb called after her. "Let me know if you need anything or if I can help."

"Bye-bye!" Iris turned and hurried from the backyard, and Judy waited until Iris was gone to turn to her mother.

"What a story, huh, Mom?"

Judy's mother answered, "She's illegal."

"*Undocumented*," Aunt Barb corrected, bristling.

"Semantics." Judy's mother scoffed. "You can go to jail for employing an illegal. I know, I looked it up online."

"Aunt Barb, Iris works for you?" Judy asked, newly confused. She had assumed that Iris was her aunt's friend, not hired help. Her aunt was a landscape architect and didn't earn that much, and since Uncle Steve's death, she'd had to sell their big house in Unionville and downsize to the rental she lived in now.

"Yes, she works for me part-time." Aunt Barb turned to Judy, touching her arm. "Sorry, honey, I kept it private, I guess because of her status. She used to clean houses, but now she works at one of the mushroom growers."

"How does she work for them if she doesn't have any papers?" Judy started thinking like a lawyer, an occupational hazard.

"The big mushroom growers like Phillips hire only workers with papers, but some of the independents don't. There's a lot of undocumented workers in Chester County, in the mushroom industry and horse farms."

"When did she start working for you?"

"As long as you've known about her."

"How did you meet her?"

"When your uncle got sick, I hired an agency to clean house and she came, every week. One day she mentioned to me that she could weed for me, too. I hadn't gotten to it, taking care of your uncle." Aunt Barb frowned, pained. "I thought that was so nice, that she noticed the garden was being neglected. I hated looking out the window and seeing the weeds popping up. She began to care for it, and she did a wonderful job, and during chemo, she brought me chocolate milkshakes and cheese goldfish because I had a craving for them. There was a time when that was all I could keep down and—"

"She's not even a nurse," Judy's mother interrupted.

"I don't *need* a nurse. I just need someone I can rely on."

Judy's mother scoffed. "You could have called me, Judy, or any one of your friends from work, like Colleen Connor. We would have helped."

"Colleen's busy with young kids, and Iris has become a friend." Aunt Barb gestured at the platter of chocolate chip cookies. "She baked cookies because she knew I was having my family in. She cares about me."

Judy's mother rolled her eyes. "Stop paying her and see how much she cares."

Aunt Barb pursed her lips. "I pay her, but she *cares.*"

"She doesn't pay taxes, none of them do. They burden the system."

"She'd love to become a citizen, but she can't. She's not a political issue, she's a *person.*" Aunt Barb raised her voice, though it sounded reedy and thin. "She goes to church every Sunday, and actually, I go with her. I began going when Steve got sick, and it comforted me."

"What?" Judy's mother arched an eyebrow. "You go to a Spanish church?"

Judy cringed. "Mom, don't—"

"Judy, please, stay out of it," her mother shot back. "This is between Barb and me."

Judy clammed up, torn between disagreeing with her mother and upsetting her aunt, their sisterly disagreements in the very DNA of sibling rivalry.

Aunt Barb pursed her lips. "Yes, the congregation is mostly Latino, but so what? Both priests, Father Keenan and Father Vega, have welcomed me. They're kind and wonderful people."

Judy's mother frowned. "So you're not a Protestant anymore? You're Catholic now?"

"Do you have to label it?" Aunt Barb shot back, angering. "Nothing gets you to church like a cancer diagnosis, and now I have one of my own. Are you seriously blaming me? And why is it any business of yours, how or where I pray? It's a very vibrant congregation. In fact, they performed 467 baptisms last year, the most in the Archdiocese."

Judy's mother pursed her lips. "Sorry if I'm not overjoyed that they have so many children, because they'll be in the schools, which I'll have to pay for."

"That's not what's bothering you, Delia. Not really."

"Of course it is."

"Bull." Aunt Barb turned to face Judy, her thin skin mottled with emotion. "Your mother and I had a fight before you came today, because I would like Iris to help me recuperate after my mastectomy. Your mother wants to do it instead, but I think she should go home after the mastectomy."

Judy's mother pursed her lips. "Iris isn't family."

Aunt Barb frowned. "She's a friend."

"Stop saying that. Friends have things in common."

"We do." Aunt Barb threw up her hands. "We're about the same age, both widows, no children, and we love to garden and bake. She's teaching me Spanish, and I'm teaching her English. We have fun, and I can depend on her."

Judy's mother snorted. "You can depend on me, Barb. When have you *not* been able to depend on me?"

Judy couldn't take it anymore. "Mom, enough, let's not fuss. Aunt Barb, I think we can all help, but either way, we should make a truce right here and now. No more quarreling. We need to pull together. Don't you agree, ladies?"

Judy's mother fell stone silent.

Aunt Barb only looked worriedly away, where Iris had gone.

Chapter Four

After dinner, Judy ducked out of the kitchen to make some phone calls, leaving her mother and Aunt Barb at the kitchen table over mugs of tea. The afternoon had passed without event, and their interactions had been limited to getting ready for the hospital and making the small talk that came easily to blood relatives. Judy couldn't help but sense that Aunt Barb's illness loomed over their heads all day and she had learned from her experience with her uncle that a cancer diagnosis changed the very air in a room, present but invisible. She'd learned, too, that for all the upbeat chatter about clear nodes and early detection, cancer could be cruelly unpredictable; her Uncle Steve's lymphocytic leukemia had been in remission when it morphed like a shape-shifter into the deadly Richter's Syndrome, striking him down within weeks. She prayed she wouldn't lose her aunt to the disease.

Judy tried to shake off her anxiety but couldn't, and she headed into the living room for the couch, seeing Aunt Barb's hand everywhere. The living room was tiny but super-cozy, with a loveseat and an easy chair with faded chintz slipcovers, piled with woven jacquard blankets that she collected. Her framed floral needlepoints covered the walls, which were of white plaster, and her gardening books filled the white-painted shelves. A rustic brick fireplace with a blackened surround left a permanently charred, woodsy smell in the air.

Judy slid her phone out of her back pocket, scrolled to her phone log, and pressed the number to return Linda Adler's call. It rang and rang, but the call went to voicemail and she left a message. Next she pressed in the number for her boyfriend Frank, whom she had already called on the drive to her aunt's, but he hadn't called back. He liked Aunt Barb, and Judy knew he would be upset by the news about her cancer, which was why she hadn't left it on his voicemail or sent him a text.

"What's up, babe!" Frank shouted, when the call connected. The background was noisy shouting and laughing, punctuated by the *thwap thwap thwap* of basketballs hitting a gym floor.

"Where are you? Did you get my messages?" Judy tried to swallow her annoyance. He hadn't listened to her messages, because he never did, which drove her crazy.

"I can't, I'm filling in on a round-robin tournament!"

"You're not supposed to be playing basketball." Judy didn't bother to disguise her dismay. Frank had broken his hand on the job and was wearing a cloth brace for two more weeks.

"Don't sweat it, babe! It's not a problem!"

"Frank, think. Of course it's a problem. It's crazy."

"Don't worry! I know what I'm doing! I shoot with my right hand!"

"Are you serious? What if your hand gets bumped? Or you fall? What about your brace?"

"I removed it! That's why it's removable!" Frank burst into laughter, which got drowned out by wild cheering. "It's an emergency!"

"A basketball emergency?"

"Relax, Mom!"

"I *am* relaxed." Judy tried not to act like his mother, but it was difficult when he acted like a child. "And what about the dog? Could the vet dip her?"

"I couldn't take her because the guys needed me, Joey got sick! I can't talk now! We're about to hit the court! Call you later!"

"No, wait, listen." Judy worried she would be overheard by her mother or Aunt Barb, so she got up and walked around the couch, cupping her hand over her phone. "I won't be home tonight. I'm staying at Aunt Barb's—"

"What did you say? I can't hear you!"

Judy went to the front door, twisted the knob, and went outside, closing the door behind her. It had gotten dark and cold, but she hugged herself. "Aunt Barb's cancer is stage II—"

"Babe!" Frank shouted, impatient. "Can't you talk louder? There's too much noise! I can't hear you, I gotta go!"

"This is important!" Judy gritted her teeth. "I want to talk to you about—"

"Sorry, babe, I really gotta go! We're up! Text me!" The line went dead.

Judy pressed END, but wasn't ready to go inside. She sank onto the front step, holding on to her phone while Frank's photo faded from the screen. She eyed the sky, in thought. There was no moon tonight, only a starless black blanket that illuminated nothing. She'd learned today that life really was short, and it wasn't just a cliché. Her biological clock was ticking, and she wondered if she was as happy as she used to be with Frank. He was so terrific and fun when times were easy, but in the rough patches, he seemed to fade away. She didn't know if he was selfish or if she'd trained him wrong, being basically independent. And she didn't know if she had to do anything about it, necessarily.

Suddenly, her attention was drawn by a black police cruiser

driving slowly down the street, its high beams on. It paused at the houses, then stopped in front of her aunt's house.

Judy straightened up, surprised. The cruiser's powerful engine rumbled into silence, and two uniformed officers emerged, alighting from the driver's side and passenger seats. The cops met in front of her aunt's house, then walked up her walkway toward the front door. Judy couldn't see their features in the dim light, but they made similar silhouettes, about the same size and build. She rose to greet them. "Hello, Officers, can I help you?"

"Good evening, I'm Officer Bart Hoffman, and this is my partner Officer Paul Ramirez of the East Grove Police Department. Are you Barb Moyer?"

"No," Judy answered. "That's my aunt."

"Is she here?" Officer Hoffman's jaw set in a grim line, but that was all Judy could see of him under the patent bill of his cap.

"Yes, she's inside."

"We'll need to talk to her."

Chapter Five

The policemen stood in front of the couch, their black Wind-breakers and thick black gun-and-radio belts incongruous in the chintzy vibe of the cottage. Both men had taken off their black caps and held them almost identically, in the crook of their elbows.

Judy gestured. "Aunt Barb, this is Officer Hoffman and Officer Ramirez. Gentlemen, Barb Moyer, and my mother, Delia Carrier."

"Ladies, pleased to meet you." Officer Hoffman was the older of the two, forty-something with cool slate-blue eyes and a skinny face, his hair buzzed into an old-school cut. Officer Ramirez was much younger, with warm brown eyes, a wide-open face, and light acne scars pitting his cheeks. He was bald but it looked as if he shaved his head, not came by it naturally.

"So, Officers," Aunt Barb said, blinking. "What can I do for you?"

"We'd like to talk to you for a moment or two." Officer Hoffman nodded. "Do you mind if we sit down?"

"Not at all. Please, have a seat." Aunt Barb eased into the

club chair, and Judy stood next to her, hovering protectively at her elbow.

Officer Hoffman cleared his throat. "I'm sorry, but we have to inform you that we found Rita Lopez deceased this evening, in her vehicle in East Grove. The coroner hasn't yet determined the cause of death, but it appears that it was a natural death, a heart attack. Please accept our condolences."

For a minute, nobody said anything. Officer Hoffman looked tense. Aunt Barb blinked. Judy didn't recognize the name, so she stood mute next to her mother.

"This is awkward, Officers." Aunt Barb frowned slightly. "I don't know anyone named Rita Lopez. Are you sure you have the right house?"

Officer Hoffman pursed his lips, which were thin. "Your name and address were listed as her emergency contact in a card in her wallet."

"I was?" Aunt Barb asked, taken aback. "May I see the card?"

"Sorry, we don't have it with us. Hang on a sec." Officer Hoffman extracted a skinny notebook from his back pocket, then produced a ballpoint pen from inside his Windbreaker. He flipped through the pages of his notebook, then read off a phone number. "Is that your cell-phone number?"

"Why, yes, it is."

Officer Hoffman made another note, then looked up. "The deceased had a Pennsylvania driver's license in her wallet, under the name Rita Lopez. The photo was a match, but grainy." He flipped back a few pages in his notepad. "The vehicle she was found in had Pennsylvania plates, TAJ 3039. Is that your friend's license plate?"

"I don't know."

Officer Hoffman flipped a few pages back again. "The vehicle was registered in Arizona under the name of Anna Martinez,

387 Canary Lane, in Mesa. Do you know anyone by that name, Ms. Moyer?"

"No, I don't." Aunt Barb tugged on her head scarf.

"It's possible that Rita Lopez isn't her real name or the name that you know her by." Officer Hoffman checked his notebook. "The deceased is a Hispanic female, mid-fifties, with short dark hair. Height about 5'1", weight about 150 pounds. She was wearing an Eagles T-shirt and jeans."

"*Iris?*" Aunt Barb recoiled, her hand flying to her cheek.

Judy gasped, horrified. She flashed on Iris, wearing her Eagles T-shirt and jeans, then looked over at her mother, whose mouth had dropped open, her lips parted in surprise.

"Officer. No, wait." Aunt Barb was shaking her head. "It can't be Iris. She's at work now."

Officer Hoffman consulted his notebook again. "The deceased was found this evening, at about 8:05 P.M., in a vehicle by the side of the road, on Brandywine Way, facing west. The vehicle was a brown Honda, two-door, 1984."

Aunt Barb kept shaking her head. "That's Iris's car, but it can't be her. Somebody must've stolen her car."

"What is Iris's last name and her address?"

"Wait, hold on." Aunt Barb paused, flushing. "I'm not sure I should tell you that. That's her personal business."

"Did your friend enter the country legally or illegally?"

"Why?" Aunt Barb pursed her lips.

"If she entered legally and we know the point of entry, we could check her fingerprints, on file there. Usually the undocumented carry a *MICA* or a *matricula,* an identity card from the Mexican consulate, but she didn't." Officer Hoffman paused. "Ms. Moyer, we're not Immigration, we're the East Grove Police. Our only interest is identifying the deceased, notifying her next of kin, and liaising with the county coroner to return her body to her loved ones."

"I don't know."

Judy swallowed hard, listening. She didn't like Aunt Barb's lying to the police, but she understood that her aunt was just protecting her friend. She hoped Iris was alive, but even if somebody had stolen Iris's car, there was no explanation for how they got her clothes, too. Plenty of people in the Philadelphia suburbs wore Eagles' regalia, but it was too coincidental that her aunt's name, address, and cell number were on a card in the wallet.

Judy's mother returned with a glass of water and offered it to Aunt Barb. "Here we go, honey. Have some."

"Thanks." Aunt Barb set the glass down on the wooden coffee table, untouched.

"We do need to get a personal ID." Officer Hoffman hesitated. "We have an email photograph of the deceased, taken at the scene. We can show it to you."

"Why didn't you say so?" Aunt Barb held out her hand. "Let me see that picture. We can settle this here and now."

Judy squeezed her aunt's arm. "Aunt Barb, let me look instead. You don't want to see that."

"I'm okay." Aunt Barb faced Officer Hoffman. "Please, let me see the photo."

Officer Hoffman exchanged a look with Officer Ramirez, who pulled a BlackBerry from his Windbreaker pocket, hit a few buttons, and presumably downloaded the photo, pausing before he handed it over.

Aunt Barb accepted the phone and looked down. "No," she whispered, hushed. "No, it's not possible. Iris?"

"Aunt Barb, I'm so sorry." Judy put an arm around her aunt's shoulders, feeling a wave of sympathy.

"Oh no, no, no. This can't . . . be." Aunt Barb burst into tears and buried her face in her hands, dropping the phone.

Judy's mother grabbed some Kleenexes from a box on the

table and handed them to Judy for Aunt Barb, then picked up the phone and handed it to Officer Hoffman.

Aunt Barb sobbed, hoarse sobs racking her frail frame. "She should have been . . . at work. Why wasn't she . . . at work?"

Judy hugged her aunt close. "Maybe she wasn't feeling well, so she left work and went home?"

Judy's mother nodded, dry-eyed, taking her place behind the chair. "That's probably what it was, Barb. You never know, she could have been nauseated. Nausea is a sign of heart attack. Jaw pain, too. Shoulder pain. Women often mistake warning signs. They think the problem is the flu, but it's not. Did you know that?"

Judy knew her mother was talking only to fill the silence, so she didn't answer, but kept rubbing her aunt's back.

"No, no . . . this is too awful, it can't be. It just can't be. I just can't believe . . . it's her."

"Ladies, excuse us." Officer Hoffman rose quietly, and Officer Ramirez followed suit. "We'll leave now and give you some privacy."

"Officers, no, wait." Aunt Barb lifted her face from her palms. Tears filled her eyes, her brow collapsed into deep furrows, and her downturned mouth made a mournful gash. "I want to go, I want to . . . see her. Where is she?"

"What?" Judy asked, aghast. She couldn't imagine her aunt's going to the scene and seeing the body.

Judy's mother frowned. "Barb, no, you're not thinking clearly. You've had a shock. Stay home, please. You have so much to do. Your friends from work have been calling. You have to call them back."

Office Hoffman blinked. "Mrs. Moyer, there's no need for you to go to the scene. A photo ID suffices for a personal ID, for our purposes."

"I *want* to see her." Aunt Barb took a long final sniffle, but her lips trembled, curling into a miserably wiggly line.

"Aunt Barb, this is too awful to do—"

"No, it's not, I can do it." Her aunt shook her head, stricken. "I know what death looks like. I saw my parents. I saw Steve, I was with him. I held his hand." Aunt Barb pursed her lips, as if what she was about to say physically pained her. "Iris carried my name and number in her wallet. She thought I was there for her. Now I will be. I'm going. I'll just get my purse, Officer."

Judy sighed inwardly. Her aunt may have been the baby of the family, but when she wanted to do something, there was no stopping her. It was no accident that she could grow the notoriously tricky heirloom roses. "Aunt Barb, let me go with you then."

"I'd love that, if you don't mind."

Chapter Six

Judy parked her tomato-red Volkswagen Beetle behind the police cruiser, on a long, straight stretch of Brandywine Way, a single-lane backroad through acres of shorn hayfields, which would have been pitch black except for the police activity. Uniformed police officers and men in ties and jackets stood in the street, talking in groups. Several police cruisers parked, with their red, white, and blue lights flashing silently from a light bar atop their roofs. Red flares marked a perimeter, sending smoke trailing into the air, where it vanished. In the center of the scene, its front bumper buried in a huge hay roll, sat an old brown Honda.

Judy looked over at her aunt, who had sobbed softly during most of the ride. "Aunt Barb?" she said, touching her arm. "We're here."

"Okay." Her aunt dabbed her nose, then put her Kleenex away in the pocket of her parka. She had on a red knit cap and seemed lost in her maroon parka, which dwarfed her since she'd lost weight. Her skin looked pale even in the dim interior, lighted only by the flashing lights of the police cruiser in front of them. "Thanks for taking me. I just want to see her, for myself."

"I understand." Judy patted her aunt's arm, stuffed in the thick parka.

"I know she's gone, but I don't know, in a way. It's unreal to me, it's abstract. Does that make any sense?"

"Sure," Judy answered, meaning it. She knew-but-didn't-know so many things in her life. She knew-but-didn't-know that she wouldn't marry Frank. She knew-but-didn't-know that she wanted to be a partner. She knew-but-didn't-know that she wanted to be closer to her mother. She knew-but-didn't-know that Aunt Barb could die. "I think it's good that we came."

"Thanks." Aunt Barb closed her eyes, and a tear rolled down her cheek, illuminated by the flashing lights. She wiped it away quickly. "Iris was my best friend. I didn't want to say so before, in front of your mother. I was afraid that she—or my friends at work, whoever—would judge me."

"I wouldn't have," Judy said softly.

"I know that, but shame on me. Iris has such a good heart. She always understood how I was feeling, even when Steve died. She was there." Aunt Barb frowned, blinking wetly. "Please don't take that the wrong way. You and your mom were there, too. But after the funeral, when everybody went home and the casseroles were eaten and the phone calls stopped, Iris was there." Tears brimmed in Aunt Barb's eyes, threatening to spill over again. "I told everybody at work that my garden healed me after Steve passed, but it was really her." Aunt Barb's lower lip puckered, her tears pooled in her eyes. "She's my best friend. I never even said so, before now. I never even told her, and now it's too late."

Judy's heart broke for her. "Aunt Barb, I'm sure she knew."

"But still, I should have told her, or you or your mom and people at work. Why didn't I?" Aunt Barb wiped her eyes, shaking her head. "Because I was ashamed? Was it class or race? Or money? What's the difference? I'm a moral coward. We got along great. We talked about everything. We laughed and laughed." Aunt Barb wiped her cheeks and eyes, then seemed to will her tears to subside. "I'll find a way to make it up to her. I will bury her and I will mourn her."

Judy touched her arm again. "I'll help you."

"I knew you would." Aunt Barb managed a sad smile. "You know who my emergency contact is, now that your uncle is gone?"

"My mom?"

"No. *You.*"

"Aw, thanks." Judy felt tears come to her eyes, but blinked them away. She prayed that Aunt Barb recovered from her awful disease and there was no need for her to have an emergency contact for many, many years.

"Look, here comes the police." Aunt Barb shifted up in her seat, and Judy turned to see Officer Hoffman striding toward them, bulky in his jacket and gun belt, carrying a clipboard. He had his cap back on, his Windbreaker was buttoned up, and his mouth made a grim line.

Judy lowered her car window, letting in a blast of brisk air. "Should we get out?"

"Yes, please." Officer Hoffman stood aside, taking a pen from inside his Windbreaker, and Judy got out of the car, checking to see if her aunt needed help, but it didn't look like she did. Aunt Barb walked over to Officer Hoffman, plunging her hands into her pockets and standing in the headlights from the Volkswagen.

"Ms. Carrier." Officer Hoffman gave Judy the clipboard, which had a pen under the silver clasp at the top. "Please initial here, on this line." He pointed at a grid with a thick finger. "This is our case log, which shows who visited the scene and when. It's for our records."

"No problem." Judy wrote her initials in the block and handed the clipboard back to Officer Hoffman.

"Ladies, you won't be permitted inside the perimeter. Just stay with me, outside the flares."

Aunt Barb frowned. "But that's so far from the car."

"No civilians inside the perimeter, that's our procedure. We didn't ask you down here, the ID is already made. If you want to be here, you have to follow procedure. Ladies, follow me and stay with me."

Officer Hoffman turned away, Judy took Aunt Barb's arm, and they walked together outside of the flares, past the group of police and administrative personnel, then farther down the road. A uniformed police officer stood off to the side of the street, his orange flashlight in hand, ready to redirect traffic, but the only cars and people were official. They got closer to the Honda, and a fire-department truck was parked at its front, where several sets of bright white klieglights had been set up, top-heavy on spindly metallic stalks, with tripod feet.

A gleaming blue van with the white symbol for the county coroner sat behind the Honda. Its back doors had reflective chevrons and were hanging open, so Judy assumed that the van hadn't been loaded yet. Iris's body must still be inside the Honda. A photographer took pictures inside the car, and his electronic flash fired at irregular intervals, visible through the windows, which were rolled down on the driver's side. Shadowy silhouettes moved around inside the Honda, but it was too far to see anything clearly.

Judy sighed inwardly, the sight making her profoundly sad. It seemed wrong that someone could die in such a mundane way, a heart attack while driving, sitting for hours strapped into a car seat, surrounded only by people whose job it was to see to it that she was examined, investigated, photographed, documented, and carted away in a van, to be taken to a morgue. Judy guessed that there would have to be an autopsy because it was an unattended death, and somehow that made it worse, that in a few hours or maybe even the next day, another stranger would invade the very corpus, slice a Y-incision into her chest, then extract, examine, measure, and weigh her organs, record her demise in triplicate, and issue a death certificate.

They reached the point directly across from the Honda, so that they were lined up with a clear view of the front seat. They stopped, and Aunt Barb's attention riveted on the Honda, where silhouettes were still moving around inside the car. There did appear to be a figure in the front seat, but it was too far away to see clearly, for which Judy was secretly grateful.

Aunt Barb craned her neck, standing on tiptoe. "What's going on, Officer? What are they doing in there?"

"That would be the coroner and the deputy coroner, performing the last stages of their investigation. They and the evidence technicians examine the body and make sure it gets photographed the way it was found." Officer Hoffman gestured to the group of police officers. "The department already has uniformed officers interviewing neighbors, to see if they saw the vehicle pull over or anything else unusual or out of the ordinary. We ask them if they know the deceased or recognize the vehicle, and if they've had any strange events in the area."

Aunt Barb frowned, but didn't look away from the Honda. "There are no neighbors."

Judy nodded. "And it's not as if it's a crime scene."

"No matter, crime scene or no." Officer Hoffman shrugged in his heavy Windbreaker. "We follow the same procedure. It's an apparently natural death, but we still investigate as if it's a crime scene. An assistant from the D.A.'s Office is here, and so are two of the county detectives."

Judy eyed the clump of men. "Are the detectives the ones in suits and ties?"

"Yes. In addition to the interviews, we have uniformed officers patrolling the perimeter, looking for anything suspicious or out of the ordinary on the ground, near the vehicle, or even in the hayfield."

Aunt Barb shivered slightly, her eyes glued to the Honda. Grief etched lines into the pale skin of her face, stretched thin across her gaunt cheekbones. The tip of her nose was turning red, though it wasn't that cold.

Judy talked to fill in the silences, her mother's daughter. "Officer Hoffman, do you do anything differently in terms of your investigation, if the deceased is undocumented?"

"No," Officer Hoffman answered. "We do everything by the book. For example, we had an aggravated robbery last week of an undocumented worker, which unfortunately happens a lot, since they get paid in cash. We investigated and prosecuted that case the same as if that person were a citizen. We have to. Same difference if we arrest an undocumented person or if an undocumented person is our suspect. We Mirandize him, and he's entitled to the same free lawyer as a citizen."

Judy had no idea. "If you were to ascertain that someone you arrest, or a victim, was undocumented, what are your obligations to the immigration services at the federal level? Do you have to report to them?"

Officer Hoffman's blue-eyed gaze shifted slyly to her. "You're talking like a lawyer. Are you a lawyer?"

"I am." Judy smiled. "Does it show?"

"Luckily, no." Officer Hoffman permitted himself a tight smile. "Anyway, in answer to your question, I don't know if we legally have to notify the feds, but we do. It's not our first priority, but the chief will probably contact ICE tomorrow."

"What's ICE?" Judy asked.

"Immigration and Customs Enforcement. We have a small police force in East Grove, only eight uniformed officers, three evidence techs, and the chief."

"But it's fairly safe out here, isn't it?"

Officer Hoffman nodded. "Yes, the main issue in the undocumented community is robbery and theft. They can't use the banks and are always taking cash to Western Union, to be wired home. You ask me, Western Union would be out of business but for them." Officer Hoffman surveyed the scene. "It will take us a few more hours to process here. We'll probably release it tomorrow. We lucked out in that this isn't a busy road."

Meantime, Aunt Barb had fallen into a grave silence, still fixated on the Honda. "It looks like the window is down in the front seat, doesn't it, Officer?"

Officer Hoffman squinted. "Yes, it does."

Judy looked, too. "Did the coroner do that, or the evidence techs?"

Officer Hoffman shook his head. "No. We leave everything untouched, everything exactly the way it was found."

Aunt Barb was shaking her head. "Iris doesn't drive with the window open, even on a nice day. She doesn't like her hair to blow around, and I can't understand why she's on this road at all."

Judy asked, "Is it on the way home for her, from work?"

"No, not at all." Aunt Barb kept her eyes trained on the Honda. "It's a straight shot from where she works to her apartment. So if she felt nauseated at work and decided to go home, she wouldn't take this way. This is like the hypotenuse to the triangle. It would add twenty minutes to the trip. Also, remember that call she got before she left today? I wonder where her phone is."

"Hold on." Officer Hoffman motioned to the coroner's van, where there was new activity. Two young men in black uniforms emerged from the back of the van with a stretcher and carried it toward the Honda. "The coroner's office is getting ready to take her now. Some of the big departments have standup screens that you can put up, so that nobody can see anything. We don't have the budget for that."

Judy put her arm around her aunt. "Aunt Barb, you want to go back to the car?"

"No, thanks." Aunt Barb formed praying hands, which she pressed to her lips.

Uniformed personnel climbed out of the Honda's front seat, and others arrived to help. Their bodies made a crowd of dark silhouettes around the car, blocking Judy's and Aunt Barb's views, but in the next moment, two men in black uniforms lifted a body from the front seat. Then it disappeared from view again, as they must have put it on the stretcher.

Judy couldn't see the body and was sure her aunt couldn't, either. She looked over to check, but before she knew what was happening, Aunt Barb had slid out from under her arm and was charging forward, bolting between the flares, through the perimeter, and toward the Honda.

"Miss, please, stop!" Officer Hoffman called out, giving chase.

Chapter Seven

"Aunt Barb!" Judy caught her aunt by the elbow just as she almost stumbled on an electrical cord from the klieglights, which blasted the area around the stretcher with light. The crowd of police personnel turned around at the commotion, and the klieglights made harsh, contrasting shadows on their faces. Their expressions looked collectively disapproving.

Judy looked past them, stricken. Iris was laying on the stretcher, inside a black vinyl body bag that had yet to be zipped, its sides gaping open. Her eyes remained closed, but her head was to the side, showing her ear and the gold crucifix earrings. Her hands were resting together on her body, but oddly, it looked as if one or two of her nails had been broken, the red polish chipped off and some of the rhinestones missing.

"Oh, Iris, no!" her aunt cried out, collapsing, and Judy grabbed her, hugged her close, and moved her away from the sight.

"Aunt Barb, come with me, I'm sorry, so sorry."

Officer Hoffman took her aunt's other arm gently. "Ladies, you must exit the perimeter."

"No, no, no." Aunt Barb sobbed, hanging her head, sagging between the policeman and Judy, and letting them lead her away from the stretcher and back to the Volkswagen, where they eased her, sobbing, into the passenger seat and closed the door behind her.

Judy faced Officer Hoffman. "I'm sorry that happened. I didn't see that coming, but I should have."

"No need to apologize." Officer Hoffman nodded, sympathetic. "You never know how people are going to react in a situation like this. That's why we do death notifications in pairs, and why we always make sure that the next-of-kin is sitting down when we do the notification. I've had the craziest things happen during a notification. One time, I told a man that his son had been killed in an auto accident, and the man jumped up from the couch and ran clear out of the house. We had to chase him down the street."

"Oh my," Judy said, thinking that being a policeman had to be one of the most demanding jobs on the planet.

"So thank you for your cooperation. I'll make a note that your aunt made a personal identification."

"I have one question before we go." Judy couldn't get Iris's broken fingernails out of her mind, for some reason. "What happens next, to the body? Will there be an autopsy?"

"Yes, since the new D.A., we always autopsy after an auto accident to find out if there was a medical event."

"How long would that take and who would get the results?"

"Let's see, it's Saturday night, so I bet the autopsy would be Sunday or Monday. They would release the body, probably on Tuesday, to the funeral home that would be picked out by whoever claims it."

Judy thought ahead. "That might be my aunt, but I will do the arranging."

"If she claims the body, she would be responsible for the expenses at the morgue. If the body were unclaimed, then it would be cremated at the county's expense." Officer Hoffman took a step closer. "You didn't hear this from me, but we have a real problem with the undocumented bodies. The families know that if the body is unclaimed, we'll cremate it at taxpayer expense, so they wait to claim the body, let the county cremate it, then claim it."

Judy's thoughts were stuck on Iris. "What if she didn't die of natural causes? What if there's something suspicious about the death?" She gestured at the guys in ties. "Can I talk to the detective on the case?"

"Sure, I'll go get him. Stay here." Officer Hoffman turned and jogged off toward the group, and Judy opened the car door and leaned in to her aunt.

"I'm so sorry, Aunt Barb. How are you?"

"It's just so sad." Aunt Barb had stopped crying, but her eyes were filmed and bloodshot, and her knit cap tilted askew. She slumped in her too-big parka, wiping her eyes with a balled-up Kleenex.

"Do you feel up to seeing the detective on her case? Officer Hoffman went to get him, and I can talk with him alone or with you."

"Let's do it, it's important." Her aunt dabbed at her eyes again. "I'll stay in the car, though. I feel tired."

"Of course." Judy straightened up, left the passenger door open, and turned around to see Officer Hoffman approaching them with a man about six feet tall, with a bulky build, short hair, wire-rimmed aviator glasses, and crow's-feet that placed him in his mid-forties. She put on a professional smile, which was another thing she hadn't learned in law school.

Officer Hoffman gestured at the detective. "Ms. Carrier, this is Detective Raymond Boone. He's assigned to the case, and I'll take my leave now. Nice meeting you and your aunt."

"Thanks." Judy waved to him as he left, and Detective Boone extended a hammy hand.

"Ms. Carrier, I'm pleased to meet you. Thank you for coming out to make the identification."

"Thanks for your help." Judy accepted his handshake, firm enough to make her glad she worked out. "This is my aunt, Barb Moyer, who knew Iris. Iris's last name was Juarez."

Detective Boone looked down at her aunt with a sympathetic frown. "Ms. Moyer, I'm very sorry for your loss. I'm glad you asked to see me and I would've contacted you myself in a day or two, at your home."

Aunt Barb sniffled. "Detective, I want you to do everything possible to find out what happened here because Iris was a wonderful person, and my dearest friend, and she deserves everything that you can do for her."

"I certainly will." Detective Boone nodded, setting his mouth. He slipped his hand inside his dark sport coat and extracted a ballpoint pen and a skinny notepad like Officer Hoffman carried. "Now, tell me about yourself and how you know the decedent."

Aunt Barb cleared her throat. "I'm a landscape architect and I live in Kennett Square on Vaughn Road. Iris was my best friend, and she worked for me, as a gardener and as a companion, for the past three years or so."

Detective Boone flipped open the cardboard cover of his pad, clicked on his pen, and started taking notes. He looked over at Judy, blinking behind his aviator glasses, which were smudged. "Ms. Carrier, how do you know Ms. Juarez?"

"I just met her today at my aunt's house."

Aunt Barb interjected, "Iris was leaving for her shift at Mike's Exotics. She works the three-to-eleven. She came by this morning to bring me some cookies since my family is here for a visit."

Judy noted that Aunt Barb wasn't telling him about her cancer and respected that she wanted to keep it private. She let her aunt take the lead, since she had the information.

Detective Boone made another note. "Address and phone?"

Her aunt gave the phone number, then answered, "Point Breeze Avenue, Point Breeze Apartments, 1-C. Do you have her phone? She got a call today that concerned her, and I'm curious about it."

"I'll see if the phone was bagged yet."

"She seemed fine when I saw her today and she never mentioned anything about heart trouble. She's very healthy."

"Do you know who her family doctor is, if she had one?" Detective Boone cocked his head.

"I don't think she had one. She used the LCD, but she never went unless I nagged her."

Detective Boone made another note. "Officer Hoffman tells me that you're the emergency contact, and that Ms. Juarez didn't have close family or friends in the area besides you. Is that correct?"

"She didn't have family, but she did have a good friend, Daniella Gamboa. Somebody will have to notify her, about this. I never met her but Iris talked about her. They used to work together at Mike's Exotics, but Iris told me Daniella doesn't work there anymore."

"Do you have contact info for Ms. Gamboa, like an address or phone?"

"No."

"We'll find Ms. Gamboa." Detective Boone made a note. "We'll conduct our investigation in the next few days, and we'll keep you informed." He turned to Judy. "Officer Hoffman mentioned to me that you're an attorney in Philadelphia, so I expect you'll be an asset."

Judy tried to believe him, but nobody liked a Philadelphia lawyer, least of all a detective. "Thank you. I know that Officer Hoffman said that the case appears to be a natural death, and I'm sure that's true, but—"

"The manner of death does appear to be natural, because of the condition of the body and the circumstances in which the body was found." Detective Boone gestured at the Honda. "The facts suggest she had a heart attack while she was driving."

"Which facts suggest that, specifically?"

"Several. As is typical, her body slumped forward and took pressure off the gas pedal, then the car drifted off the road into a hay roll. The engine was running when we found the car. The fuel tank was almost out of gas. The air bag did not deploy. This was a low-speed collision, there's no injury or seatbelt marks that we could find."

Judy took it in. "Well, my aunt had some questions, like the phone, and also that Iris should have been at work."

Aunt Barb added, "She never misses work and is very diligent, so I can't for the life of me understand why she wasn't there."

"I see." Detective Boone made a note. "I will be sure to follow-up with the folks at Mike's Exotics."

"You know the place?" Judy asked.

"Of course." Detective Boone smiled crookedly. "East Grove isn't Philly."

Judy continued, "Plus, my aunt made the point that it doesn't make sense that Iris was on this road, at all. Apparently, it's not on the way home from work."

Aunt Barb chimed in, "This is way out of her way. There's nothing around here. I can't imagine what she was doing here, can you?"

Detective Boone scribbled in his pad. "She could've been going somewhere other than home, obviously. If she began to experience symptoms of heart attack or a stroke, such as confusion or disorientation, she wouldn't know where she was driving. But that would be just speculation."

Judy didn't know enough to agree or disagree with him. "My aunt also made the point that her window was open, and Iris didn't like to drive with the windows open because it messed up her hair."

Aunt Barb nodded. "That's true, and besides which, she only had a T-shirt on, not even a sweater. Women our age don't do that. We're always cold."

Detective Boone looked up from his pad. "We can't assume that she died in the evening hours. We don't have the time of death yet. It's certainly possible that she passed in the daytime. It was a sunny day, so she could have had the window open."

"But people would have seen her and called the police."

"Unlikely. This road isn't well-traveled, and they might not have realized she was dead."

"Detective Boone, there was one last detail that concerned me, which was that I noticed that Iris had a few broken nails."

Aunt Barb looked up. "She did?"

"Yes, they hadn't been broken earlier today, when I saw her." Judy didn't know how much more of this conversation her aunt could take. "I noticed because her nail polish was unusual, red with rhinestones. I'm not sure what it means, but I wanted to mention that to you."

Aunt Barb bit her lip. "Iris took great care of her hands and nails. She loved to do her nails. She wore gloves when she gardened because of them."

Detective Boone flipped his pad closed. "I wouldn't want to speculate on the significance of someone's breaking their nails. We have four pathologists in this county, and one of them will perform an autopsy, run toxicology tests, and do whatever else they think is indicated."

Aunt Barb gasped, horrified. "Wait. What? You're going to do an autopsy on Iris?"

"Yes." Detective Boone pursed his lips, and his jowls fell into sober lines. "I know it's, uh, distasteful, but it's standard procedure in a case like this."

"Oh no." Aunt Barb covered her face with her hands, and Judy put her hand on her aunt's shoulder, looking at Detective Boone.

"Thanks for your time. I think I'll take my aunt home now."

"Sure, sorry about your loss." Detective Boone gave a short wave, then turned away, and Judy walked around the VW, climbed into the driver's seat, and looked over at her aunt.

"I'm sorry."

"Thanks." Aunt Barb gave her nose a final blow. "Let's get out of here."

"I agree." Judy put on her shoulder harness, twisted the key in the ignition, released the brake, and hit the gas, turning the car around to put the coroner's van behind them. "I go straight, right?"

"Yes, and I'll tell you when to turn left."

"But we went straight to get here, didn't we?" Judy glanced over.

"I know, but we're not going home yet."

Chapter Eight

"Where are we going?" Judy asked, worried.

"Mike's Exotics, where Iris worked. I want to see if she went in today. I want to find out what happened."

"Do you really feel up to that, right now?"

"Yes, and I don't want to let it wait." Aunt Barb stowed her Kleenex in her pocket and straightened in the passenger seat. "She would still be on shift, so they should be there. I want to talk to her boss. His name is Julio, and I met him once when I dropped her off, because her car was in the shop." Aunt Barb pointed to the left. "This is the turn, up ahead."

"But you're tired. Maybe we should go home." Judy spotted the break in the cornfield on the left, but there was no street sign.

"No, I'm fine, and what's the point of putting it off?"

"You could sleep and get your feet under you, emotionally. You just got blindsided in the worst possible way."

"But I only have the weekend. The mastectomy is Monday."

"We can go tomorrow."

"Julio might not be on the job tomorrow and he's the one I want to talk to. I won't sleep if I don't understand what happened to her." Aunt Barb turned her face to the window, but there was nothing to see in the dark.

"What is it you think happened?" Judy turned left onto another long country road. Bugs flew from the gloom into their headlights, making *tink tink* sounds when they hit the glass.

"I don't know. I only know that what I'm hearing doesn't make sense. She didn't have any heart issues."

"What's the LCD you keep mentioning?"

"It's the health service in Kennett Square, that the undocumented use."

"So it can't be the best medical care, can it? She could have had heart issues and not known it."

"But she was strong, and able, and hard-working. And what about the car window? And the nails? And that phone call, the way she acted afterwards?"

"Those are strange little details, but they don't necessarily mean anything." Judy regretted having brought any of it up. "It's not as if there was any sign of foul play."

"I know that. I'm not saying that."

"Then what are you saying?" Judy asked, her tone gentle as they drove into the dark.

"I'm just saying that if I can ask a few more questions, so that I have answers when I put my head down on the pillow tonight, I think it makes sense to do so."

"I agree, but I think Detective Boone will follow up. It's police business, and he seemed pretty good."

"I think he will, too, but I'm not about to sit on my hands. Besides, since when do you care if something is police business? That never stopped you or Mary."

"Except that she's getting married." Judy thought back to the day, when she'd felt like Debbie Downer at the bridal shop. "Our days of excellent adventures might be over. She's a partner now, too."

"Don't worry, you two are thick as thieves. By the way, how are you and Frank doing?"

"Great, fine." Judy usually confided in her aunt, but didn't want to burden her any further, with so much already on her plate.

"Thinking about getting married?"

"Maybe."

"Take your time, there's no rush. Sometimes when your friends get married, it puts pressure, but it shouldn't." Aunt Barb paused, musing. "Though I hated it when your mother got married before me. Everybody knows I'm nicer."

Judy smiled as they passed a dark barn with a tall blue silo. "But she's older than you. She would have hated it if you got married before her, wouldn't she have?"

"Honey, let me tell you. Marriage was *not* on that girl's mind. She liked the bad boys in high school. You wouldn't know it to look at her now, but she's where you get your wild side."

Judy chuckled, then thought of her mother, waiting for them at home. "Aunt Barb, how long do you expect this will take? I'm trying to decide if we should let her know we'll be late."

"Good point, I'll text her." Aunt Barb reached for her purse and got the phone.

"What are you going to say?"

"I'll tell her we're running late and not to worry, is all." Aunt Barb texted away, as the light from the phone screen shone upward, illuminating her laugh lines, which bracketed a sly smile. "I can get you out of anything, even ballet lessons. Remember?"

"Of course." Judy chuckled at the memory, from when she was only six years old. Her mother had decided that her tomboy daughter needed some civilizing and signed her up for ballet lessons, but Judy hated every minute of them. She'd begged to quit after the first recital, in which she starred as a dancing poodle in tiara-kid makeup, a pink tutu, and a puffy pink tail. Her mother had relented and let her quit only because Aunt Barb had prevailed upon her to let Judy take drawing lessons instead, which had led to her lifelong love of art and painting.

Aunt Barb looked over. "I still remember the song from the recital. Isn't that crazy?"

"I remember it, too." Judy decided to sing it, to cheer her aunt up. " 'We are little dancing poodles, and we are here to say . . . ' "

Aunt Barb joined in, " 'We come from France, to do our dance . . . ' "

" 'But we only do ballet!' " they sang together, then laughed. Judy's throat thickened. She loved her aunt and couldn't imagine losing her, not now or ever. "I can't believe you remember that."

"Are you kidding? I still have PTSD."

Judy chuckled, then turned right and left, following her aunt's directions through corn and soybean fields and past horses grazing in rolling pastures, their outlines indistinct in the darkness and their whinnying cutting through the night air. The fields gave way to farmhouses and barns, then to trailers and smaller homes, until they spotted a small cast-iron sign that read, WELCOME TO EAST GROVE. The town was of colonial vintage like Kennett Square, and quaint brick and clapboard houses lined the road, their wooden porches just steps from the curb. Judy headed for the outskirts of town, past a check-cashing storefront and a shabby Mexican tacqueria.

Finally they came upon a long, low series of square buildings, only one story high, mere cinderblock boxes attached in a row, like railroad cars. They had no windows, so there was no way to tell if anyone was inside, and the only light came from flickering fixtures on the roofs of the buildings, which cast jittery cones of light on the worn asphalt lot.

"Here's Mike's." Aunt Barb gestured at a driveway that had

no sign, except for PRIVATE PROPERTY, NO THRU TRAFFIC. "That's the parking lot."

"Why no sign?" Judy steered into the lot, where there were a few old cars parked in a row.

"Everybody knows where Mike's is, he's one of the tiny, independent growers. He owns about ten other growers, all independent. He produces exotics."

"What's 'exotics'?" Judy turned off the ignition and put on the emergency brake, looking through the windshield and noticing for the first time that the buildings had large numbers painted on the cinderblock, in black. The building on the end, closest to them, was number seven.

"Fancier mushrooms. Portabella, mitake, shitake, cremini. But he hires the undocumented."

"How does he get away with it? What about Immigration?"

"The way the system works is that Immigration stages a raid only if there's a significant number of complaints, in relation to the size of the workforce. Bottom line, nobody complains." Aunt Barb picked up her water bottle and took a sip of water. "Immigration isn't the real problem, anyway, the IRS is. If a grower submits a list of social security numbers and they're not good, it takes the IRS three months to figure that out. So in three months, after the grower gets the IRS notice, he fires the employees and they go to another grower, or another location of the same grower, like Mike's."

"Really?"

"That's how it worked with Iris. She's worked at all of his locations for about a year now." Aunt Barb eyed the buildings. "It's like a shell game, because even workers with legitimate green cards have only six months in the country, then they have to go back. They worry they can't get back in, but plenty of them do, and they end up at one of the shadier growers."

"Was Iris afraid of being caught?"

"She worried about it constantly. She lived in fear of being deported, always looking over her shoulder. You saw her, she was so quiet, she learned to be invisible." Aunt Barb paused, and her eyes glistened anew. "There are so many undocumented workers here, and everywhere."

"But that doesn't make it right." Judy believed in the law, even if it meant siding with her mother.

"I know, but they're here, living in a parallel universe. They're an open secret."

Judy thought of the undocumented workers she'd seen in the city, the busboys smoking outside the back door of the restaurants, or the men who delivered her takeout pizza by bicycle. "We know and we-don't-know."

"Yes, and the interesting thing about an open secret is that people look the other way, literally. Iris became the kind of woman whom people looked away from. Unmemorable and marginalized, even more than the average middle-aged woman."

Judy could hear the resentment in her aunt's voice. "Where did she work before Mike's?"

"She cleaned houses for that service, which is when I met her, as I told you. She also did yard work, and she washed and mended horse blankets. At one point, she worked three jobs."

Judy slid the keys from the ignition. "Okay. So why are we here?"

"You'll see. I have a plan. Just follow my lead." Aunt Barb reached for the door handle.

And Judy wondered when it got to be so hard to keep up with someone almost twice her age.

Chapter Nine

"So what's your plan?" Judy took her aunt's arm, but she needed no help, standing straight and tall, her step fueled by a new determination.

"To see the boss and get to the bottom of this, that's what. Iris works here and she should have been here tonight." Aunt Barb gestured at the cinderblock buildings. "These are the growing rooms, and the packing area and office are behind them."

Judy grimaced at the disgusting odor of manure that permeated the air. "They really use manure to grow mushrooms?"

"Yes, horse manure and some chicken, but they call it compost. That's why there's always mushroom growers next to horse farms. Chester County produces almost half of all mushrooms grown in the United States."

"Really? How do you know that?"

"Everybody does. It's a source of local pride, and Iris used to tell me all about the business, and she gave me the inside track."

"But how did she work with this *smell*?" Judy couldn't imagine anyone breathing that stink, twenty-four/seven.

"God knows." Her aunt wrinkled her nose. "The men pick

the mushrooms, and the women pack, but it's gross in the packing room here, too."

Judy didn't know much about how mushrooms grew, except it had been a joke at her old law firm that the partners treated the associates like mushrooms—keep 'em in the dark and feed 'em shit. "How is that sanitary, to grow food in horse manure?"

"They pasteurize it. You'll see, we're going inside." Aunt Barb charged past battered trash cans and broken wooden pallets. "This place is such a dump. I don't know how they pass inspection."

"Who inspects?" Judy asked, as they approached the door to the building.

"The state and federal agencies, and the mushroom growers have their own independent council that inspects as well. Someday I'll figure out how Mike gets away with what he does." Aunt Barb reached for the metal handle on the battered door, which had a thick spring. "He must pay somebody off."

"I'll get the door," Judy said, but her aunt had already opened it and they entered the building, where the manure stink was stronger, turning Judy's stomach. They found themselves in a cold, rectangular hallway with a grimy gray utility sink and blue plastic trays scattered on a concrete floor. "It's so chilly in here."

"Because we're close to the growing rooms. Let's keep going. The office is behind the growing rooms."

"I got the door." Judy crossed to another door, also with a metal handle and a spring. Wrinkled paper signs were taped to the door in English and Spanish: HAIRNETS MUST BE WORN, REDECILLA DEBE USARESE EN ESTA AREA. NO SMOKING EATING OR DRINKING IN THIS AREA, PROHIBIDO FUMAR COMER O BEBER EN ESTA AREA.

"This is a growing room," her aunt said, charging through the door into a freezing-cold, dark room that reeked of manure. A mechanical thrumming filled the air, the sound of refrigeration units atop the building.

Judy followed, but the stench of manure overpowered her, triggering her gag reflex. Her step slowed, and she covered her mouth instinctively, trying not to throw up. She could barely see a thing, and the room was dark except for a single bare fluorescent panel on one of the wooden racks of brown mushrooms, which ran the length of the immense room, almost floor to ceiling. Narrow aisles ran between the racks, and as her eyes adjusted to the darkness, she could make out the dim outline of twenty-some figures moving up and down the aisles, hunched over the trays.

She walked past, shuddering against the cold, her eyes tearing from the manure stink. They looked like shadows instead of people, but they were men dressed for the frigid temperature in heavyweight hoodies and bulky jeans, with baseball caps over their puffy white-paper hairnets. None of them looked up, but stayed face-down as they picked small brown mushrooms from trays of thousands, seeming not to see or hear her. She realized that they all had earplugs in against the mechanical noise.

Judy felt so disturbed by what she was seeing that she found her pace quicken. She couldn't have imagined such awful working conditions, worse than hell itself, because of the manure. She caught up with her aunt, who was at a door in the back wall, with more Spanish and English signs, then one in a language she didn't recognize: **TOLONG TANGAN HALANGI PINTU! Do not block door!** Judy placed a hand on her aunt's back. "Go, please, I can't take this smell."

Aunt Barb opened the door. "This must be the packing room."

Judy followed her into another massive cold room, filled with manure smell and mechanical noise. She blinked against the sudden brightness from fluorescent panels suspended from a grimy corrugated ceiling, illuminating twenty-odd women working at a long assembly line, packing mushrooms behind a wall of heavy machinery that had huge rolls of plastic wrap.

Her aunt hurried ahead, but Judy slowed to take it in, imagining poor Iris working here. None of the women looked up, their ears plugged against the refrigeration noise, breathing in the manure smell. They were white, Hispanic, and Asian, all dressed in dark blue smocks over hoodies and wool hats over hairnets, packing mushrooms into light blue containers, positioning them in the wrapping machines, stamping them, and placing them in large, unmarked cardboard boxes. The humans worked like robots, part of the assembly line itself, and the job horrified Judy as much as the growing room. She hurried ahead to keep up with Aunt Barb, past a time clock with yellow cards in trays, and reached a scuffed swinging door, pushed it open, and entered a short hallway leading to some sort of office.

"That was awful." Judy took a deep breath, but the air was still smelly. She felt vaguely ashamed at herself, for beefing about the asbestos damages cases, but she knew that wouldn't stop her.

"Finally, the office! Let me do the talking." Aunt Barb flagged down an overweight man who looked to be in his mid-thirties, lumbering down the paneled hall toward them, a confused frown folding his fleshy face. His hair was a sparse brown, and he had on a light blue oxford shirt, loose tan work pants, and worn black sneakers.

"Ladies?" He waved back at them. "May I help you? The public isn't allowed in the—"

"I'm sorry, but we're looking for Julio," Aunt Barb answered, as they reached the man. "He's the boss, right? Or is Mike around?"

"They're not here. I'm Scott Panuc, assistant operations manager. What can I do for you?"

"Scott, my name is Barb Moyer, this is my niece Judy, and I'm a friend of Iris Juarez, who works here—"

"I'm sorry, I don't know who you're talking about." Scott folded his arms over his chubby belly.

"Look, I know that Iris worked here. She's been working here for two months on the three-to-eleven shift, in the packing room. She should've been working tonight."

"No, you have your facts wrong." Scott shook his head, sticking out his lower lip. "I don't know any Iris Juarez. Nobody works here by that name."

Judy held her tongue, only because her aunt wanted to do the talking.

"Scott," her aunt said, calmly, "I know she worked here. She started two months ago. I dropped her off here two weeks ago."

"I'm sorry, but I can't help you. I don't know what you're talking about—"

"I *know* she worked here. I picked her up here, too, the same day. That was when I met, or at least saw, Julio."

Judy interjected, "Scott, we're not from Immigration or the IRS or anything. We're just personal friends of Iris's, trying to figure out what happened to her. I don't know if you heard but she was found dead in her car today, on Brandywine Way."

"Oh no!" Scott's eyes flared, his surprise genuine. "Oh, uh, jeez, I'm sorry to hear that."

"Me, too." Aunt Barb sighed, whether from relief or fatigue, Judy couldn't tell. "Okay, so now we know. She worked here."

"Yes, she did." Scott buckled his lower lip. "I didn't know who you were, well, you know."

"I know. The police think she had a heart attack. I'm just trying to get to the bottom of it, because she should have been at work tonight."

Scott hesitated, rubbing his face. "Yes, to be honest, she should have been here, but she didn't come in today."

"So you didn't see her today at all?"

"No, she was a no-show." Scott shrugged his heavy shoulders sadly. "It's not like her, but then again, you never know."

"Did you call her when you realized she wasn't here?"

"No, I never do. I figured she moved on. They move around a lot and usually don't say where they're going. One day, they just disappear."

Judy remained silent. Nobody had to ask whom he meant by *they.*

"That wouldn't be like her, either, just to disappear without saying so." Aunt Barb seemed to slump in her parka, and Judy could feel her leaning on her arm for support.

"No, it wouldn't, but I didn't change what I usually do." Scott's face fell into lines. "Iris really is, or was, a special person. My wife and I just had our second baby, and she brought in cookies for me to bring home."

Aunt Barb smiled sadly. "That would be Iris to a T."

"I didn't know she had heart problems."

"She didn't, that I know of. That's what I'm trying to figure out, that and why she was on Brandywine Way. You have any idea why she would be down there?"

"No, not at all. There's nothing there." Scott frowned, puzzled.

"She was friends with Daniella Gamboa, and I think Daniella used to work here, didn't she?"

"Yeah, but she left."

"Do you know why?"

"No idea. Like I say, they come and go. One day last week, she didn't show up."

Judy interjected, "Was Iris friendly with any of the other women in the packing room?"

Scott shook his head. "No, there's so much moving around. They don't even know each other's names, and that's the way they like it. The only exception is when the families come up together, like cousins will work together and they stick together. But I never saw Iris with any of them."

Judy got another idea. "Did she have a locker or anything we could look through? Maybe it would contain something that would help us."

"No," Scott answered. "Like I say, there's so many changes in the workforce, we don't give them lockers. Only management has lockers. The employees keep their things in their cars or their fanny packs. They're big on fanny packs."

Judy made a mental note. "Scott, do you know who her doctor might have been?"

"No. I assumed she used the LCD. Most of them do."

Judy remembered that Aunt Barb had said the same thing. "Did she ever say she didn't feel well at work?"

"No, never. She never missed a day and she took all the extra shifts I could give her. She was a workhorse. They all are. They never complain. They're the best workers you'd ever want, the Mexicans."

Judy didn't know whether to be offended, because his tone was so favorable.

Scott smiled crookedly. "You're looking at me funny. You must not be from around here."

"No," Judy said, feeling her face flush. "I'm trying to wrap my head around the use of these undocumented workers. It's an open secret."

Scott nodded. "Oh, absolutely, but I don't think we're that different from a lot of other places in the country. I'd love to hire Americans, but they don't want to pick mushrooms. It's filthy, smelly work. We advertise on craigslist, Monster, everywhere, but nobody applies. We pay minimum wage, too, so it's not like we're exploiting anybody." Scott opened his palms, in uneasy appeal. "Listen, you have to be realistic. We need the labor, and the Mexicans are happy to have the work."

"Let me ask you one last question." Judy was still trying to understand. "We were at the scene tonight, where Iris was found, and the police said they'll follow up with you about her. Will you confirm that she worked here, or will you try to keep it quiet, like you did with us?"

"No, we cooperate with the East Grove police. They get it."

"Don't they report you for hiring undocumented workers? Do you ever get raided?"

"We don't get raided because nobody files a complaint, and the local police tend not to give us too much trouble." Scott glanced over at a clock on the wall. "Well, I better get back to the floor. Can I show you ladies out?"

"Yes, thanks." Judy put an arm around her aunt, who looked suddenly thoughtful.

"Come with me." Scott motioned toward a brown metal door near the office area. "And please, accept my condolences. Iris was a very special lady, and we'll say a prayer for her tonight."

"Yes, thanks," Aunt Barb said quietly. "Good night."

"After you, Aunt Barb." Judy opened the door to let her aunt out, and they walked together toward the car.

"I think we need to text your mother again. We'll tell her we decided to go out for an ice-cream sundae."

"What? Aren't you tired yet?" Judy chuckled, in surprise.

"Hell, no." Her aunt pulled down her knit cap and shoved her hands deep into her pockets. "I'm just getting started."

Chapter Ten

Judy pulled up, cut the ignition, and looked around. The apartment complex where Iris lived was too run-down to be well-lighted, and the only light came from a street lamp, which dimly illuminated a large, square parking lot that seemed to be the focal point of the apartments, a connected series of two-story buildings wrapped in a U shape around the lot. Old cars filled the parking spaces, some with missing hubcaps and others with dented doors, and the lights from the apartments showed people leaning on the cars and sitting on their front steps or on plastic beach chairs, visible only in silhouette, laughing, talking, or smoking, the red tips of their cigarettes glowing in the dark.

"Judy, you ready to go?"

Judy looked over. "Sure, but what are we trying to accomplish, again?"

"I told you, you're not going to talk me out of this. I have one day of freedom left. Even if the police follow up, there's things they might miss. They didn't know Iris the way I know her. And I'm sure the roommates will be much happier talking to me than the local constabulary."

"On it." Judy pulled the key out of the ignition, and they both got out of the car and walked to the driveway of the apartment complex, where she took her aunt's arm.

"I can walk, you know." Aunt Barb's gaze slid slyly to Judy under her knit cap. "My legs are fine, it's my breasts that are the problem."

"Yes, but if I hold your breasts, people will talk."

Aunt Barb laughed. "Look around you, they already are."

Judy looked at stoops and beach chairs, where heads were turning. The residents had grown quiet as the two women made their way down the center of the square parking area, and a short man nearest them flicked his cigarette into the air, where it arced like a falling star.

"It's because we're *gringas*," Aunt Barb said, lowering her voice. "By the way, like my accent?"

"Nice. How good is your Spanish?"

"Let's put it this way, your mom is the linguist, not me. But I understand it better than I can speak it."

"Which apartment did you say it was again?"

"This one, right here." Her aunt turned right between two parked cars and walked until they reached a path of cracked concrete that served as an interior sidewalk.

"Aunt Barb, do you realize they might not know about Iris's death?"

"I know. I'll do the talking, okay?"

"Fine with me. You're on a roll." Judy squeezed her arm, and they turned onto a crumbling concrete path that led to the front door of one of the buildings. Everyone on the step or the beach chairs fell silent, and in the lights from inside the first-floor apartments, Judy could see that they were younger than she had realized, maybe in their twenties and thirties, a group of men and women, all of them Hispanic, in an array of T-shirts, sweatshirts, and jeans.

Her aunt stopped short in the middle of the path. "Hello, my name is Barb Moyer and this is my niece Judy. I'm a friend of Iris's and I'm here to see her roommates Maria Elena or Hermenia."

"I'm Maria Elena," said one of the women, in slightly accented English. She was sitting in a beach chair, holding a phone and wearing a white sweatshirt and jeans, but it was too dark to see her facial features. She sounded young, and her long, glossy curls shone in the light from the window.

"Maria Elena, would you mind if we went inside and talked a minute, about Iris?"

"She's not home."

"I know, I'm a friend of hers, and—"

"Oh, wait, I know who you are!" Maria Elena's tone warmed up. "You're the lady with the roses. Iris told me about you."

"Yes, that's me."

"What about Iris?"

Aunt Barb hesitated. "I'm afraid I have bad news. I'm very sorry, but I'm here to tell you that she has . . . passed. She was found tonight in her car, on Brandywine Way."

Maria Elena gasped, and everyone burst into shocked Spanish chatter, and Judy caught the words *morte* and *accidente*.

Her aunt said, "No, not a car accident. They think she had a heart attack."

"No." Maria Elena moaned, and another wave of chatter went through the crowd, which grew somber, and an older man made the sign of the cross on his chest.

"Do you think we can go inside? There's just some things I want to talk to you about."

"Sure, of course." Maria Elena rose, made her way through the crowd, and led them to the front door and inside the building. They walked down a long, dimly lighted hall, and at the end was a door, which Maria Elena unlocked and pushed open, flicking on a stark overhead light. "Come in, please."

"Thank you," Aunt Barb responded, and they entered a neat, if small, living room that was modestly furnished with an old brown couch, a red plaid chair, and a wooden rocker set around a battered coffee table. A tiny galley kitchen was on the right part of the room, but there was no dining-room table, and two closed doors off the room presumably led to the bedrooms.

"I can't believe this happened, are you sure it's true?" Maria Elena frowned sadly, pocketing her keys. In the bright light, Judy could see that her warm brown eyes had filmed, dampening her mascaraed lashes. She was pretty, with a small nose and heart-shaped lips, slick with gloss.

"Yes, it's true," her aunt answered. "I'm so sorry. The police came to me because she has my name as her emergency contact."

"So she's really . . . dead?" Maria Elena sank onto the plaid chair, linking her fingers between her knees, absorbing the shock. Her nails were polished red with white chevrons at the squared-off tips, reminding Judy again of Iris's broken fingernail.

"Yes, it's true. I identified her."

"That's terrible." Maria Elena shook her head, numbly, and wiped her eyes. "This makes me so sad. That hurts my heart."

"I'm so sorry. And her family at home, it's all gone?"

"Yes."

"Do you know Daniella Gamboa?"

"I meet her once or twice."

"Do you have her cell phone or address?"

"No." Maria Elena sniffed, brushing a tear away before it started to spill down her cheek. "Iris is so quiet, like, to herself, but she is so sweet, she has such a sweet heart. She's older, you know, she act like my mother. She is always baking cookies and cakes, to get us to eat, and she is so religious, all the time she want us to go to church with her. She says we drink too much beer. She tells us, like, all the time." Maria Elena wagged her finger, with a mock-comic frown. " 'Ladies should not drink too much, never out of the bottle.' She wants us to make a *jurma-mentos*."

Judy interjected, "What does that mean?"

"Is a special thing, like, you go to church with her and make a promise to God that we don't drink for, like, two weeks." Maria Elena chuckled. "She wants us to, anyway, but we don't do it."

"How long have you lived together?" Aunt Barb asked, but she was beginning to sound tired again.

"About six months. She take us both in, her other roommates go home. Me and Hermenia, she's out with her boyfriend. Iris meets us at the mission and she takes us in. She get us jobs."

Judy interjected again, "What's the mission?"

"You know, the church mission, they give out clothes and toys for free."

Her aunt asked, "Do you know why she didn't go to work today? When she left my house this afternoon, that's where she said she was going."

Maria Elena shook her head, blinking away her new tears. "No, I don't know. I work the morning shift today and she's gone when I got home."

Aunt Barb asked, "Do you work at Mike's, too?"

"Not anymore. I work in a restaurant and I clean houses." Maria Elena wrinkled her pretty nose. "I don't want to do the mushrooms anymore, even though they pay good. That smell, I can't take it. It gets on your clothes and your hair." Maria Elena turned to Judy. "You know what I'm saying, you can't get the stink out. It's like *on* you, like, all the time. I won't have no boyfriends if I smell like that. That's why Iris use the perfume, so much."

Her aunt asked, "Maria Elena, was Iris sick lately? Did she mention anything about her chest hurting or not feeling well?"

"No."

"Do you know who Iris uses for a doctor? Does she have a doctor?"

"I guess she goes to LCD, but I don't know."

"Do you know any reason why she'd be on Brandywine Way? Do you know where that is?"

"I know where it is. I don't know, like, why she was there." Maria Elena tossed her head, and her curls bounced.

"Did you text her today?"

"No."

"Do you mind if I go in her room? I just want to look around and see if there's anything to explain why she missed work today." Aunt Barb emitted a small sigh. "I should get some clothes to bury her in."

"Oh right." Maria Elena rose. "Come on."

"Thanks," Aunt Barb said, and they crossed the living room to the kitchen side, where Maria Elena opened the door onto a room that was barely big enough for a single bed, neatly made with a blue comforter, and a beat-up, fake-wood chest of drawers. A pair of old pink flip-flops sat beside the bed on the floor, ready and waiting for a woman who would never come home.

"She has the smallest room, that's why she doesn't share." Maria Elena tried to press the door open all the way, but it banged into the wall. "We share. Also it works out better because she doesn't stay out late, like us."

They entered the tiny room, barely able to fit the three of them, with Judy feeling strange, having just come from seeing Iris's lifeless body on the stretcher. A large crucifix hung on white walls, and the dresser held an old-fashioned runner of white cotton, on which rested a few bottles of nail polish, perfume, a ceramic statue of the Virgin Mary, a plastic white crucifix, a multicolored clay plate that held gold-toned hoops and necklaces, and a yellow shaker of athlete's foot powder.

"Where's the closet?" Aunt Barb asked, turning on her heel, but Maria Elena shook her head.

"She don't have one."

"Where does she put her dresses?"

"In the drawers. She only has two dresses, that she wears to church."

"But that can't be. I gave her dresses, and sweaters and shirts, too. Jewelry." Aunt Barb frowned, puzzled, looking around. "I don't see any of the stuff I gave her here. There were shoes and rain boots, too."

Maria Elena shook her head. "I don't know, maybe she give them to the mission. She's always after me to give my things to the mission, too. When I meet her at the mission, the first day, she isn't there to *get,* she is there to *give.* She always says, 'Maria Elena, God wants you to take care of people,' but I tell her, 'Iris, it's not like I have so much.' She wants us to give our *money* to the mission, too!" Maria Elena's eyes flared open, incredulous. "I tell her, '*mami,* you can give your money away, but me, no. God don't want me broke.'"

"Oh my, what a wonderful spirit she had." Aunt Barb rested a hand on the dresser, seeming to steady herself. "Judy, can you look through these drawers and find a nice dress for her?"

"Sure." Judy went to the dresser and opened the top drawer, which contained folded underwear, bras, and a Bible. "Do we need underwear?"

"No, funeral homes usually have that."

"Good." Judy opened the second drawer, of neatly folded T-shirts that looked as if they had been ironed, which for some reason caught her in the throat. "I don't think there's anything useful in here."

"I help." Maria Elena squeezed past Judy, went to the dresser, and opened the third drawer. "I know the dress she like the most."

"Thanks." Judy looked into the third drawer, which held pressed jeans, sweatpants, and two folded shift-type dresses, both a flowered pattern, with a light blue sweater, also carefully folded.

"This one." Maria Elena picked up a dress with pink flowers, her eyes glistening anew.

"Thank you." Judy accepted the clothes and took a look at her aunt's heartbroken expression, which told her it was time to go home.

And that their questions about Iris's death would have to be answered another day.

Chapter Eleven

They hit the road in silence, with Judy following GPS directions home, and her aunt turned away, to the window. They wound through the dark outskirts of Kennett Square, passing check-cashing agencies, a tacqueria, and a Mexican restaurant until they reached the town proper, with its charming brick houses, mullioned windows, and gas streetlights. A quiet sniffle came from the passenger seat, and Judy patted her aunt's arm.

"I love you, Aunt Barb. I'm sorry about Iris."

"Thanks," her aunt said, without turning her head from the window.

"She sounds like she really was an amazing person, giving everything away."

"I know, I had no idea. I always wondered what she did with the money she earned, because I know she didn't have anybody to send money home to." Aunt Barb sniffled again. "I guess she kept what she needed to live on and gave the rest to the mission. What a wonderful person."

"I'll say."

"Thanks for indulging me, too. I don't know why I'm running us ragged tonight. I guess it was so I didn't have to think about the fact that she was . . ." Aunt Barb's voice trailed off, and in the sudden silence, the GPS said:

"Prepare to make a left turn in one hundred feet."

Judy switched into the left lane, ready to make the turn, and it occurred to her that life should come with a GPS, to tell you to prepare for the twists and turns on the way, big ones or little ones, like that a beloved aunt would have cancer, or your boyfriend would forget to drop the dog off to get flea-dipped, or that seventy-five asbestos cases would come from New York to suck the life from your practice. The trip through the growing room at the mushroom farm made the damages cases look like a first-world problem, but problems were problems.

"It doesn't make sense, but death never makes sense." Aunt Barb rummaged in her parka pocket and produced her balled-up Kleenex. "In a way, it was just like Steve. Even though I knew he was going to die, I still couldn't believe it when it happened. Just like her, he was so vital and healthy, he did everything right."

"I remember." Judy had loved her uncle, an accountant. A reserved and careful man, he'd taught her chess, not only the game itself but the exotic names of the various openings, like the Sicilian Defense and the Queen's Gambit, as well as chess notation, which was like some mysterious language that only they spoke, Ne4 Nge7. Judy always got special attention from her uncle and aunt, because she was their only niece and they'd never had children of their own.

"I'm feeling him tonight, too. Maybe that's why I went crazy, running hither and yon. It's funny, when you get older, one death kicks up all the other deaths."

"I bet that's right." Judy noted that her aunt hadn't mentioned the possibility of her own death, though it had to be uppermost in her mind.

Aunt Barb blew her nose. "I guess we can't really know what

Iris was doing today. It seems strange that she didn't tell me, though. She never lied to me before."

"She didn't lie to you exactly, did she? You just assumed she was going to work, but she didn't go to work."

"That's true, but still."

"Like the clothes and shoes you gave her. You didn't know she was giving them to the mission, you just assumed she kept them."

"Yes, that's true, too." Aunt Barb nodded. "So what do you think she was doing then, on Brandywine Way?"

"We don't know enough about her life, to say. Maybe somebody told her they had some stuff for the mission so she went to pick it up before work, that's possible." Judy heard herself say it. "The detective will let us know, but I'm thinking that the police probably took her cell phone. That's how they found the wallet and came to your house."

"Oh, right."

"And like the cop said, fingernails break all the time, and because it was a nice day, she decided to drive with the window open. All of that is completely possible."

"I suppose so, but I want to see what the police come up with, don't you?"

"Yes." Judy didn't mention the autopsy, but she didn't need to.

"You know the most ironic thing is that Iris was so worried about me with my cancer. She wanted me to go to church with her tomorrow morning, to say a prayer before the mastectomy."

"That's very sweet," Judy said, meaning it. The GPS was about to tell her to turn left, but she turned it off.

"I'm going to go myself and say a prayer for her, and I suppose I should talk to the priest and arrange for her burial."

"You're going to the Spanish church?"

"Yes."

Judy turned left. "I'll go with you."

"You don't have to."

"I know, but I want to."

"Thanks." Her aunt looked over with a smile, her wan face barely illuminated. "And then there's only one more thing I want to do before Monday morning, for Iris."

"What's that?"

"I want to plant a rosebush for her. I have a cutting that came in the mail from the nursery, and we were going to put it in together on Sunday."

"I'll help you do that, too," Judy said, touched. Her aunt was always thoughtful, her actions straight from the heart. Judy would never forget that when it was time to outfit her dorm room at college, she and her mother had gone shopping for all of the practical items: a small refrigerator, a microwave, a mesh hamper, and a pair of flip-flops to prevent athlete's foot in the showers. But Aunt Barb had taken Judy antiquing, and together they'd found a beautiful old quilt, hand-stitched in a flower-garden pattern, that made the dorm room homey. That very quilt was still at the foot of her bed, to this day.

"Thanks, honey."

"It would be my pleasure, Aunt Barb." Judy turned onto her aunt's street, cruised past the houses, and turned into the driveway and cut the ignition. The dashboard clock read 10:48, so she knew her mother would be waiting up, probably tapping her foot.

"God, I'm tired."

"Why don't you go up to bed, and I'll deal with my mother? It'll take a law degree to survive the cross-examination we're about to get."

Aunt Barb chuckled and picked up her purse. "I'll be right in. I have to get the cutting from the garage and bring it in the house. It would probably be fine, but it's supposed to be cold tonight and I don't want to lose it."

"I'll get it. Tell me where it is."

"You don't mind?"

"Believe me, I'm getting the easier job. You deal with my mother, I'll deal with the plant." Judy yanked the key from the ignition, and grabbed her purse. "Meanwhile, I don't even know what a cutting looks like. Is it big?"

"No, not at all. It's just a cane. It should still be in the box from the nursery, I didn't take it out."

"What's a cane?"

"A cane is the term for the stem on a rosebush."

"Of course it is."

Her aunt snorted, opening the car door. "Like a lawyer has the right to complain about obscure terminology."

"Okay, a fair point." Judy got out of the car, chirped it closed, and cleared her head with a lungful of fresh, cool air. She glanced at the house and saw through the window that the living room was empty. "She must be upstairs already. You want me to come in and be your lawyer?"

"Ha! I can handle my own sister." Her aunt took out her keys, unlocked the door, and handed the set to Judy. "Take this, you need them to unlock the garage. It's the little key with the red surround. Can you lock it when you're finished?"

"Sure. You lock the garage, in this neighborhood?"

"It was Iris's idea, after I got the electric mower. She heard people were stealing equipment, so I figured it was better to be safe than sorry."

"Right, so what am I looking for? A cardboard box near some gardening equipment?"

"Exactly, I think I put it on the far wall, next to the tools. You'll see that I have the blue carryall and Iris has the purple. I think it's in between them. I wanted it as far from the door as possible, to avoid the draft. The light switch will be on your right side when you go in."

"Got it. Good luck with Mom."

"Pssh. Child's play."

"Ha!" Judy let her aunt inside the house, then turned and continued down the driveway, the gravel crunching under her clogs. Weariness washed over her, and she slid her phone from her purse and checked the screen to see if Frank had called, but he hadn't, which was par for the course. She was always the one doing the calling, making sure he was on track to come home, to meet her, or to run errands. If they got married and had a baby, it would be redundant.

A motion-detector light went on when she reached the garage, and she found the red key, unlocked the handle, and pulled the old metal door upward, rattling in its tracks. Her aunt's yellow Mini Cooper sat parked in the darkness, and Judy went to the right doorjamb, fumbled for the switch, and turned it on. A bright fluorescent panel in the ceiling came to life, but she didn't see a cardboard box. She walked beside the car to the far wall, where there was a red gardening cart with two wheels, with a rake, shovel, and a spade with a long handle. Suddenly, the fluorescent light flickered and phased off, plunging her in darkness.

"Perfect," Judy said to herself, reaching for her phone, flicking on the flashlight function, and aiming it at the far wall, walking over to look for the box. A cone of intense brightness traveled over a green heavy-duty hose, a bag of Miracle-Gro potting soil, yellow jugs of Preen and white of Roundup, a stinky spray bottle of rabbit and deer repellent, and a red jug of something called Sevin, with a label that showed creepy pictures of ticks, worms, and God knows what.

"Gross." Judy pointed the flashlight along the floor to the right and spotted a large purple plastic chest next to the same type of chest in blue, but still didn't see the damn box. She went over to the wall and started rummaging around, juggling the flashlight to search through a dirty assortment of trowels, hand spades, and a weird tool that looked like it could dislodge an eyeball. But still no box. The flashlight's beam fell on the plastic chests, which were large, and she considered that maybe the cardboard box was inside one of them. She couldn't remember whether her aunt's chest was the purple one or the blue, but no matter. She went over to the blue one, opened the lid, and aimed the flashlight inside, but all it contained was a pair of messy knee pads, a red Phillies cap, a kneeling pad, and a bunch of mismatched gardening gloves in wacky patterns like kittens, puppies, and daisies. The chest was such a happy clutter that it had to belong to her aunt.

She closed the lid, and just to be thorough, went over and opened the lid to what had to be Iris's chest. She aimed the flashlight inside, but no cardboard box was there either, only a pair of oversized white cotton gloves, sitting neatly folded atop a clean trowel and spade, and underneath that was a book entitled *Roses for the Beginner,* with a greeting card sticking out from the cover, on top of some old newspapers. She reached for the book, opened the cover, and inside was a birthday card. Judy opened it to find her aunt's handwriting:

Iris, You are already a better gardener than this guy! Happy Birthday, from B!

Touched, Judy replaced the card, closed the book, and was about to put it back when she noticed a large white envelope sticking out from underneath the old newspapers. She picked up the envelope, which was heavy and bulky but unsealed. She lifted up the flap, looked inside, and couldn't believe what she was seeing. It must've been the flashlight, playing tricks on her eyes.

She knelt on the garage floor, set her flashlight on the edge of the chest so that it cast light on the envelope, and slid out its contents.

In her hand was a thick stack of cash, bound with a rubber band.

Chapter Twelve

Judy entered her aunt's house with a cardboard box of the rose cutting and an old needlepoint bag she'd found in the garage, which contained the cash from Iris's gardening chest. The living room was empty, for which she was grateful, because she needed a moment to compose herself. She estimated the cash to be about $10,000, though she hadn't taken the time to count it.

She set the box, bag, and her purse down, her thoughts racing. She didn't know if the cash belonged to Iris, or if her aunt knew about it, or why it was in the garage. She reasoned that it probably belonged to Iris because it had been in her gardening chest, and also that her aunt didn't know about it, because Aunt Barb wouldn't have kept cash in the garage. Judy remembered what her aunt had said, about Iris wanting to keep the garage locked. Evidently, she wasn't worried about somebody's stealing the new lawnmower.

"Judy?" her mother asked, coming downstairs in Aunt Barb's pink chenille bathrobe, covered with whimsical flowers. "What took you so long?"

"Sorry." Judy moved the needlepoint bag behind the couch, with her foot. Nobody needed more drama before the mastectomy Monday morning. "The light went off in the garage and I couldn't find the box Aunt Barb wanted me to bring in. It was on the other side of the car."

"No, I mean tonight. What took you so long tonight? You two were out for hours." Her mother reached the bottom of the stairs, with a frown. She'd washed off her makeup but her hair was still up in its topknot, though it was slipping. "Your aunt said you went for a drive, but she didn't say where and she just fell asleep in her clothes, exhausted. You couldn't have gone for an ice cream because nothing around here is open late."

Judy decided to tell the truth because the only lies she told her mother was that she was eating healthy, getting enough sleep, and not working too hard. "We made two stops, one to Iris's job to find out if she'd gone in today, which she hadn't, and the other to her apartment, to talk to her roommates and get some clothes to bury her in."

Her mother's frown took up permanent residence. "Why didn't you call me?"

"We texted," Judy said, but even she knew it sounded weak.

"You couldn't pick up the phone and talk to me? Why did you leave me hanging?"

"Sorry, we should have called. Hold on, let me get something to eat." Judy felt starved all of a sudden, so she walked into the darkened kitchen and flicked on the light. It had been too long a day, capped off with the discovery of the hidden money. It got her thinking that Iris might not be the saint that she'd seemed to be. "Is there any leftover chicken?"

"Please don't make a mess in the kitchen." Her mother followed her inside, leaning on the archway, her arms still folded. "It's eleven o'clock. The kitchen's closed for the night."

"I'm not going to make a mess." Judy had forgotten her mother had a kitchen-closed rule, a necessity with four kids, but less so tonight. Even so, to keep the peace, she bypassed the refrigerator, went into the cabinet, grabbed a glass, and filled it with water.

"You didn't answer my question."

"What question?"

"Why didn't you call me?"

"Mom, we should have, and I apologized." Judy sipped the water, but it did nothing to satisfy her hunger, which only made her cranky.

"I'll tell you why you didn't call. You didn't call because you knew I would tell you not to do it. Your aunt needs to rest and take care of herself. She isn't a well woman, don't you know that?"

"Yes, but she wanted to get it done before her operation on Monday."

"You shouldn't have listened."

"Mom, what was I supposed to do? She's a big girl, and Iris was her best friend."

Her mother scoffed. "Iris wasn't her *best* friend. She was a paid companion. They didn't know each other that well."

Judy realized her mother might be right, if the secret money meant anything. "Still, Aunt Barb says she was her best friend. She told me in the car, at the scene."

"That's ridiculous! I would have known if she was her best friend!"

"She didn't want to tell us because we might not approve." Judy didn't need to add, *And she was right.*

"How can they be best friends? They don't even speak the same language."

"They find a way to talk to each other, it's not impossible." Judy couldn't resist adding, "You're the linguist, right? People can learn a new language."

"Oh please. The woman is illiterate." Her mother gave a quick shake of the head. "In any event, I'm very disappointed in you."

"What? Why?" Judy moved to put the glass in the dishwasher, but it was already running. She reached for the Palmolive, twisted on the faucet, and began to wash the glass in the sink.

"I think you encouraged your aunt, going to the scene with her. She has things to do, people like Myra who called here for her. She must've turned off her cell, so they called here. What were you thinking?"

Judy recoiled, surprised. "I didn't have any choice. I wasn't going to let her go alone."

"Why not? You should've said you wouldn't go, like I did."

"Why?" Judy twisted off the faucet, slipped a dishrag off the hook, and dried off the stupid glass. "What purpose would that have served?"

"She might not have gone. She could've identified Iris from the picture on the email. Even I could see it was Iris, and I only met the woman once. I said I wouldn't go, but you undermined me, and the two of you went traipsing off." Her mother gestured vaguely to the door.

"Mom, please don't blow it out of proportion. I was just trying to be nice to her. She's lost her best friend right before her mastectomy. Does it get any worse? I was just thinking of her."

"And I'm not?" Her mother's blue eyes flared, her anger growing.

"I didn't say you weren't." Judy felt nonplussed. She didn't want to fight, but she didn't see a way to head it off. "I think we're both trying to help her, you and me, each of us in our own way—"

"Honey, take your cues from me right now. Follow my lead. Your aunt is at sixes and sevens, more upset about the procedure than you know."

"Did she say that?"

"No, but she doesn't know what she wants right now. We have to call the shots for her."

"No we don't, Mom."

"Yes we do." Her mother folded her arms in the thick bathrobe, and Judy's chest tightened.

"She's not a child."

"The chemo makes her thinking foggy. It clouds the brain. I read that in the books. You heard what she said this afternoon."

"She's not on the chemo now."

"It's still in her system."

Judy suppressed an eye-roll. "Why don't we not go there? Neither of us are doctors."

"The correct verb is *is,* and you don't have to be a doctor. It's common sense. Open your eyes. You saw her tonight, she's very emotional. She's all over the place. She doesn't know her own mind right now."

"Mom, she's having a mastectomy, not a lobotomy. She has cancer, not schizophrenia."

"What's that supposed to mean?"

"It means she's not crazy, she knows her own mind. Tomorrow she wants to go to church and plant a rosebush for Iris. Am I supposed to go with her or not?"

"Church?" Her mother frowned in confusion. "When was the last time she went to church?"

"It's not for her. She's going to Iris's church and she wants to talk to the priest about funeral plans."

"She's *burying* her now?" her mother asked, incredulous. "Where's she going to get the money?"

"I don't know," Judy answered, thinking of the ten grand in the needlepoint bag.

"And I suppose you think you're going with her to this church?"

"I was going to. You should, too."

"Where is it?"

"Who cares? Mom, it's *church*. What could your possible objection be?"

"Have you been listening to me at all?" Veins popped out in her mother's lovely forehead. "I don't think she should go, or you either, driving around. She should stay home and rest. Pack a go-bag, like it says in the books. We need to make sure she has her front-closure shirts, slip-on shoes, ice packs, and alcohol pads for her drains. Also the compression bras, we didn't get to talk about that yet."

"Can't I get those things for her, Monday afternoon? She says she has one day of freedom left. If she wants to go to church, she should go to church."

"Why do you have to talk to me this way?"

"What way?"

"Is this a lawyer thing? You turn everything into an argument."

"I'm not, you are!" Judy couldn't help but raise her voice.

"What are you talking about?" Her mother shook her head. "You're the one who ran off, sending funny texts instead of calling. What is it with you two? Did you have your fun?"

"*Fun?*" Judy felt her own anger give way. "Do you think it was *fun* to go identify Iris tonight? Do you think we were having a good time, trying to understand how she died? You know, Mom, I don't understand you. It's like you're jealous."

Her mother's lips parted, and she stepped backwards. "Jealous of what?"

"You're jealous of me and Aunt Barb. You're even jealous of Iris and Aunt Barb." Judy regretted that the words had slipped out of her mouth, but it was too late to stop now. "Why aren't you happy that Aunt Barb has a best friend in Iris? Why aren't you happy that Aunt Barb is close to me? You should be happy for her! She's your sister!"

"How *dare* you speak to me that way!" Her mother's eyes widened in outrage, but Judy could see a flicker of pain cross her forehead and realized that she had just answered her own question. It was because Aunt Barb *was* her sister that her mother wanted to be the one who was closer to her. But Judy had no way to take the words back or to change their truth. Still her mother didn't need it thrown in her face, and Judy felt a wave of shame.

"Mom, I'm sorry—" she said, her cheeks aflame, but her mother had already turned away, hurrying from the kitchen.

Chapter Thirteen

Sunday morning, Judy and her Aunt Barb found themselves completely out of place in the crowd heading from the parking lot to the church. Judy was the only blonde, and they were taller than everyone by a foot, so they stood out like walking lighthouses. Besides that, everyone seemed to know each other, greeting each other with hugs and kisses, and there were kids of all ages holding hands, jumping up and down, laughing and talking, filling the air with Spanish and English, making a collectively happy bubble of families flowing toward the tall, arched doors of the church.

"It's such a pretty church, isn't it?" Aunt Barb said pleasantly, as they approached.

"It sure is." Judy tucked her aunt's arm under hers, a spontaneous burst of affection. Her aunt had come downstairs this morning determined to go, even though Judy could see that her eyes were puffy, undoubtedly from crying. It had been a tense breakfast, with Judy's mother characteristically reserved toward her, just short of the silent treatment. If Aunt Barb had noticed, she kept it to herself, and her mother had surprised no one by deciding that she wouldn't go to church with them, but instead would pack the go-bag.

"The church is relatively new and looks it, doesn't it?"

"Yes, it does," Judy said, as they reached the sidewalk that led to the doors. The church was a lovely structure, and its tan stucco exterior, arched windows, and rounded bell tower topped with red tiles, suggested its Spanish design.

"Have you ever been to a Catholic church?"

"No." Judy wished Mary were here, her guide to all things Catholic. "Will the service be in Spanish?"

"Yes, and this is the one we always went to," her aunt answered, as they filed in behind the line. "Father Keegan performs it, and your mother would be happy to know he's Irish, complete with freckles. He always jokes that they keep him here as a token, but he's not white, he's pink."

Judy smiled, but flashed on the $10,000 cash. Her aunt would have mentioned it if she had known about its existence, and Judy didn't want to tell her about it yet, because she didn't want to upset her before her operation. "By the way, remember when you were talking about how you used to give Iris clothes and things?"

"Sure, yes."

"Do you think she ever sold them?"

"No, of course not."

"Why not?" Judy inched up as the line toward the entrance shifted forward. "Do you know what her financial situation was like?"

"Not really. I paid her well, and she never complained about money. I knew she could live well enough to take care of herself, and she was careful about her money."

"How so?"

"Whenever we ran an errand, like to the garden center, she never bought anything for herself. Same thing when we went for chemo. I would treat her in the coffee shop. She never spent money."

Judy doubted that Iris could've saved as much money as had been in the garage. "Did she have a bank account, or anything?"

"No," her aunt answered, lowering her voice as they entered the church. "Generally, you need a passport or a Social Security number for a bank account. I don't think she had either."

"So she kept it in cash?" Judy passed through an anteroom with buttery yellow walls and a warm, orange-tiled floor, containing a carved wooden angel, and a blue-cloaked Virgin Mary standing next to the American flag.

"I really don't know."

"I know it's none of my business, but did you ever give Iris money?"

"Sure, as gifts, when I could get her to take it. Why do you ask?"

Judy thought fast, lying even as she walked past a marble stand that held a bowl of holy water. "I'm thinking about her estate, now that she's gone. I'm wondering if I should try to follow up with that."

"I doubt that there's much money in it, but that's a good idea. Perhaps next week you could try to locate it. Iris's friend Daniella might be able to help. Thanks so much for thinking of it."

"You're welcome," Judy told her, feeling guilty for keeping the discovery of the money from her aunt, a material omission in front of a painted plaster bust of a smiling Pope Francis, resting on a windowsill. A bank of candles flickered in red glasses below a primitive wooden crucifix, and a bronze plaque on the wall read **Madre de Dios Church,** with the names of benefactors and supporters.

They walked through a large, tiled lobby where everyone milled about greeting each other, and nuns with blue aprons over their gray habits threaded their way through the crowd, with rosary beads hanging from their waists. One of the young nuns emerged from the crowd, took Judy's hand, and shook it. "Welcome, ladies," the nun said in accented English, her brown eyes friendly.

"Thank you," Judy said, and the nun greeted her aunt, then they passed through modern glass doors into one of the loveliest churches Judy had ever seen. The vaulted ceiling was a full two stories tall, and the walls were of buttery yellow lined with stained-glass windows, but the altar caught her eye. It was white and large, spanning all the way to the ceiling, and its curved shape echoed the exterior of the church itself. A crucifix hung at its apex, and along its right and left sides were painted pictures of men and women farmers, which would have been equally at home in America or Mexico.

The church was packed, and Judy and her aunt slid into the last oak pew and sat down, which was when she realized that everybody else knelt and crossed themselves before they went into the pews. She watched fascinated as one family made double and triple crosses over their foreheads and mouths before they took their seats, and she tried not to feel like a total Spanish-Catholic rookie.

The congregation settled down as Father Keegan swept to the altar, took the oak lectern, and opened his palms, then began speaking in rapid Spanish. He was dressed in white robes with a green overlay, and looked to be middle-aged, with wire-rimmed glasses, graying hair, and a ready smile. Judy got the gist of what he was saying, which was to thank everybody for coming, tell them that God loves them, and that they should have faith in him.

Suddenly Father Keegan's expression saddened. He continued speaking, but had spotted Aunt Barb and Judy, making eye contact with them. Father Keegan said the name Iris Juarez, and Judy's aunt nodded, her eyes filming as she whispered to

Judy, "He's telling everybody that Iris died yesterday, of a heart attack. He's asking everyone to pray for her soul."

"Oh my," Judy said under her breath, as murmuring, sniffling, and tears rippled through the congregation. She put her arm around her aunt, who bent her head as Father Keegan began to lead the congregation in prayer, evidently for Iris. The church echoed with the sibilant softness of the Spanish language, and Aunt Barb began to cry, resting her head on Judy's shoulder.

Judy listened to Father Keegan conduct the Mass, then watched everyone line up to receive Holy Communion, but all the time she was wondering about the $10,000 in the garage. The Mass ended shortly thereafter, and the congregation rose to leave, and by the time she and her aunt stood up, Judy was already getting an idea. "Aunt Barb, why don't we go see Father Keegan? I think it would be nice to thank him for remembering Iris in the service."

"I was thinking the same thing, honey." Her aunt smiled at her, and Judy felt another guilty pang for lying. They walked up the center aisle as the congregation filed past them, the parents falling into conversation and the children skipping ahead in groups. They reached the front of the church and waited their turn to speak with Father Keegan, who was standing beside the lectern talking with an older woman. When his conversation was over, the priest motioned them forward, broke into a sad smile, and extended a hand to Aunt Barb.

"Barb, I'm so sorry about Iris," Father Keegan said, shaking her hand. "What a terrible shock, for all of us. You saw for yourself the reaction of the congregation. The community is praying for her soul. You have my deepest sympathies."

"Thank you, so much, Father Keegan." Aunt Barb's lips trembled, suppressing her emotion. "I thought the world of her, you know that, and you know she loved you and this church. She talked about you, and how much you've done for the community.

"This is my niece Judy Carrier."

Judy shook the priest's hand. "Pleased to meet you."

"And you, too." Father Keegan smiled, and up close his eyes were a lively blue and his skin actually was freckled.

Father Keegan turned again to her aunt. "Iris was one of our most devoted parishioners, and I was so shocked to hear what happened. It's a loss for all of us."

"It certainly is. I will be responsible for seeing that she receives a proper burial."

"That's very kind of you. Let me know when you receive her remains from the coroner, and we will have a Mass for her."

"Thank you."

Judy interjected, "Father Keegan, may I ask, how did you find out about her passing?"

"I got a telephone call last night from Detective Boone. He's in charge of the matter."

Judy took the lead. "He is, and we had a question or two about her death, like why she didn't go to work that day. We asked at Mike's Exotics, and they said she just didn't show up. Can you shed any light on that?"

Father Keegan shook his head. "No, and that's what I told the detective. It did seem unusual to me. It wouldn't be like Iris."

Judy continued, "We're not sure why she was on Brandywine Way in the first place. Do you have any ideas about that?"

"I can't help you there, either." Father Keegan shook his head.

"Could she have been visiting someone, a friend perhaps? Daniella? We spoke with her roommates, but they don't know."

"Not that I know of. Iris had Daniella, but not many close friends." Father Keegan's gaze shifted to Judy's aunt. "Mrs. Moyer, I think you were her closest friend."

Aunt Barb swallowed visibly.

Judy glossed over the painful moment, taking over the conversation. "Do you have the names and addresses of any of her cousins in Mexico? We were wondering about what to do with any monies remaining in her estate."

Father Keegan cocked his head. "I don't know any of them, unfortunately. I doubt that she had much money, a will, or anything of that sort."

"Father Keegan, was Daniella here today?"

"No, she wasn't, but she isn't as devoted as Iris."

"Do you know where we can find her? We don't even know if she knows that Iris has passed."

"I'm sure she does. Word travels fast in this community. Daniella would be at the mission. She works there, too."

"Is that nearby?" Judy asked, thinking ahead.

Chapter Fourteen

"Damn, we should've gotten the address." Judy drove back and forth on the same two-lane road, trying to find the mission, but they kept getting lost. "Then I could have plugged it into the GPS."

"Father Keegan said it was next to the firehouse," Aunt Barb said, her face to the window. "There's the firehouse straight ahead, and the only thing next to it is that strip mall."

Judy stopped at a traffic light, eyeing the run-down strip mall of three crappy storefronts, one of which had a handmade going-out-of-business sign. "Can you have a mission in a storefront?"

"Pull in. Let's see." Aunt Barb clucked. "You know, I've been down this road a bunch of times, but I've never seen a mission. It's as if all of this existed around me, but I never noticed it before."

"I know what you mean." Judy was thinking about how much her Aunt Barb hadn't noticed about Iris. The hidden cash made her feel uneasy, and it seemed to mirror what her aunt was saying about the neighborhood; there were things in plain sight that they should have seen, but they'd missed.

"The light's green," her aunt said, pulling Judy out of her reverie. She cruised forward, crossed the intersection, and turned into the crappy strip mall, which held a tiny parking lot in front of the stores. She spotted a battered Hyundai leaving the strip mall from the back.

"Maybe it's behind the stores. Again, no sign."

"Evidently, everybody who needs it knows where it is."

"Right." Judy steered around the back, entered a littered back lot, and hit the brakes quickly, surprised to find small children running around, playing on old upholstered couches, used card tables, scattered mattresses. "Yikes, good thing I was going slow."

"I'll say."

"I guess this is it." Judy eyed a rusty white Dumpster that read SOCIETY OF ST. VINCENT DE PAUL. The back of the building was a dingy gray stucco cluttered with electric meters and heating units next to an unmarked glass door, which stood open, propped up by a cinderblock.

"Hey, that's my ottoman!" Aunt Barb exclaimed, opening the door.

"What do you mean?" Judy cut the ignition, took her purse, and got out of the car.

"That flowery ottoman, next to the maroon couch." Aunt Barb pointed, climbing out of the passenger seat.

"I don't remember that ottoman."

"You wouldn't. It's from the old house, and I kept it in the garage because it didn't go with the new furniture. I always thought I'd get it reupholstered but I never got around to it. I gave it to Iris when we cleaned out the garage. She said it was pretty, and I thought she could use it."

"When did you clean out the garage?" Judy's ears pricked up, wondering when Iris had put the money in her storage chest.

"About a week ago. I was feeling better and I wanted to clear the decks before my mastectomy."

"Was it your idea to clean the garage?"

"Yes, and I totally forgot about the ottoman when we went to Iris's apartment. She didn't have the room for it, so she must've brought it here." Aunt Barb shook her head when they reached the ottoman. "An ottoman is a rich-people thing, when you think about it. It requires room. Space. I'm not rich by any means, but I have room for an ottoman. I assumed she did, too." Aunt Barb sighed. "I don't know what I was thinking. I've been so insensitive, living in my own little world."

"That's not true. You didn't know."

"Maybe I didn't want to know, or maybe I should have known. Isn't that the height of insensitivity? That you just didn't know, because you couldn't imagine that people lived a different life from the one you do?" Aunt Barb kept shaking her head. "Isn't that the very definition of insensitivity? Of selfishness?"

"Not at all. You were being generous, and you can't find a negative in that." Judy guided her aunt toward the open door. "Aunt Barb, when I was in the garage last night, I noticed that there were two plastic chests, the same type but different colors. Was one of those Iris's?"

"Yes, I gave it to her. The purple one, for Iris. Get it?"

Judy had missed that. "What's it for?"

"I got her my favorite gardening tools, a trowel, a spade, and the best fork for weeding. There's only one that works really well." Her aunt's face fell. "Poor Iris. I don't think I could bring myself to see that chest now."

"You ever go in the chest?"

"No, why would I? I have my own tools."

Judy felt reassured. "Do you want me to take it away?"

"No, not at all. I want it to stay just the way it is. I still have your uncle's jackets in the closet."

"That's okay, whatever you want." Judy squeezed her arm, and they entered the building, their eyes adjusting to the cramped, dimly lighted room. Women speaking Spanish looked over briefly, then returned to going through cardboard boxes of used toys, books, and children's shoes. Kids played underneath metal rolling racks stuffed with clothes, and Judy recognized one of the little girls from church.

"Judy, look over there." Aunt Barb gestured at one of the racks. "I see two of the dresses I gave her, hanging up, and some of the shoes, too. So this must be where she brought it. She gave it to the mission, like Maria Elena said. How nice is she? I mean, was."

Judy saw grief cross her aunt's face. "She was nice, but I wonder why she didn't tell you."

"I bet she thought it would hurt my feelings."

"That's probably why," Judy said, wondering what other reasons Iris could have had for keeping secrets, as well as how she got the money and why she stowed it in her aunt's garage.

"There's the counter." Aunt Barb led the way toward an ancient cash register on a plywood counter. Behind it, shoes, rain boots, and work boots sat stacked on old wooden shelves, next to a random array that included an old bicycle, floor lamps without shades, and a push lawnmower that was missing a blade. They lingered at the counter, then one of the women came over from the far side of the room, with a smile. She was in her thirties, but heavily pregnant, and her belly strained both her sweatshirt and jeans.

"Hello, ladies," she said in English, with only the hint of an accent. "Is there something I can do for you?"

"Yes," Aunt Barb answered. "My name is Barb Moyer, and this is my niece Judy. We were friends of Iris Juarez's."

"Oh no." The woman's face creased with sadness, and she extended a small hand. "I'm Maria. I'm so sorry about Iris. We all loved her."

"Thank you, and I'm sorry for your loss." Aunt Barb released her hand. "We're looking for Daniella. Father Keegan sent us."

Maria blinked. "Daniella isn't here."

"Oh, I got the impression she worked here on Sundays."

"She does, usually. Sometimes with Iris."

"But Daniella didn't come in today?"

"No, they called me this morning to come in for her, so I came in. Sunday is a busy day for us, after Mass. We have to open."

"Why didn't she come in? Is she sick?"

"No."

"Do you know where Daniella is, where she lives? We'd like to go talk with her."

Maria hesitated, and Judy became aware that the women had stopped talking in the background, evidently eavesdropping as they looked through the clothes and shoes. "She went home."

"Where? Kennett Square?"

"No, home to Mexico."

"Really?" Aunt Barb frowned, puzzled.

Judy hid her surprise that Daniella would leave the country, on the same weekend her friend turned up dead. "When did she leave?"

"I don't know."

"When was the last time she worked here?"

"Friday, I think." Maria scratched her cheek, her manner suddenly hesitant.

Aunt Barb rested a hand on the counter, seemingly tired again, so Judy took over.

"Maria, who told you to come in today? Who called you?"

"Lupe."

"Who's she?"

"She's, like, the boss."

"What did she say?"

Maria pursed her lips. "She said I had to come to work because Daniella went home."

"Did she say when Daniella went home?"

"No."

"Did she say why?"

"No."

"How did she know?"

"I don't know. I don't know anything more than she told me." Maria averted her dark eyes.

"What's Lupe's phone number?"

"I don't know."

"What's Lupe's last name?"

"Why?" Maria edged backwards, resting a hand on her pregnant belly.

"Maria, we're just friends of Iris's, and there's no hidden agenda here. It would really help us if we could talk to Lupe. If she called you on your cell phone, you could just look at the phone to get her number."

Maria shook her head. "I . . . don't feel good telling you her number."

"I understand." Judy didn't want to give up. "Maria, how about you tell us Lupe's last name then? We're just trying to talk to her about Iris's death. They were friends, and somebody should tell Daniella that Iris died, don't you think?"

"I don't know."

"Please?" Judy smiled in a way that she hoped looked reassuring. Suddenly her phone began ringing in her back pocket. "We'll keep the information to ourselves, I promise. How about you tell me her last name and I'll get the number myself?"

"No, no." Maria backed away from the counter. "I don't feel . . . comfortable."

"But we could get that information anywhere. Father Keegan

would tell us her last name. You would just be saving us the trouble of asking him."

"Then ask him. Please, ask him."

"Really?" Judy's phone kept ringing, and Aunt Barb took her arm, looking at her with pained eyes.

"Judy, let's go. I don't want to upset anybody. That's not the point."

"You want to leave?"

"Yes, please." Aunt Barb gestured at the ringing phone. "And you should answer that. I bet it's your mom, and we don't need to make her angrier than she already is."

"She can wait."

"It could be an emergency."

"All right, I hear you." Judy checked her phone on the fly.

As it turned out, it wasn't her mother.

But it *was* an emergency, of sorts.

Chapter Fifteen

Judy hustled to the counter of the modern octagonal desk that dominated the busy emergency room, which was staffed with medical personnel, hustling this way and that. She had been sent back into the ER by the department's receptionist, who hadn't known which examining room Frank was in. Evidently, he'd reinjured his wrist in his basketball game, and Judy was hoping that it wasn't broken, because she wanted to break it herself.

"Excuse me, I'm looking for Frank Lucia." Judy addressed the medical personnel in general, because she didn't know which one to talk to. The doctor was on the phone, but both nurses looked up at her, one from the computer keyboard and the other from the printer.

"And you are . . . ?" asked the nurse at the printer, standing with an open palm as a document eked out of the tray. She was pretty, with cropped red hair and green eyes so bright they could've been contacts. Fabric daisies curled around the rubbery black stem of her stethoscope, and her scrubs were Barbie pink.

"I'm Judy Carrier. His girlfriend." Judy caught a quick exchange of glances between the two nurses, sensing their collective disappointment that Frank had a girlfriend, a familiar reaction.

"Great." The nurse flashed a smile that tried but failed. "He's in room seven. I'm Melanie, his nurse, and he's ready to be discharged if you can drive him. He can't drive himself because of the Percocet."

"Was he in pain?" Judy tried not to sound hopeful.

"Initially, he had some discomfort."

"Poor thing," Judy said, but she really meant *good*. She was hoping he was very uncomfortable. "What was the injury exactly? He wasn't very specific on the phone. Did he reinjure it?"

"Yes, there was no new fracture, but the doctor had to reset the bone, so it would heal properly. We gave him another cast."

Judy wanted to give him a new cast, right in the face. "So playing basketball caused the bone to shift?"

"Yes, and the soft tissue in his wrist swelled during the night. He narrowly avoided another surgery."

"So does that mean the healing process has to start over from the beginning? Are we talking eight to twelve weeks?"

"Yes, and I explained to him that he has to be patient. He can engage in only limited activity. I know that won't be easy for him, seeing as how he makes his living with his hands."

Judy couldn't suppress her eye-roll. "Or maybe people who make a living with their hands shouldn't play so much basketball. Do you think concert pianists shoot a lot of hoops?"

"Ha!" The nurse laughed lightly. "Everybody needs to have fun."

"Do they? I'm a lawyer. I don't believe in fun."

"All work and no play makes Jack a dull boy."

"I wouldn't know," Judy shot back, then realized it sounded harsher than she felt. Or maybe it was exactly how she felt and she didn't know how harshly she felt until this very moment. But the nurses were exchanging significant glances again.

"I'll be right in with his prescription and discharge papers."

"Thanks." Judy turned away, her chest tight. She walked down the gleaming hall until she found the right examining room, pushed aside the privacy curtain, and went in.

"Babe?" Frank grinned in a loopy way, lying fully clothed on the bed, his eyes at a druggy half-mast. His left arm was back in its familiar blue cotton sling, and a fresh blue nylon cast covered his wrist to the knuckles. His skin was uncharacteristically pale, his hair disheveled, and his gray logo fleece and jeans looked rumpled enough to have come from the hamper, which they probably did. Judy felt herself softening and went to him.

"How are you feeling?"

"I feel great, I feel awesome! I love you!" Frank hugged her close, then threw up his arms like he'd scored a touchdown, or maybe a three-pointer. "Life is good!"

"Good." Judy gave him a grudging kiss on his grizzly cheek. His breath smelled like onions, but luckily, she loved onions.

"Thanks for coming to get me!"

"No problem, thanks for playing basketball." Judy couldn't help her sarcasm. She'd had to race back to Aunt Barb's house and drop her off, leaving her aunt to face Iris's death, Daniella's disappearance, and her impending mastectomy, with only Judy's mom for company. The entire weekend had been cut short because Judy wouldn't have time to go back to Kennett Square tonight and still be at work tomorrow morning.

"Uh-oh. Are you pissed at me?" Frank pouted comically, his reaction exaggerated by pharmaceuticals.

"Let's go home, Frank." Judy retrieved his puffy black jacket from the chair. "Sit up please, and I'll help you on with your coat."

"Don't be mad. I didn't do it on purpose." Frank sat up groggily, and Judy held his shoulder to support him.

"Of course you didn't. Nobody hurts himself on purpose."

"Right! Then why are you pissed?"

Judy picked up his right hand and began stuffing it in the sleeve of his coat. "You decided to play basketball with an already-injured hand, so it was completely foreseeable that you'd hurt yourself."

"Wow, you sounded like such a lawyer just then!" Frank broke into a grin. "It's because you said 'foreseeable.' Lawyers say that. Also Judge Judy."

Judy draped the coat over his bad arm, thinking that it didn't seem right that Frank kept doing dumb things and sticking her with a mess. Maybe that's what was bothering her, the very injustice of their relationship. She turned when she heard a noise behind her, and the nurse entered the room, carrying a few sheets of paper.

"Here are your discharge papers, Frank."

"Hi, Melissa!" Frank stood up, then listed to the left. "Whoa. My stomach feels funny."

"That's the Percs." The nurse smiled at him, her eyes soft with sympathy. "Can you sign these for me?"

"Uh, sure, Melissa. Then again, maybe not." Frank sank down into the bed, and Judy took the pen and papers from the nurse's hand.

"I'll sign. Drunky McDrunkerson is losing his sea legs." Judy scribbled Frank's name, handed back the pen and papers, and managed to get them both out of the ER and through the hospital exit doors onto a busy Seventh Street, where she took Frank's arm. "You feel well enough to walk? I'm parked in the garage."

"Totally," Frank answered, though he leaned heavily on her

arm as they waited for traffic to let up, then crossed the street. The morning sun had vanished, and gray clouds gathered in the sky. The city air smelled gritty and damp, after the freshness of the countryside.

"So you drove here?"

"Yeah, my truck's in the garage. So we'll have to come back for it tomorrow morning. I need it for work. I have to go out to Jersey to bid on a job tomorrow."

Great, Judy thought to herself, as they went through the door to the garage, found the grimy elevator, climbed alone into a cab with filthy corrugated walls, and watched the broken floor numbers light up. She was in no mood to talk, and Frank had fallen uncharacteristically silent. They got out of the elevator, and when they reached her car, Judy chirped it open and stowed Frank in the passenger seat, where he listed to the left, with a grateful smile.

"Thanks, babe. You take such good care of me."

"No worries. Put on your seat belt." Judy closed the door, then went around the car, tossed her bag in the back and climbed into the driver's seat, then closed the door behind her.

"You're mad at me, I know. I really am sorry."

"Forget it," Judy said, without meaning it. This wasn't the time or the place to talk about anything that mattered, and she had to sort out her thoughts. She put on her seat belt, started the engine, and reversed out of the spot. The garage was dark and cramped even by Philly standards, and she steered toward the exit ramp, where they corkscrewed their way downward in darkness.

"Babe. You want to say I-told-you-so, so you should just go ahead and say it."

"I don't want to say I-told-you-so." Judy navigated with care, if only to avoid his eye.

"Yes you do. Say it."

"I wish I could get you to understand this, but I don't want to be right. I just want you to do the right thing."

"But it was an accident."

"It was an accident when you injured it the first time." Judy twisted the steering wheel, hugging the concrete center of the down ramp, like a descent into urban hell. "It's not an accident when you injure it the second time, because you're not supposed to be playing basketball."

"What was I supposed to do? They didn't have enough guys for a team. They couldn't have entered the tournament."

"You know why they didn't have enough guys?" Judy finally reached the first floor, where she followed exit signs to the cashier. "Because most of the guys are doing what grown-ups do on a Saturday, not playing basketball."

"What are you talking about? You can still be grown-up and play basketball." Frank's tone sounded hurt, but Judy didn't look over. The cashier's booth was coming up, and her purse was in the backseat. She'd forgotten to take her wallet out for parking money.

"Do you have any cash on you?" Judy asked, though she knew the answer. "I only need about ten bucks."

"No."

"How about a card?" Judy slid the parking ticket from the visor, knowing that answer, too.

"I maxed it out on supplies, so I shouldn't use it."

Of course you did, Judy thought but didn't say, simmering. She braked in the line at the booth, twisted around, and grappled in the backseat for her purse.

"Anyway, grown-ups play basketball. What do you think the NBA is?"

"That's not the point." Judy yanked open her purse, retrieved her wallet, and found her credit card. "You need to take care of yourself better. You need to think of yourself."

"That's selfish."

"No, it isn't."

"Yes, it is. They needed me."

"I needed you, too, Frank," Judy said, her voice catching. She slid out her VISA card and gave the car some gas. She still couldn't meet his eye.

"What did you need me for? Why?"

"Lots of reasons." Judy hesitated to tell him, not wanting to make him feel guilty, which was ridiculous. He was in the wrong, so he should feel guilty about it, but she had trained him to think she didn't need him. She steered to the booth, where she handed her credit card and ticket to an older man behind the thick, smudged glass. "Here we go, sir."

"Like what, babe? What did you need me for?"

"I was in Kennett because Aunt Barb has breast cancer. She's having a mastectomy tomorrow morning. My mom is already there, with her."

"Oh no, I'm sorry." Frank sounded genuinely shocked, and Judy felt her chest tighten.

"I know, and it's terrible for her."

"Is she going to be okay?"

"I hope so."

"I'm sure she will."

"It's stage II, Frank. Not everybody gets better."

"She will." Frank patted her hand on the stick shift, and Judy glanced over. His eyes looked pained, if unfocused, but he seemed suddenly pale under his grizzly stubble.

"You okay?"

"I don't feel so good. My stomach."

Judy wanted to explain about the chemo and Iris's death,

but he was too sick to listen. "So, just rest. We'll be home soon."

"Okay, I think I need to." Frank leaned back against the headrest and closed his eyes. "I'm sorry about Barb, but she's a strong woman, like you. She'll be okay, I know it. Don't worry."

"I'm sure she will be," Judy said, but she didn't believe her own words. She took her credit card back from the cashier, steered out of the lot, and motored onto Seventh, where she stopped at the traffic light. It had just turned green when her phone rang in her pocket, and she pulled it out quickly. The screen showed a photo of a grinning Mary, and Judy hit a button to talk, but kept her voice low. "Hi Mare, I'm driving."

"Okay, I won't keep you. Did you decide about the cases?"

"What cases?" Judy felt suddenly teary at the sound of Mary's voice.

"The damages trials."

"Arg. I haven't had a chance. Sorry. Can we talk about it tomorrow?"

"Fine, but what's the matter? You don't sound good."

"It's not me. It's my aunt Barb. She has cancer."

"No! Not Aunt Barb!"

"I know. She's having a mastectomy tomorrow." Judy still found it hard to say. "We're trying to be optimistic. She's optimistic."

"Oh God. I'll say a prayer and so will my mom."

"Thanks," Judy said, but she didn't know if prayer helped. She wished she had Mary's faith. She wished she had anybody's faith. She could use a credible God, right about now.

"What can I do?"

"Nothing, thanks."

"Where are you now?"

"Back in the city, heading home."

"I'm at the office. I can be there in five minutes. We can hang."

"No, I'm fine, thanks."

"So is that why your mom came in?"

"Yes, I was in Kennett Square until today."

"Oh no. Poor Barb. She's so nice. You sure you don't need help?"

"No, I'm fine."

"Take the time off if you need to, this week. I'll cover your desk. You're not in court or anything, are you?"

"I'll be in tomorrow. I have a deposition in the morning."

"Judy, don't. Cancel it. Take the day off. Go be with Barb and your mom."

"I wanted to, but they told me to go to work. I'll see them on Monday afternoon, after the dep." Judy glanced at Frank, who had fallen asleep, his head bobbing as they drove over the cobblestones in the historic section of the city. She braked slightly, slowing the car so he wouldn't wake up. "I should go, I just picked Frank up at the ER. He reinjured his hand, playing basketball."

"Oh no."

"Oh yes. Apparently he's in the NBA."

Mary snorted. "I guess he can't wash the dog now."

"Bingo. It's all part of his plan, no doubt." Judy had completely forgotten about the dog, who probably needed to be walked, too. "So I'll be doing flea laundry all night, and I think I'm out of Wisk. Whatever. Gotta go, okay?"

"Okay. Sure. Bye."

"Bye." Judy hung up, pressing the screen to end the call, then steered the rest of the way home, trying to sort out her emotions. She hated to think of the chores that lay ahead tonight, washing the dog, vacuuming the rugs, and doing the laundry. She had no idea how she'd get the time to go back for Frank's truck. Even so, she knew that worrying about mundane tasks was easier than worrying about her Aunt Barb, Iris, or her mother, but by the time she reached their street, her heart was nonetheless heavy.

She reached their neighborhood in artsy Old City, its narrow streets limned with art and photo galleries, cool boutiques, and brick rowhomes of a colonial vintage, which had been converted to apartments. She turned onto her street and took the first parking space that she saw, a few doors from their apartment. She cut the ignition, and was about to wake Frank up when she looked over at her building.

Standing on her front step was a smiling Mary DiNunzio.

And in her hand was a red plastic jug of Wisk.

Chapter Sixteen

"Here's my question," Judy began to say, as she stuffed a sheet into the washing machine. Frank had gone upstairs to bed, and she was standing with Mary in the hallway that passed for a laundry room, because the washer-dryer could be covered by a louvered door. "Why can't my boyfriend be as awesome as my girlfriend?"

"It's the boy part." Mary smiled, looking adorable in a Penn sweatshirt, jeans, and ponytail. She had on the tortoiseshell glasses she wore when she wasn't at work, but she was even cuter in glasses than contacts, every inch The Girl Most Likely.

"No, I mean it." Judy slammed the washer door closed, for emphasis. "You're so awesome to show up on my doorstep, just when I'm feeling the worst ever. I can't thank you enough for that."

"Honey, you don't have to thank me."

"No, you're amazing. You don't even have to be asked, you just know what I need." Judy cranked the big dial on top of the washing machine to HEAVY LOAD, because even a single sheet overwhelmed the tiny washer-dryer. Or maybe she was feeling sorry for herself and suddenly everything seemed like a Heavy Load.

"You sounded bummed on the phone, and we need to catch up. I've been so crazy lately, with the wedding and all. And it's nothing to come over, I'm only uptown."

"No, it's *everything*. Your coming over here, it's why you're the best friend ever in the history of friends. You know what I need even before I do."

Mary chuckled. "All right already, so what's your point about Frank? You have to cut him a break. He's not at his best right now."

"Oh please. He's not on Percocet all the time, and he wouldn't be on Percocet this time if he made better decisions." Judy uncapped the new Wisk jug and poured a blue stream into the little opening in the machine.

"Aren't you going to measure the detergent?"

"No, I live dangerously."

"I always measure."

"I know, and that's why I have a sucky boyfriend and you have a great boyfriend. Sorry, I mean fiancé." Judy set the heavy Wisk jug on the washer with a *thump*. "Jeez, this thing is a lethal instrument."

"You were saying . . ." Mary cued her as usual, and Judy wondered where she'd be without her best friend to keep her on conversational track.

"I was saying, you don't have to be responsible about *everything*. Maybe I'm putting in too much detergent, but so what? *That* you can take a chance with. But playing basketball with a broken hand isn't the kind of thing that smart people take chances with. Agree?"

"Yes."

"So what's his deal? Is he stupid?" Judy waited to hear the

washing cycle start, and when it did, she shut the louvered door. "Now let's go find the dog. She hides when it's bath time."

"Of course he's not stupid. He runs his own company."

"Exactly, so why can't he figure this out? Penny! Penny!" Judy padded into the living room in her stocking feet. "It's not rocket science."

Mary followed her, with a confused frown. "What can't he figure out, again?"

"That I need help." Judy glanced around, but her dog was nowhere in sight. Their small living room looked sweet—two floor-to-ceiling windows facing south, a funky purple velvet sectional with a flea-market Victorian coffee table, and all four walls covered with her bright, abstract oil paintings—except that Frank had left his sweat socks and running sneakers on the ottoman, an open bag of hard pretzels and a Coors can on the end table without a coaster, and the remote control on the floor beside the couch. "See? Look around. Would you leave the place like this?"

"He was going to the ER. He was in pain."

"He lifted his beer, didn't he? I always have to get after him to clean up. And where's the dog? Penny, Penny! Come!"

"Is she upstairs?"

"No, I bet the coat closet. Meanwhile, he was supposed to take the dog to be dipped, but he forgot, so now I have to wash her myself again, because I just did all the sheets." Judy headed for the entrance hall. "Anyway, if he can't figure it out himself, why can't he just watch you? Why can't he just do what you do? Why can't he just *copy* you? Or *copy me*? If he did for me what I do for him, we'd get along great!"

"He's a fun-loving, happy guy. He's the kind of guy that takes you out to dinner on the spur of the moment."

"So does that mean he's not an adult? Can't you be a fun-loving adult? We are!" Judy opened the door to the coat closet, flicked on the light, and found Penny trembling under the coats, a chubby golden retriever trying to make herself invisible. "Penny, come out. I mean, honestly! He's a sucky boyfriend!"

"He's not sucky. You love him, don't you?"

"Yes, but the problem is that he's sucky, sometimes. Penny, please come out!" Judy went inside the closet, grabbed the dog by the collar, and slid her out on the floor. The dog's toenails scraped the hardwood, and her eyes went as round as brown marbles, so Judy stroked her back. "It's okay, honey, you need a bath. You don't want fleas, do you?"

"He's not sucky all the time."

"No, but is that the standard? Penny, come on, sweetie, let's go." Judy coaxed the dog to the stairwell, where she balked, but the only bathtub was upstairs. "Mary, believe me when I tell you, a guy who's sucky sometimes might as well be sucky all the time."

"Why? That doesn't follow."

"Yes it does. Think about it." Judy tried to budge the dog, but Penny crouched on all fours, her hackles shaking and her fluffy head hanging. "Bottom line, I can't rely on him. I have to take care of him. And when I need anything, he's not there because he's not used to me asking."

"You didn't train him."

"Exactly what I've been thinking!" Judy tugged at the dog. "Anthony would never pull this crap. He's responsible."

"I can't take credit, his mother trained him. He never poops on the rug anymore."

Judy gave up on moving Penny. "I'm gonna have to carry her upstairs. I hate that. She weighs a ton."

"I'll take the front, and you take the butt."

"You don't mind? You've already qualified for sainthood."

"No, I haven't. A saint would take the butt."

"Thanks." Judy picked up the dog's hind, and Mary came around to the head and shoulders.

"Hi, Penny. So, you're upset."

"Me or the dog?" Judy started climbing with Mary behind her, so that Penny traveled backwards up the stairs.

"Maybe this isn't the best plan. It's literally ass-backwards."

"Welcome to my world."

"You seem so bummed, honey. Are you saying you want to break up with him?"

"I don't know, but we can't talk about it anymore anyway." Judy worried that Frank might hear them as they got closer to the second floor, so she flared her eyes meaningfully at Mary, who understood instantly, since all women understood Meaningful Eye Flarings.

"So talk to me about Aunt Barb. You're worried about her."

"I am, but it's not only that." Judy struggled to not drop the soft, heavy dog, as she squirmed. "So much happened this weekend, I don't know where to start. Her best friend died, and it seems really hinky. Plus I found ten grand in cash money hidden in her garage."

"*What?*" Mary asked, incredulous, and Judy told her the whole story, from meeting Iris, to hearing about her death from the police, to visiting the scene on Brandywine Road, then Mike's Exotics, Iris's apartment, and finally the church and the mission, with Daniella's disappearance. There was so much to tell that the story lasted the entire time they washed, toweled off, and blow-dried the shaking dog, then put in a new load of laundry, and finally left to go pick up Frank's truck. They took Judy's car, with Penny asleep in the backseat, in some form of doggie shock.

"You know what I think?" Judy asked, as she steered through the dark city streets to the hospital garage. It was drizzling, and droplets dotted her windshield, but there was no traffic. Sunday nights in Philadelphia, everyone was home, depressed about work the next day. "I think something fishy is going on, considering everything as a whole."

"What do you mean?"

"We have Iris found dead, out of nowhere, and her best friend leaves to go back to Mexico, and there's secret money stashed in my aunt's garage. Considering the totality of the circumstances, as the lawyers say, it raises a lot of questions."

"Like what?"

"Like where did she get the money? Why did she hide it from my aunt? Why did her best friend leave, even before her funeral? Who was that call from that she got? And is any of it connected to the hidden money?" Judy felt good to be talking things over with Mary the way she always did. It wasn't about men all the time, just most of the time. "I don't think she was murdered, there were no signs of violence. I saw the body, I know." Judy shuddered at the memory. "If there had been signs of a violent death, or a weapon, I would say the broken nails were a defensive wound."

"But there wasn't."

"I know. Right. I can't wait to see what the coroner turns up, but what if she was murdered, and the money had something to do with it?" Judy steered into the darkness, switching on the windshield wipers. "We've handled murder cases before, and if this happened in Philly, we'd put two and two together. Secret money, a sudden disappearance, and a mysterious death? What more does it take?"

"It's not a mysterious death. Don't get carried away."

"But we love to get carried away, and there are legit questions."

Mary snorted. "So what are you thinking? Who would kill Iris, and why?"

"I'm not sure. A few things are possible. I liked Iris and—"

"Stop. Assume you don't know Iris. Because you don't."

"I do, kind of." Judy flashed on Iris's shy smile, in the rose garden. "I've been hearing about her for a while. Plus Aunt Barb adores her and she's an excellent judge of character."

"Would she if she knew that Iris was keeping some mighty big secrets from her? Hiding money in her house?"

"A good point." Judy stopped at a streetlight, its redness fragmented by the raindrops on the windshield. "So we'll put out of our mind that we think Iris is a nice person."

"Exactly, and if so, the most likely possibility is that she either stole the money or was mixed up with something unlawful that generated cash."

"Why do you say it's from something unlawful?"

"Because you said she was in the country three years, and she probably made minimum wage at her jobs, if that. You can't save that much money that quickly, so she had to come by it another way."

"Hmm." Judy thought about it. "And she would've hidden it because she has no other place to put it. She can't get a bank account because she doesn't have a Social Security number, and she can't leave it at her apartment because of the risk of theft. Her roommate told us there's a lot of theft in the undocumented community, so did the cops."

"Of course, because nobody can use a bank. My mother was the same way, when she came over from Italy. She always felt like an outsider. She didn't trust the banks, she wouldn't even use a credit card. She kept the money under the mattress."

"People really do that?"

"Italians do, big-time. Also, our sleep number is ten grand." Judy smiled.

"She still hides money in coffee cans and her sewing kits. Plus five bucks in her bra."

Judy laughed. "But your mom came in legally. There's no analogy."

"Doesn't matter. It's an immigrant mentality, and these are the new immigrants, and if they're illegal, they're essentially fugitives. They don't trust anybody or anything, they can't call the police. They live in a lawless world. That's why they come and go without a word, like the guy at Mike's told you. They don't play by the same rules."

"What's your point?"

"So, it's not that strange that Daniella would leave, or Iris would hide money, or she couldn't confide in your aunt. She doesn't trust anybody, she can't."

"So the question is, what was she up to? My aunt didn't give her that much, and I don't think she works for anyone else, except Mike's."

"Maybe she stole it from the office or petty cash, something like that?"

"I doubt that. I saw Mike's and it doesn't look like the kind of business that has ten grand lying around."

"Okay, what about selling the stuff your aunt gave her?"

"Like an eBay freak? It wouldn't amount to ten grand."

"Prostitution?"

"Yuck, out of the question." Judy shook her head. "Trust me. She had crucifix earrings."

"Ever hear of Mary Magdalene?" Mary chuckled.

"Stop."

"What about something having to do with her immigration status? Could she have been helping people across the border for money?"

"Human trafficking? Are you kidding?" Judy scoffed, braking at a stop light. "She was a cute little lady, a baker and a gardener."

"Oh, in that case forget it. No criminals bake."

Judy smiled.

"Okay, then what about selling drugs?"

"She didn't seem like that type, either."

"Not all drug dealers seem like the type, and if she goes back and forth to Mexico, you never know."

Judy braked at the next light, traveling up Lombard. "It's hard to imagine her selling drugs, given how religious she was, and what her roommates and Father Keegan had said about her."

"Means nothing. You need to buy into the premise that she's two-faced, leads a secret life, all that. If you ask me, she was up to no good, then died of a heart attack. I think that's what happened."

"They seemed surprised she wasn't at work, too."

"So she keeps secrets from them, too." Mary leaned over, putting a hand on Judy's arm. "Anyway you're missing the point. Do you know what really worries me?"

"What?" Judy glanced over to new gravity in Mary's voice.

"What if someone comes looking for the cash at your aunt's house? If Iris is in cahoots with anybody, they'll know it's there. And even if she's not, you're telling me it's a tight community, and it's possible that someone else knows about the cash and also knows that Iris is dead. So they might come and try to steal it."

"Oh no." Judy gripped the steering wheel in alarm. "I didn't think of that."

"Where's the money now?"

"I had packed it up, but I was too worried my mom would find it, so put it back in the garage, in Iris's chest." Judy was kicking herself. "I wasn't sure what to do with it. Was that dumb?"

"No, that's what I would've done. It wasn't yours to take."

"But I don't think we should leave it there, especially with my aunt going into the hospital and leaving the house unattended." Judy's mouth went dry. "They could get broken into."

"It's possible."

"What should I do? Call and tell them?"

"No, not over the phone."

"Go get it?" Judy checked the dashboard clock, which read 7:35. "And do what with it? Tell my aunt, the day before her operation? How much more can she take?"

"Hit the gas, and we'll figure it out on the way."

Chapter Seventeen

Judy steered the car onto her aunt's street, driving past a quaint cluster of older brick homes. Everything was quiet and still, now that the rain had stopped. The trees dripped water, humidity grayed the air, and the asphalt shone with wetness. Warm light glowed from the mullioned windows of the houses, from behind spiny evergreens and tall oak trees.

Mary shifted up in her seat, looking around. "I'm not moving to the suburbs, even when we have kids. There's not enough graffiti."

"Ha." Judy cruised toward her aunt's house, noticing that her mother's rental car was taking up the driveway, so they'd have to park on the street. She scanned for a space, and Penny popped her head between the front seats, panting.

"Whoa, does the dog know where we're going?"

"Yep, she comes to life on this street, every time." Judy spotted a parking space in front of the house next door to her aunt's and made a beeline for it. "She loves Aunt Barb."

"Judy, don't worry, I really think your aunt will pull through this."

"Thanks, I hope so."

"Also I put my mother on novena patrol, and she's got the juice."

Judy smiled. "So how much are we going to tell her and my mother about the money? I don't love the idea of upsetting Aunt Barb before her operation, but by the same token, I don't like hiding things from her." Judy braked and reversed into the parking space, then cut the ignition. Penny started skittering back and forth in the backseat, wagging her tail in excitement.

"So you're going to come clean?"

"Yes, and my aunt might be able to help. What if she gave Iris the money or knows how she got it? In fact, for all we know, my aunt could know that the money's in her garage, but isn't telling me." Judy slid the key out of the ignition, engaged the emergency brake, and popped off her seat belt, which triggered Penny's whimpering and pawing at the window of the backseat.

"You really believe that?"

"No," Judy answered, talking louder to be heard over Penny. "But I'm trying to keep an open mind. Let's get outta here. The dog's about to explode."

"Is she always like this?" Mary glanced back, and Penny began barking at the car window, her attention riveted on the house.

"Not really, but I haven't taken her here in a while." Judy could barely hear herself over Penny's barking, reverberating in the small car. "Can you get my purse, and I'll get the dog?"

Mary reached into the seat well and picked up the handbags, while Judy pocketed the keys, climbed out of the car, closed her door, and went to the backseat.

"Penny, settle down! Settle!" Judy opened the back door and reached for Penny's leash, but the dog shot out of the car and raced down the sidewalk to her aunt's house, her leash flying behind her. "Penny, no!"

"Wow, she's fast!"

"Penny, come!" Judy jogged after the dog, surprised. It wasn't like Penny to run off unless she'd seen a squirrel. "Penny, no!"

"Penny!" Mary called behind her, sounding distant.

Judy tore down the sidewalk and across the neighbor's wet lawn, giving chase. Luckily the neighbors weren't home and their house was dark, but the lack of lights made it hard to see.

"Penny!" Judy followed the noise of the dog's frantic barking, reached her aunt's driveway, and bolted past her garage to her backyard, praying that Penny wasn't destroying the beds of Aunt Barb's roses. Judy raced into her aunt's backyard, which plunged her into darkness. The kitchen lights weren't on inside the house, so there was nothing to illuminate the backyard. She lost sight of Penny, and the barking sounded farther and farther away.

Whoomp! Judy startled at a rushing sound, a rapid movement in the air around her, too fast to be anything natural. A large figure zoomed into her, a shadowy blur streaking from the darkness.

Judy felt a sudden blow to her head, stunning her. She cried out in confusion and fear. Pain arced through her skull. She heard a grunting sound. She caught a whiff of beer.

Judy whirled around, knocked off-balance. Her arms flew upward reflexively. She collapsed to the ground. She hit hard on her side, unable to break her fall. The shock of the impact traveled throughout her body and rattled her bones. Her face planted in the cold, wet grass.

The shadow vanished. She heard heavy footsteps splashing through the grass, running off. Penny's barking sounded far away, echoing in the night. The air went still around Judy. The only sound was her own panting. Her heart beat wildly.

"Judy!" Mary appeared at her side, but Judy couldn't see more than her outline against the cloudy sky.

"Somebody hit me . . ."

"Oh my God!" Mary threw herself on the ground and put her hands on Judy's face. "Are you okay? Stay awake! Is there blood?"

"I'm fine, I'm okay." Judy waved Mary off. "Get the guy. Find the guy. Find Penny . . ."

"Are you really okay?" Mary cradled Judy's upper body, and Judy reached for her shoulder, trying to get to her feet.

"Let me get up, I'm okay. I have to find Penny."

"She'll be fine, just be still. You could have a concussion. Where did he punch you?"

"No, he hit me in my head, with something." Judy struggled to stand up, and a light went on in the kitchen in the back of her aunt's house, illuminating the backyard.

"Judy, is that you?" her mother called out, opening the back door. "What's going on? What are you doing here?"

"Mrs. Carrier!" Mary shouted, panicky. "Come here quick! Somebody hit Judy!"

"Oh no!" her mother wailed. "Mary, is that you? Be right there!"

Judy scrambled to her feet, weaving slightly. Her head pounded. She couldn't hear Penny barking anymore, and it terrified her to think that something had happened to the dog. "Penny! Penny!"

"Honey?" Her mother hurried toward her with Aunt Barb, both of them in bathrobes.

"Judy, what's happening?" Aunt Barb reached her and helped her up by the arm. "Are you okay?"

"I'm fine, really." Judy stood up, leaning on Mary. She looked around wildly. The backyard was empty. The rosebushes drooped with rainwater, their fading blooms glistening in the light from the window. The man was gone and so was Penny. "There must have been two men."

"How do you know?" Mary asked, urgent.

"Two *what*?" her mother joined in, shocked. The back porch lights went on in the house whose backyard bordered Aunt Barb's, then the house next to it, as the ruckus roused the neighbors.

"Two men." Judy struggled to piece it together through the pain. "Penny saw them before I did. That must be why she freaked out in the car. I didn't see him until he hit me."

"*Hit you?*" her mother repeated.

Aunt Barb gasped. "Two *men,* in my backyard? Sweet Jesus!"

"What did he look like?" Mary gripped Judy's arm, steadying her.

"I didn't see him, I couldn't tell." Judy felt shaken, trying to process what just happened. "That must have been what Penny chased after. Not a squirrel, a person. Otherwise she would have stayed with me. There must've been another man who hit me, then ran away. So there were two men."

"I don't see anyone around." Mary swiveled her head left and right. "I don't hear a car starting. They must've gone."

"We can't let them get away." Judy took off toward the street, but wobbled, dizzy.

"Judy, stop, no, you're hurt." Mary hurried after and caught her arm. "We have to take care of you first."

"But we could see the car or a license plate." Judy tried to go, but Mary held her back.

"No, it's too dangerous. We're lawyers, not cops."

"Then call 911. My phone's in my purse." Judy steadied herself, touching her head where she'd been hit. A lump swelled under her fingertips. She hadn't seen what he'd hit her with. A rock? It hurt like hell, and when she pulled her hand away, her fingertips glistened darkly.

Aunt Barb said, "Your forehead's bleeding, honey! Oh my God!"

"Let's get in the house!" Her mother came to her side. "They could still be out here."

"No, wait, I'm worried about Penny." Judy felt the warm wetness sliding down her forehead, but she'd never forgive herself if anything happened to the dog, who'd been trying to protect her. "Hold on a sec, okay?"

Aunt Barb squeezed her other arm. "Penny will come back. She knows where the house is."

"Penny!" Judy hollered, turning. Suddenly she heard barking and faced the direction of the sound, beyond the privet hedge that bordered her aunt's property. "Penny, come!"

"I think I see her!" Mary yelled.

"Me, too!" Judy almost cried with happiness when she spotted the golden retriever racing toward them from the neighbor's backyard, trailing her leash. Penny bounded panting to Judy, then jumped up on her, almost knocking her to the ground all over again.

"Thank God!" Judy buried her knuckles deep in the dog's thick ruff, curly with sweat. Penny didn't look injured, but she emitted a weird, primal smell.

"Hurry, please let's go inside." Her mother led the way, and Mary came around her other side.

"Judy, come on. We'd better call 911."

Chapter Eighteen

Half an hour later, a line of black-and-white Kennett Square police cruisers parked out front of Aunt Barb's house, their light bars flashing silently. Wooden sawhorses cordoned off her aunt's section of the street, and a few neighbors stood outside the perimeter, drawn by the unaccustomed activity in this quiet section of town. Uniformed police officers searched Aunt Barb's house, as well as her garage, backyard, and the environs, carrying long-handled Maglites that flashed jittery cones of high-intensity light over the heirloom roses and privet hedges.

Officers Hoffman and Ramirez flanked the front door, and Detective Boone sat on the couch opposite Judy, Mary, and Aunt Barb, taking notes in a skinny pad. Judy's mother bustled around, supplying everybody with mugs of coffee and freshening the ice in the Ziploc bag for Judy's forehead, which had already stopped bleeding. She had a goose egg above her hairline, but it would be hidden in her hair, and even her aunt didn't think she needed stitches.

Iris's gardening chest sat in the middle of the living-room floor, its secret cash exposed while Judy explained how she'd discovered it to an astonished Aunt Barb, who slumped in a chintz wing chair, her hand covering her mouth almost the entire time. Judy felt terrible for her, having to deal with this shock the night before her operation.

"So Aunt Barb, you didn't know anything about this money," Judy stated the obvious for the record, in lawyer mode.

"Not a thing." Her aunt shook her head, stricken.

"That's what I thought." Judy faced Detective Boone. "I want it absolutely clear that my aunt wasn't involved in any way with whatever crimes Iris may have committed in connection with this money."

"Understood." Detective Boone blinked behind his wire-rimmed glasses, his pen over his notebook. "We've just begun our investigation, but at this point, I doubt the assistant district attorney would consider charging your aunt with anything."

"Excellent." Judy went into a mental at-ease, and Aunt Barb shot her a grateful, if shaky, smile. "How much cash do you think it is?"

"I would say $7,000 to $9,000."

"I thought it was more."

"I know, most people do. Money takes up a lot of space. It always looks like more than it actually is." Detective Boone frowned slightly. "So, did you see who hit you?"

"No."

"Did you get any description at all? Height, weight?"

"No, I don't know."

"Was it a big guy, a fat guy?"

"Biggish, I think. It was pitch black out there and it was so, well, unexpected."

"White, black, Hispanic?"

"No idea. I feel sure that it was a guy, because I heard the grunt and it sounded deep." Judy racked her brain for a description, but she just kept coming up empty. "It was a man, and as I said, I smelled beer."

"Did he say anything? Call you a name or anything?"

"No." Judy could have kicked herself. "I feel so dumb."

"Don't blame yourself. It's frightening to be assaulted."

"Do you know what he hit me with? Did they find anything where he hit me, like a rock?"

"No not yet, but they'll keep looking. A punch can feel like a rock."

"It wasn't a hand. It was an object." Judy had the random thought that it could have been a gun, but she wasn't about to freak out her aunt and mother.

"Uniforms are canvassing the neighbors to ask if they saw anything suspicious, like anybody who doesn't belong here or a car they didn't recognize. You never know, we could get lucky."

"Great."

"And you didn't see the second man, did you?"

"No, I made a deduction that there was a second man because the dog didn't stay with me." Judy scratched Penny's side with her foot, since the dog was asleep on the rug beside her.

"Let me get this straight." Detective Boone pursed his thin lips. "You found the cash in your aunt's garage and nobody knew anything about it, is that what you're telling me?"

"Exactly. Mary and I came out here tonight because we were worried that if somebody knew about the money, they might come after it, and evidently we were right."

"That's not necessarily true, as long as we're talking about logic and deductions." Detective Boone cocked his neat head of close-cut sandy hair. "We have had reports of a prowler in this area, and we don't have any evidence to connect your assault to the cash in the garage."

"Oh come on," Judy said, skeptical. "It's too coincidental, Detective. I spent one morning at church and could see that everybody knew Iris. It's likely they could know more about her than we do. Obviously, there's more to this situation than we thought."

Mary chimed in, "Besides, if it's a random prowler, why didn't he just run? Why did he hit her?"

Detective Boone made a note. "She's tall and strong. He had to prevent her from giving chase. He wasn't taking any chances."

Judy still wasn't buying it, but she had a more urgent concern. "Look, right now, what's worrying me is my aunt's safety, and my mother's. What can you do to protect them in the event that these guys come back?"

Aunt Barb shifted in her chair. "That's what's worrying me, too. I do have surgery tomorrow morning and I have to be at home, recovering. My sister is going to stay with me."

Detective Boone looked from Aunt Barb to Judy's mother, who was standing beside the wing chair. "Ladies, the police can patrol the neighborhood, but they can't guarantee your safety. We don't have the manpower. If it's going to concern you, and I understand why it would, I suggest you stay in a hotel."

Aunt Barb's face fell. "A hotel? I won't feel at home in a hotel, and it might be weeks."

"You can stay with me, at my house," Judy offered, meaning it. She'd love to have her aunt under her roof, and she'd find a way to tolerate her mother. The only problem was the fleas, but nobody had to know about that.

Her mother lifted an eyebrow. "We'll stay in a hotel. We'll be more comfortable."

Judy tried not to feel hurt. "Mom, that's not as homey, for Aunt Barb." She turned to her aunt. "Aunt Barb, please stay with me. The hospital's right in town, so it's actually more convenient, and for your doctor's appointments, too. And I'd be able to see you after work and help out. What do you say? You like the city."

"Yes, but I hate to impose." Aunt Barb smiled slowly, and Judy knew she was winning the battle.

"You wouldn't be imposing at all. You and Mom can have my bed, which is a king, and I can sleep on the daybed in my office."

"What about Frank?" Aunt Barb asked, and Judy felt a twinge, realizing she hadn't even thought about her boyfriend, who shared her bed.

"He can stay at his grandfather's in South Philly. He's over there all the time."

Suddenly a heavyset uniformed officer opened the front door. "Detective Boone?" he said, stepping inside the living room. "Uh, got a minute?"

"Not now." Detective Boone gestured at Judy, frowning. "I'm taking a victim statement."

"Captain said to let you know if we found anything in the garage, and we did."

"What did you find?" Detective Boone turned to the cop, and Judy's ears pricked up.

"Money." The cop lumbered into the room. "In an old trunk in the corner, under some other stuff. About thirteen grand."

"Oh my God!" Judy said, shocked.

"Oh no!" Aunt Barb moaned.

Judy's mother pursed her lips in a knowing line. "This is awful, just awful."

Detective Boone rose. "What did you do with it?"

"We left it where it was. Cap said to ask you." The cop shrugged. "He said if the homeowner wants us to move it out, we will."

Judy got up, turning to her aunt. "Aunt Barb, don't you want them to bring it inside? We can't leave it in the garage."

Aunt Barb blinked. "It's not mine. It's Iris's. I don't know what to do with it. Put it in the bank?"

The cop grinned. "Give it to me, I know what to do with it."

"I do, too!" Officer Ramirez said at the door, and next to him, Officer Hoffman slapped him five.

Judy's mother asked the detective, "But isn't it evidence?"

Judy suppressed an eye-roll. "Mom, it's not evidence because there's no crime."

Her mother sniffed. "I asked the detective."

Detective Boone shook his head. "Your daughter's correct, Mrs. Carrier. I can't say I've had this situation before. I'll double-check with the A.D.A., but my sense is we'll leave to you what to do with the money. It's not police business."

Judy looked at Mary. "I'm sure we can set up a trust account for Iris's estate."

Mary nodded. "Right, and in the meantime, we can put it in the firm's safe."

"The firm has a safe?" Judy asked, surprised. "Who knew that? Is that something you have to be a partner to know?"

"Yeah." Mary chuckled. "Like the secret handshake."

Suddenly there was a commotion from the policemen upstairs, who were coming down the staircase, the footsteps heavy. "Detective?" called the first cop, coming into view.

"What is it?" Detective Boone turned to the stairwell.

"You know that pink bedroom in the back?" The cop gestured to the back of the house, his dark eyes animated under the patent bill of his cap. "Well, we found more cash."

Judy gasped, catching Mary's incredulous eye. "What are you talking about?"

"It's like a bank in there." The first cop shook his head, marveling, and the one behind him nodded. "There's money in shoeboxes in the closet and a cedar chest. Plus, on the far side of the bed, you can see where somebody cut the floorboards. I bet there's money under the floor, but we didn't go there. We only found it because the rug looked messed up on the far side."

Detective Boone frowned with disapproval. "Officers, why were you looking in the cedar chest? That wasn't your orders."

"Sorry, but we played a hunch. We cleared it with the captain, so you can take it up with him."

"What was the hunch?" Judy interjected, glossing over the awkward moment.

"We knew there was dough in the garage, and we figured that the motherload had to be in the house. If it were me, common sense, I'd hide money in the house first, then use the garage second, like, for the leftover. It's safer."

"You're right." Judy kicked herself for not thinking of it herself.

"What the hell?" Judy's mother turned to Aunt Barb, who was sinking into the wing chair. "Barb, how can this happen? Did you just give that woman your guest bedroom?"

"Yes, totally. Why wouldn't I?" Aunt Barb turned her palms up, in appeal. "She slept over whenever she took me for chemo. I told her to make herself comfortable in there, to consider my home, her home."

Judy's mother *tsk-tsk*ed. "But still, it's your house. Didn't you ever go in there? Didn't you notice anything unusual?"

Judy interjected, "Mom, it's not her fault."

Aunt Barb held up a palm, signaling to Judy to stop. "Thanks honey, but I can explain." She turned to Judy's mother. "Delia, nobody else used that guest room for years, until Friday, when you came. *You* didn't see anything unusual, did you?"

Judy's mother flushed. "I'm hardly unpacked. But I bet I would have found the money, sooner rather than later."

"Delia, I trusted her. She stayed over when she helped me, for nights in a row. I would never dream of going into her room and searching it, for heaven's sake. I respected her privacy."

Detective Boone glanced uncomfortably at his feet, which

didn't stop Judy's mother. "But Barb, what about when you clean? Didn't you see anything?"

Aunt Barb shook her head. "Iris did all the cleaning, every two weeks."

Judy's mother laughed, without mirth. "You're too trusting, honey. That woman had a perfect plan. She had you all figured out. The only question is, how much more money did she hide in your house?"

"Mom, please, enough." Judy met Mary's eye, with a Meaningful Flare. "It looks like we have our work cut out for us. Time for a treasure hunt, eh, girl?"

"Let's get busy," Mary answered, with a grim smile.

Chapter Nineteen

Judy and Mary zoomed toward Philly on a Schuylkill Express-way slick with rainwater. They had packed all the cash they could find in a duffel bag, and it came to about $50,000. Judy had driven the whole way home paranoid that they would get in an accident or be carjacked. The duffel was in the trunk of her car, which meant the total worth of her vehicle was $55,000.

Judy checked the rearview mirror again, and all was well. Her aunt and her mother dozed in the backseat, with Penny sleeping between them like a furry demilitarized zone. The two sisters had reached an uneasy truce while they packed Aunt Barb's luggage to move to Judy's apartment, but Judy felt preoc-cupied the whole time, worrying about the secret money and her aunt's mastectomy.

"You all right?" Mary asked quietly. "I've been yapping away about the wedding again. The dress, the band, the hall, and the pigs in a blanket. Sorry if the wedding is taking over my life."

"No, it should, and it's fine. It's good to talk about something happy." Judy managed a smile as the city skyline popped into view in the distance, its modern neon lights outlining the ziggu-rat of Liberty Place and the pointed spike of the Mellon Center.

"But what's up?"

"I just want my aunt to be okay. I can't believe this strain is good for her."

"It can't be helped, and you heard what she said, that it took her mind off of everything."

"I guess." Judy took the Montgomery Drive exit.

"I think it's a good idea for them to stay at your apartment, unless it comes to fisticuffs."

Judy smiled. The best thing about Mary was that she could always cheer her up, no matter what the circumstances. "Thanks so much for all you did tonight."

"No problem. I'm glad I was there." Mary checked her phone, and a quick flash of light illuminated her face. "It's getting late. Bennie said to text her when we get close to the office. She's in, getting ready for trial."

"I'll pull up in front of the building, and my mother and aunt can wait in the car. It won't take that long, will it?"

"No. The kids are asleep, right?" Mary glanced behind her in the backseat. "I didn't want to say this in front of them, but your getting attacked tonight made me rethink my theory about Iris's death."

"Me too." Judy swung the car onto the West River Drive, which bordered the winding Schuylkill River. Tall, leafy oaks lined the riverbank, but the dark river glistened like a winding black python. "I can't wait to see those autopsy results. It's just too coincidental that these alleged prowlers were there tonight. I wonder if they were staking out the house, waiting for me to leave. I was there last night, and this is the first night without me. I'm thinking she was in business with them."

"What kind of business? Drugs?"

"What else could it be, right? Maybe the autopsy will show a drug overdose or that she did have a heart attack, but it was caused by a drug overdose, or there were drugs in her system. It wouldn't have to be hard drugs like heroin or cocaine, it could just be something like prescription pills. Iris could have been using her own supply. That would explain her death and also the presence of the money."

"Why was she on the road then? Why did she miss work?"

"She was making a delivery or picking up a supply. She got a mystery call, maybe that was it. Either way, it's clear by now that she was living a secret life, isn't it? And with something like drug dealing, she'd come in contact with a lot of unsavory people. Dangerous people, thugs." Judy shuddered to think that thugs were in her aunt's backyard, maybe with a gun. "It was a lucky break that we went there tonight, wasn't it?"

"Yes, but tomorrow, you're going to need foundation."

Judy managed a smile, but was still shaken. She didn't want to believe that Iris was guilty of drug dealing, but tonight had almost changed her mind. "Still, it's so hard to believe, if you had seen Iris. Really, she was a cute little person."

"Get real, Jude. You say the undocumented community is very close, and there have to be people who sell it drugs. That must be what she was up to, and Daniella, too."

"A fine friend she turned out to be, huh? She leaves town before Iris is even buried."

Mary snorted. "I'll never do that to you when we start our drug business."

"One way or another, we'll be partners." Judy steered around the curve past Chamonix Drive, practically devoid of traffic. The tires rumbled on the wet asphalt.

"Right! Meanwhile, you have to go home and throw boyfriend out of bed."

"I know. I texted him, but he didn't text me back. Either he's asleep or he's mad."

"You texted him about your head and he didn't write you back?"

"No, I didn't mention my head."

"Why not?" Mary frowned. "You were *assaulted*."

"Why, do you think he'd rush to my aid?"

"You didn't give him the chance."

"Trust me, he wouldn't."

"You don't know that."

Judy looked over in the dark car. "You're supposed to be on my side."

Mary shook her head. "I am, but I have to be honest. You're being hard on him. The guy can't win."

"I hate when we disagree."

"You and him?"

"No, me and you." Judy steered past the Victorian boathouses on the opposite bank of the river, which usually made a picturesque backdrop, but tonight were shrouded in darkness and fog. "I'm trying to lighten up on him, but I can't. Or every time I do, he just does something else to make me mad. I don't think it's the worst thing that he stays at his grandfather's for a week or two."

"It's going to be longer than that."

"Whatever, the break will do us good." Judy had been thinking as much all night, but it was one thing to mull it over and another to say it out loud. "I want him to miss me. He's taking too much for granted. Anyway, it can't be helped."

"You sound like you're falling out of love. Are you falling out of love, honey?"

Judy thought about it. "No, I'm still in love. But I'm falling out of like."

"That's worse," Mary said softly.

"I know." Judy hit the gas, and the VW zoomed past the Art Museum, its Grecian columns lighted from beneath.

"When I called Bennie, I told her what happened tonight, and she's wondering what's going on with you." Mary paused. "She mentioned that a client named Linda Adler called her because you didn't return her call."

"Oh no." Judy kicked herself. "Linda is the plaintiff in a sex-discrimination case Bennie gave me. We traded calls, but I dropped the ball, it's true."

"She says it's not like you, not to return a client's call. Maybe you should tell Bennie about your aunt, huh? That's the reason, isn't it?"

"I'm not going to pimp out Aunt Barb's mastectomy as an excuse for my mistake. It's my aunt's personal business."

"I didn't mean it that way, and Bennie really is worried."

"Worried enough to save me from the lawyer hell of asbestos damages? I'm dreading working those cases." Judy shook her head, driving toward the city. "What's the value of a human life? Do I really want to think about that right now? How much would I get for Uncle Steve? Or my aunt? I mean, there are worse jobs, like picking mushrooms, but is that the test?"

Mary's tone brightened. "You know, you could even use Allegra. It would give her something to cut her teeth on."

"I like Allegra too much to put her on these cases," Judy said, meaning it. Allegra Gardner was their teenaged intern, a genius-level prodigy who had actually been their client, having hired the Rosato firm to investigate her theory that the man convicted of murdering her sister was actually innocent. That she'd turned out to be right surprised everyone but the girl genius. Judy sighed, driving toward the city. "Mary, everybody hates asbestos cases. Remember Stalling and Webb? They lost associates in droves."

"We won't lose you."

"No, of course not," Judy rushed to say, though she wondered if she meant it. "But I've been thinking about it, and I'm going to ask Bennie to decline the representation."

Mary looked over in disbelief. "She already accepted it, and she won't turn down that much business."

"It's not worth the money. Let them go kill somebody else's soul."

"We don't have a choice, as a firm." Mary frowned, her mouth tilting down unhappily at the corners.

"Yes we do. We have free will. We choose how we make money in this world. Who knows how long any of us will be alive?" Judy was thinking again of Aunt Barb, even Uncle Steve. "You can't give up your life to earn a living. All you have is your integrity. Did we forget that?"

"No, but we have to be realistic. We can't lose that business."

"Don't take this the wrong way, but *I* can lose that business. It's not my firm, as an associate, but it is my practice and my life." Judy made a decision. "I'm going to talk to Bennie."

"Okay." Mary's tone grew gentler. "But do yourself a favor. Wait until her trial's over, your chances are better. She should be finished Wednesday morning."

"You think it can wait?"

"Sure. It'll take a while to get those cases and files. You want me to go in with you? I'll be your co-counsel."

"No, thanks."

"How about I soften her up first?"

"Is that even possible?" Judy couldn't help but crack wise.

"Good point."

"Text her, will you, Mare? We're almost there."

Chapter Twenty

"I can't wait to get rid of this dough." Judy rode up in the elevator with Mary, holding the duffel bag of cash and feeling as if their floor couldn't come fast enough. "It stresses me out. I almost confessed to the security guard and I didn't even do anything."

Mary smiled. "You'd make a lame drug dealer."

"I know. How do they do it?"

"They have guns."

"I'm surprised you're not nervous. You're always more worried than I am." Judy watched the floor numbers change above the elevator doors.

"The wedding cured me. Nothing is as stressful as planning a wedding."

"How about a pregnancy test?" Judy asked, and they both laughed. The elevator *ping*ed when they reached their floor, and the doors slid open, parting to reveal a reception room filled with exhibits and cardboard boxes that hadn't been there Friday.

"Poor Bennie," Mary said, stepping off the elevator. "She told me her trial was a monster."

"That's a helluva record." Judy followed Mary past a wall of cardboard boxes, stacked five high.

"Oh geez, there's more." Mary turned right down the hallway, and Judy followed, surprised at the sight. The hallway was lined with cardboard boxes that ran the entire length of the baseboard, stretching all the way to Bennie's office at the end of the corridor. There had to be a hundred boxes or more.

"Yikes, I feel sorry for her." Judy followed Mary to Bennie's door, where they both stopped at the threshold of her office, unnoticed by the boss, who sat working at her desk. Her large blue eyes focused on her laptop and her curly blond hair had been twisted into an unruly knot by a ballpoint pen. She had on her trademark white oxford shirt and khaki suit, which Judy assumed she had been born in.

"Hi Bennie," Judy and Mary said, in unfortunate unison.

"Ladies, good to see you." Bennie looked up with a concerned frown. "Carrier, is that the bump?"

"It looks worse than it is."

"Sheesh, sit down. You, too, DiNunzio." Bennie waved them into the patterned chairs opposite her desk. Files, notes, and documents sat stacked around her, and the cherrywood shelves lining the office were filled with crystal awards and fancy bowls that she had earned over a long career, as one of the best trial lawyers in the country.

"Thanks, but we can't," Judy told her. "My aunt and mom are waiting in the car. Can we get this money into the safe?"

"Sure. Follow me." Bennie rose quickly and came around the desk, eyeing Judy's injury. "Is this why you didn't call Linda Adler back? I got a message she was trying to reach you. If so, it's a good excuse."

"Right, sorry," Judy answered, without elaborating. "We keep missing each other, but I'll follow up."

"Good. So, tell me what happened to you guys. Who jumped

you? Do the cops have a suspect?" Bennie left her office, and Judy and Mary followed her down the hall.

"Not so far."

"Carrier, about this money you're bringing me, you have to get it out of the safe tomorrow. Overnight is fine, but not longer."

"Why?" Judy hadn't even thought about what to do with the money, after tonight. All she could think about for tomorrow was Aunt Barb's mastectomy and a deposition in *Adler* that she was going to try to postpone. "I can't tomorrow. I have a deposition in *Adler,* I'm deposing Govinda from PennBank. That's what Linda was calling about."

"We can't have that amount of money here. You've made yourself the de facto custodian of these funds, which puts you in an unethical position vis-à-vis the Code. It looks like we're commingling funds, which we aren't." Bennie barreled ahead. "Get yourself an estates lawyer, tonight. It needs to go into an IOLTA account, tomorrow."

"Okay," Judy said, though she had no idea what an IOLTA account was. She had an old friend from law school who was an estates lawyer and she made a mental note to email him.

"By the way, we can't have these boxes in the hallway and reception area. You'll need to get them into a war room tomorrow." Bennie gestured to the wall of cardboard boxes, as they walked past.

"Wait. What? These boxes are mine?" Judy tried to catch up, the duffel bag bumping against her leg. "I thought they were your trial record."

"No." Bennie charged down the hallway. "The boxes are from Singer Crenheim. It's those new matters in *Bendaflex.*"

"The damages trials, so soon?" Judy looked over at Mary, whose mouth dropped open in surprise. They followed Bennie left into the law library, a cozy room lined with tan lawbooks surrounding a round mahogany table. More cardboard boxes sat piled on the table and floor. "Yikes, are these mine, too?"

"Sure." Bennie glanced back, smiling. "It's a real coup to get that much referral business from a firm like Crenheim. They picked us over every firm in Philly."

"But how did you get the files so fast?" Judy swallowed hard, because it looked like a done deal. "We only talked about this on Friday."

"I know, but it's New York." Bennie led them through the library, down the hall toward the file room and the office safe. "They don't waste any time, and I told him to have the documents couriered to us on Saturday. I knew I'd be in the office."

Judy steeled herself. "Bennie, I'm not sure we should take these cases. I want to talk it over with you."

"What's to talk about?" Bennie tossed over her shoulder. "Also, they're paying us on a flat fee, not an hourly basis, which is typical for this work. Fifty grand a case is all we get. I figure each case is a three-to-five day trial, and if you staff it with a paralegal and Allegra, you can bring each case in at thirty-five grand. Make that happen, so we keep a profit margin."

Mary interjected, "Bennie, I think Judy deserves a say—"

"Got it, Mary." Judy waved her off, because it was time for the big-girl panties. "Bennie, before we even talk fees, this is such a big commitment of time that—"

"I know, I love it." Bennie led them to the file room, opened the door, and flicked on the light, illuminating a grayish Formica counter and the rolling shelves of active case files beyond. "Marc said there were seventy-five or seventy-six different trials. That will take us two to three years down the line. Guaranteed billings every quarter, totaling 3.75 million. Wow!"

"I'm worried it will consume my entire practice."

"You're damn right it will." Bennie led them down the aisle toward the supply room. "It's a game-changer for you."

"That's exactly my problem."

"You have a problem?"

"Yes, I have a problem."

Bennie stopped in her tracks and did an about-face in the aisle, with a mystified smile. "Are you serious?"

"Bennie, I don't want to work those cases." Judy didn't dare look over at Mary, who stood aside in stunned silence. "I'm dreading the subject matter, the time, it's all too much—"

"You won't have to do it by yourself. We'll crunch the numbers and see how many people you can hire." Bennie brightened, grinning as if she'd gotten a great idea. "In fact, wait, I take that back. You run it by yourself, the whole shebang. Personnel and all. You decide whom you want to hire and whom you can fit in the budget, considering the billings you're bringing in. Run the litigation like a partner. Run it efficiently. Lean. Don't hire a lot of expensive experts. Make us 20 percent."

"But I'd be chiseling away at how much a guilty company should pay someone they wronged. It's not justice. Hell, it's not even law."

"It *is* justice." Bennie frowned, puzzled. "The punishment should fit the crime. It's about fairness. No company should pay more than someone was harmed. That's why they hired us, and they'll pay us well."

"They hired us because they don't want to do it."

Bennie pursed her lips. "They hired us because it's too expensive for them to try the cases in Philly and put up a bunch of associates in a hotel."

"But it's soul-killing. We're on the wrong side of the question."

"What are you talking about?" Bennie looked at Judy like she was crazy. "We defend the law. Everybody's entitled to a defense, even asbestos manufacturers."

"Bennie, let's be real. This isn't first-rate legal work." Judy knew it was politically incorrect to say so, but it was true. "We always get the best cases, referred or not. Antitrust, First Amendment, civil rights, constitutional law, high-profile murder defense, big-stakes commercial litigation. We're a quality shop."

"We're a *business*." Bennie's eyes flashed, but her tone remained cool. "We make law and we make money. There's no shame in taking those asbestos cases, and it keeps the lights on. Don't be a law snob. Furthermore, it's an opportunity for you. If you do a good job, and you will, they'll send us more."

"What, more damages cases?" Judy threw up her hands. "Why not other mass torts? Yaz. Pradaxa. Coumadin. Hip implants. It's a no-win for me. If I do a good cleanup job, I'll get more to clean up."

"You want to be real? I'll be real." Bennie met her gaze with naked frankness. "Carrier. You're a brilliant lawyer, a *lawyer's* lawyer. If I need a legal scholar, you're my first choice. If I need an elegant brief, you're my first choice. If I need cutting-edge case analysis, you're my first choice. I truly value what you do here, as an associate. Your litigation strategy is aggressive and creative. That's why I give you my cases, to work. Do you hear me?"

"Yes." Judy knew Bennie meant this as high praise, even though it came off like criticism.

"But you don't have a client base, and you can't make partner without a client base. You understand that's what's holding you back, don't you?"

"Yes," Judy answered, honestly. She worked on cases that Bennie brought in and was the hired gun on some work she got herself, but she didn't have the bread-and-butter client base that Mary did, getting repeat cases from small businesses all over South and West Philly.

"You don't need me to tell you that the legal business has changed. That you can't make partner in any law firm in this city without being a rainmaker. And Bendaflex is your best chance at starting your own client base."

Judy wished she could give in, but she'd come this far, so she couldn't. "What if I don't like the work?"

"Seriously?" Bennie's eyes flared an incredulous blue. "Are you really telling me you don't like what's for dinner, when I'm the one who left the cave, shot the beast, cooked it, and served it to you?"

"I'm not saying I don't appreciate it." Judy's chest constricted. "But what if I can build a client base another way? Can't you hire someone else to do the cases? Isn't that my decision?"

"In a word, no."

"*No?*" Judy repeated, blinking.

"I've heard you out, but you have to go with my decision. You're not a partner, you're still an associate, and as such, you'll do the work we give you. End of discussion." Bennie turned on her heel and walked away. "The safe's this way."

Judy stood red-faced, next to Mary, who looked stricken. The space between them widened to a corporate chasm.

Judy's goose egg started to throb, but that could have been her imagination.

Chapter Twenty-one

"Frank?" Judy said, opening the door to the apartment, with her mother, Aunt Barb, and Penny behind her. Through the crack in the door came the unmistakable sound of a football game on TV, the stench of cigar smoke, and the hooting and hollering of American men losing their damn minds.

Judy's heart sank at the scene in her living room. The mega-TV was on full blast, and the coffee table was cluttered with open pizza boxes, bags of hard pretzels, and beer cans. Frank and his two best friends were jumping up and down in front of the couch, cheering. She couldn't be mad at Frank for feeling better and enjoying himself, but she knew her mother and Aunt Barb wanted to get to bed.

"Come on in." Judy took the bags from her aunt and mother, setting them down in the small entrance room while Penny bounded into the living room, heading for the carbohydrates.

"TOUCHDOWN!" Frank yelled, raising his good arm. He had evidently recovered from his trip to the hospital, and was sitting in the middle of the couch, his bare feet on the coffee table, amid the clutter.

"I smell overtime!" shouted his chubby friend Eric Gordon,

jumping to his sneakers. They called him Cartman because of his unfortunate resemblance to the round kid on *South Park,* and he demonstrated the same wardrobe choices, namely a T-shirt, blue jeans, and omnipresent knit cap.

"Yes! Yes! Yes!" shouted Adam Dalrymple, a tall, thin, crazy straw of a hipster, who taught music at a city high school by day and played guitar with an indie rock band by night. All three men had been friends since high school, and though Cartman and Adam were married, Frank would never be, at least not to Judy, because he hadn't even noticed that she and her family were standing in the room.

"Frank?" she called out, and he turned, then did a double-take.

"Oh, hi everybody." Frank grinned, set down his beer, and came over, with a glance back at the television, undoubtedly to see if they got the extra point. The game went to commercial, and he did a double-take when he spotted Judy's bump. "Whoa, babe, what's that on your face?"

"It's a long story, I'm fine," Judy answered, testy. "Say hello to my mom and aunt."

"Hello, Delia, long time, no see." Frank hugged her mother warmly.

"You, too, Frank," her mother said, with a smile. "I heard you hurt your hand. What a shame!"

"Oh, it's nothing. Hello, Barb, great to see you!" Frank gave her aunt an obviously heartfelt hug. "Listen, I heard you're not feeling well, but I know you're going to pull through this, I just do."

"Thanks, Frank." Aunt Barb released him with a weary smile, her knit cap askew. "I'm sorry to put you out. I promise I'll keep this stay as short as possible."

"Stay?" Frank asked lightly, and behind him, Cartman and Adam started cheering and jumping up and down again.

"They got it!" Cartman yelled. "We're going into overtime, baby!"

"Yes!" Adam slapped him five. "I beat the spread! Woohoo!"

"Penny, no!" Judy shouted, trying vainly to stop the dog from grabbing a pizza crust.

"Excuse me, honey." Aunt Barb touched Judy's arm. "Can I use the bathroom?"

"Me, too," her mother chimed in. "We're middle-aged women, remember?"

"Sure, go ahead, I'll be up with the bags in a minute." Judy gestured to the stairwell.

"Thanks," Aunt Barb said, heading to the stairwell with her mother.

"Frank, meet me in the kitchen, okay?" Judy headed for the kitchen, but when she looked back, he was heading back to the living room. "Frank, can you come with me a second?"

"Right now? The overtime's about to start."

"Please, it's important." Judy went ahead into the kitchen, which was a mess. Open takeout containers of Chinese food dotted the counter, dirty dishes sat stacked in the sink, and the entire room reeked of chicken curry.

"I'm going to clean it up, so don't worry." Frank hurried in with a sheepish smile. "I didn't know you were coming home, and we didn't get the chance. But don't worry, you know I'm going to do it."

"Why don't you just clean it up as you go, Frank?" Judy couldn't keep the irritability from her tone.

"The guys brought the takeout over for the first game, but now we're on the third game. I'll do it before we go to bed."

"Also, please tell me you're not chasing Percocets with beer."

"I had one beer, and my wrist feels a hell of a lot better."

"Forget it." Judy knew she was giving him a hard time, but she couldn't help it. She was still frazzled from the confrontation with Bennie. "I called you but you didn't call back. I texted you, too."

"Sorry, I forgot to plug in my phone and the battery wore down." Frank glanced back to the living room, impatiently. "The commercial's over. What is it you want to talk about?"

"It's kind of obvious, isn't it? My mother, my aunt?" Judy gestured upstairs. "Remember, I told you today that my aunt is having a mastectomy tomorrow. I had to bring her in town to stay with us because tonight, at her house, there were two men—"

"FRANK, GET IN HERE!" Cartman hollered from the living room. "IT'S STARTING! YOU'RE GONNA MISS IT!"

"Babe, let me just go see what's going on."

"Penny, no!" Judy said, forgetting who she was talking to. "Frank, no. Don't go. Wait a minute."

"Can we talk when the game is over, honey?" Frank's brown eyes turned pleading.

"No, because you can't stay here until the game is over. That's what I'm trying to tell you."

"What are you talking about? The game will be over any minute, as soon as somebody scores."

"No it won't. Football time is different from normal time." Judy had learned the hard way that sports had its own time zone. "In football, two minutes means ten minutes, ten minutes means twenty minutes, and a single overtime can turn into double overtime, right?"

Frank's eyes lit up. "Your lips to God's ears."

"No, that's the problem. You have to leave the apartment. That's what I would've told you if you'd called me back." Judy skipped the part about her getting attacked, because evidently it wasn't as important as a stupid football game. "My aunt needs to get to bed, and she's going to stay with us. She and my mother have to sleep in our bed because that's the nicest, and

I am going to stay on the daybed. You have go to your grandfather's for a few weeks. I'm sorry, but it can't be helped—"

"What, why?" Frank looked at her like she was crazy, and Judy was losing track of how often that had been happening lately.

"Because, randomly, her house isn't safe. A friend of hers was stowing all this secret money in it, which we put in a safe at work. It's an emergency, and I really need you to work with me on this."

"On what?" Frank edged to the right so he could still see the TV, and Judy was beginning to lose patience.

"Are you listening to me? She has to be at the hospital at six in the morning, and she needs to get to bed. She obviously can't sleep with this noise level. You guys have to go somewhere else to watch the game."

"No way!" Frank's eyes flew open. "We can't leave now. We'll miss the overtime."

"Go to Cartman's. He lives close."

"But his car's parked all the way over on Arch Street. He couldn't get a space any closer. We'll never make it in time."

"Then go to that sports bar on Pine."

"There's no time for that either. What are we supposed to do, run?"

"I don't know, DVR the end of the game and don't watch it till tomorrow."

"What are you, kidding? It's not *Glee*, it's a football game." Frank snorted. "Let her go upstairs to bed. We'll keep it down. We can be quiet."

"FRANK YOU EFFING DOUCHE!" Cartman shouted, cackling. "GET IN HERE!"

"Like that?" Judy shot him a Meaningful Flare, but he didn't speak the language. "Frank, it's not even the Eagles, is it?"

"No, but we need to know who wins because we have a shot at the wild card and—"

"Forget it," Judy snapped, cutting him off. She had long ago given up trying to understand the complexities of NFL play-offs, which made the United States Tax Code look like a cake-walk. "Can't you work with me on this?"

"Babe, you need to chill. Let us watch the overtime, then we'll go."

"Frank, have a heart!" Judy raised her voice. "It's almost midnight. My aunt, whom I love, is exhausted and scared. She's going through hell."

"I know, and I love Barb, too. She loves me. She'll understand." Frank frowned, testy, and he glanced over his shoulder again.

"I don't want to ask her to understand. I want to put her first. She's been understanding all day long, and she needs us to take care of her now."

"FRANK, THEY'RE AT THE FORTY! THEY'RE SENDING IN THE KICKER!"

Frank threw up his hands. "I know, and I will. She's welcome to stay in the apartment, even in my bed. I'll stay away as long as you want me to, if you give me fifteen more minutes."

"Frank, don't you get it? The woman needs to sleep! She's having a *mastectomy* tomorrow!"

"I know that!" Frank shouted back. "What's the big deal? It's fifteen more minutes!"

"What's the *big deal*? The big deal is she has *breast cancer*! The big deal is *she could die*." Judy shouted back, but suddenly she looked over. Standing in the shadows near the kitchen threshold were Aunt Barb and her mother. And from the stricken expression on Aunt Barb's face, she had obviously heard every word.

"FRANK, YOU DOUCHE! THEY SCORED!"

Chapter Twenty-two

"How do you feel?" Judy asked, at her aunt's bedside at the hospital, waiting to be called to surgery. Her mother sat on the other side of the bed holding a plastic Patient's Belongings bag, and the room was rectangular, containing several other rolling beds, all empty. Nurses in blue scrubs and covered shoes padded noiselessly back and forth, carrying clipboards and plastic trays of medication and supplies, evidently getting ready for the day's procedures.

"Please don't worry," Aunt Barb said, but her face looked drawn, her cheeks hollow, and there were dark circles under her eyes. She had changed into a wrinkly hospital gown and a transparent blue plastic cap. A light cotton blanket was tucked underneath her legs, and compression socks and booties covered her legs and feet. A plastic port taped to the back of her hand hooked her up to an IV bag hanging above the bed, and a sensor on her index finger wired her to a monitor that tracked her vital signs.

"I love you, that's all," Judy said, then stopped herself from saying more, because it was hard to say something comforting when she was so scared. Seeing her aunt in hospital garb, attached to tubes and monitors, made Judy sick to her stomach with fear. She had barely slept for worrying about her and feeling guilt-ridden for what she'd said in the kitchen, within her earshot. They had all glossed over the awful moment last night, but Judy knew that it must've terrified her aunt, in addition to infuriating her mother.

Her mother glanced at her wristwatch. "The anesthesiologist said the surgeon is supposed to come in and talk to you. I wonder what's keeping him. You have to sign the consent forms, and we want to make clear that you're not consenting to residents or fellows performing the procedure."

"He's probably busy." Aunt Barb rested her head on the thin pillow.

Judy's mother sniffed. "You're the first surgery of the day. What can he be busy with?"

"Getting ready for me, I assume." Aunt Barb shrugged her knobby shoulders, and her hospital gown slipped slightly, revealing a collarbone that was too prominent to give Judy any comfort. She adjusted her aunt's gown, but didn't know whether she was hiding the collarbone or keeping her aunt warm.

"Aunt Barb, he's probably mixing your gin and tonic as we speak. Did you tell him you only like Tanqueray?"

"My court jester." Her aunt smiled, patting Judy's hand.

"Ha!" Judy smiled back. "You should see me at work, I provide comic relief."

"I doubt that very much."

"Don't." Her mother lifted an eyebrow. "Did you see when she dyed her hair orange, Barb? Enough said."

"Mom, be nice," Judy said, stung.

"Delia, don't be so crabby." Aunt Barb patted Judy's hand again, and a mischievous twinkle appeared in her eyes. "Now, if I croak in this operation, you two better start getting along."

Judy gasped. "Aunt Barb, don't even joke about that. That's *not* going to happen."

Judy's mother pursed her lips. "Of course not. I read online that this hospital performs more mastectomies than any other in the tri-state area."

Aunt Barb burst into dry laughter, and Judy joined her.

"Mom, way to miss the point."

Aunt Barb's smile faded, and she looked at Judy. "Don't you have to be at work, honey?"

"No, I don't. The dep doesn't start until nine o'clock, so I have time. By the way, I had emailed opposing counsel telling him I had a family emergency and asking him to postpone the deposition, but he said no."

"You didn't have to do that."

Her mother glanced at her watch again. "It's already seven o'clock. This is ridiculous. I don't know why they had us here at the crack of dawn if they were going to make us wait. There's nothing I hate more than hurry-up-and-wait."

Aunt Barb looked at Judy with concern. "Feel free to go, when you need to, if you have to prepare. I'll see you at the end of the workday. That would be great."

"No, I'll come back after the deposition, no worries. It should be by mid-afternoon, at the latest."

"One last thing." Aunt Barb's expression fell into grave lines, deepening the folds that draped her mouth. "There's something important I want to talk to you about, what you said last night, to Frank. When you said I could die."

Judy shuddered, especially in this grim context. "Aunt Barb, I'm so sorry. Really, I feel horrible."

"It's okay, sweetie." Aunt Barb kept her gaze on Judy's face, her eyes steady and even serene. "It was true, and it's something we should say to each other. I hadn't known how to bring it up, but you did, so it's time we talked about it."

"We don't have anything to talk about," her mother said, averting her eyes.

"Delia, you don't have to take part in the conversation. You can just listen or don't, as you wish. I'll talk to Judy."

"Hmph." Judy's mother folded her arms, and Judy squeezed her Aunt Barb's hand.

"What is it, Aunt Barb?"

"We say in group that the one with the cancer is never the one who has the hardest time talking about death, and that's true." A smile returned to Aunt Barb's face, but it looked forced. "But that doesn't mean it's easy for me to talk about, which is why I hid it from you both. I realize now that I made a mistake. I regret that decision. I'm sorry about that. I apologized last night to your mother, and now I'm apologizing to you."

"You don't have to be sorry," Judy said, from the heart.

"I do, because I think it made all of this"—Aunt Barb gestured to the examining room—"more shocking to you and your mother, more sudden. You're both thrown for a loop, I can see, and it's because I didn't tell you about it before."

"That's okay, we're up to speed now. We're quick studies, and we love you."

"You're such a sweetheart, and I love you, too." Aunt Barb's eyes filmed, but she blinked them clear. "What's important is the truth, and what you said last night was the truth. That's why I'm grateful to you. The fact is that I don't know if, after all of this, I'll beat my cancer, or if it will beat me. I don't know if I'm going to die, but I have to admit the possibility."

Judy swallowed hard, trying not to cry.

Her mother *tsk-tsk*ed. "I don't know what the point of this is. This talk is negative and morose. Morbid. Melodramatic."

"Delia, it may be dramatic, but it's not melodramatic. I'm talking about life and death. There's drama in that, and I don't apologize for it."

Judy shot her mother a pleading look. "Let her talk, Mom. Like she said, if you don't want to talk, then don't talk, but don't silence her. This is about her, not you or me."

"It's such negative thinking!" her mother shot back. "She's about to go into an operation. She has to believe she's going to get better or she *won't* get better."

"Mom, that's not true," Judy said, though she could see fear, not criticism, flashing through her mother's eyes.

Aunt Barb turned to Judy's mother with a deep frown. "No, it's *not* true. That's what I hate the most, that burden. We talk about that in our support group, too. How we put that burden on ourselves, or our family does. I put it on myself for so long."

"What burden do you mean?" Judy asked gently.

"The burden that if I don't get better, it's my fault." Aunt Barb emitted a quiet huff of frustration. "That if I just tried harder, or thought more positively, the chemo would have worked. That I practically caused my own cancer, which I *didn't*. My cancer wasn't caused by my bad attitude, my poor decisions, my eating too many processed foods, or my past sins."

"We know," Judy said, trying to soothe her, but her aunt seemed not to hear, glaring at Judy's mother.

"Delia, it's okay for me to tell the truth, and the truth didn't cause my cancer. My cancer was caused by bad luck, and no, I don't carry some horrible mutation in my cells, like the BRCA mutations. You know, Delia, we don't even have a family history of cancer." Aunt Barb kept her gaze glued to Judy's mother. "I'm trying my damnedest to save my own life. I don't know if I'll succeed. But if I don't, it won't be because I don't want to. Trust me, I *want to*, and I'm *trying to*."

"Mrs. Moyer, excuse me," said a man's voice from behind them, and Judy turned around to see a youngish African-American doctor with gold-rimmed glasses and a kind smile. "Good morning, I'm your surgeon, Jim Winston."

"Oh, hello," Aunt Barb said, recovering enough to manage a polite smile, and Judy stood up to let the doctor through. Aunt Barb introduced Judy and her mother, and the surgeon explained the procedure, answered everybody's questions, and had Aunt Barb sign several informed-consent forms, which was when a nurse came in to start a sedative, Versed, administered through the IV bag. In time, her aunt began to doze, but Judy couldn't bring herself to say good-bye.

"Judy," her mother said quietly, "you should be on your way now. She's resting comfortably."

"Right." Judy rose and kissed her on the cheek, touching her shoulder, fleetingly reassured by the warmth of her aunt's skin through the thin gown. "Aunt Barb, I'm going to go now. I love you."

"Love you, too," her aunt said, drowsily. Her eyelids fluttered, and she smiled. "See you later."

"See you later," Judy said, too, because good-bye sounded too final. Tears came to her eyes, and she was glad that her aunt didn't see. She picked up her handbag and messenger bag, then gave her mother a quick wave. "Call me as soon as you know anything, okay, Mom?"

"Sure, don't worry." Her mother flashed her a brittle smile, and Judy turned away and walked the gleaming corridor to the elevator. She got off the elevator on the lobby floor, and the stainless steel doors rattled open onto a crowd of hospital staff, doctors, nurses, and visiting family. She was just about to step off when her cell phone started ringing.

"Excuse me." Judy wedged her way through the crowd, digging in her purse for her phone. She worried it was a nurse or doctor upstairs, or even opposing counsel calling about the deposition. "Hello?"

"Judy, it's Father Keegan. Do you remember me from Madre de Dios Church in Kennett Square?"

"Of course, Father," Judy answered, relieved. "How are you?"

"Fine, but my question is how you are. I read on the local patch online that you were assaulted at your aunt's house last night. Is that true?"

"Yes, thanks, but it wasn't serious. Thank you for asking." Judy switched mental gears, crossing the lobby and leaving the hospital for the bustling street. People hurried this way and that, heading to work, and Seventh Street was clogged with traffic. Pewter clouds covered the sky, and the air was chilly.

"Do the police have any suspects?"

"No, not that I've heard yet." Judy looked around for a cab, wondering how much to fill him in on about Iris. "They think that it was prowlers in the area, but I'm not so sure."

"Why not?"

"We made an unfortunate discovery, that Iris seems to have been hiding a large amount of cash in my aunt's house." Judy went to the curb to hail a cab, but there was none in the rush-hour stream of cars and buses.

"Really?" Father Keegan said, his tone hushed. "I find that hard to believe."

"It's true. I saw with my own eyes." Judy had to get going if she wanted to prepare for the deposition. "I don't like to speak ill of the dead, but I'm afraid that Iris might not be as innocent as we all thought she was."

"She is, I know her."

"We're talking about $50,000 in cash, Father."

Father Keegan gasped. "Something's wrong. I've known Iris for as long as she's been in the country."

"I hear you, and I had a better impression of her, too. So did my aunt. She's heartsick over this, betrayed by a dear friend, and it comes at a difficult time for her."

"I'm sorry, but you must be mistaken. Judy, something is very wrong with this situation. There's another reason I called you this morning." Father Keegan's tone turned grave. "It was to let you know that last night, someone broke into Iris's apartment on Point Breeze."

"Oh no," Judy said, surprised. "Was anybody hurt? What about her roommates?"

"No one was home."

"Thank God. What time did this happen?" Judy spotted a Yellow cab in the distance and hustled toward it, waving.

"Maria Elena came home around eight o'clock, and the place was a mess. The lock had been broken on the exterior door, and the interior door was broken, too."

"So that must've been directly before they went to my aunt's place." Judy's thoughts raced. The cab flashed its headlights at her. "They tried Iris's apartment first, then my aunt's. Was anything taken?"

"Some of the girls' jewelry, but it wasn't valuable. Iris's bedroom and the entire apartment had been ransacked."

"They were looking for something. The money." Judy reached the cab, her thoughts racing. "So this confirms what I suspected. That no matter what the police say, the prowlers at my aunt's house were not random. Iris was involved with some very bad actors, who must have known she was hiding money. Now that she's gone, they're trying to find the cash."

"That can't be what's going on."

"It is." Judy climbed into the cab and closed the door behind her. She reached into her wallet, slid out a business card, and handed it to the older cabbie, so she wouldn't have to interrupt Father Keegan. "What do the police say?"

"They don't know, of course. Maria Elena didn't report it."

Judy realized belatedly that her question was naïve. "How did you find out about it then?"

"Through the grapevine, then I confirmed it with Maria Elena, whom I think you met."

"Were there any witnesses? Did anybody see anything?"

"If they did, nobody's telling Maria Elena. This is not a community that snitches. They're afraid of retaliation. It's like the inner-city, even though it doesn't look like the inner-city."

"Father, you should tell Maria Elena and the other roommate to get out of that apartment. Whoever Iris was in cahoots with hasn't found the money yet. They might come back or even hurt those girls."

"That isn't possible," Father Keegan said, incredulous. "Iris would never break any law. She wasn't in cahoots with anyone. What do you believe she was involved in, exactly?"

"I have no idea. I'm guessing it was some sort of drug dealing, if not hard drugs like heroin, then prescription pills, or maybe just trafficking in pills that you could buy cheaper in Mexico and bringing them into the United States. How often did she go back home?"

"Never," Father Keegan shot back, firming his tone. "She never missed Mass, and she was always working at the mission. Your theory is simply wrong. You don't have any proof, do you?"

"No, but I have $50,000 in cash I can't explain, and she endangered my aunt and my mother." Judy could hear in the priest's voice that he simply didn't believe her, but she understood that. It was his nature and calling to believe the best in people. He had faith.

"Where is the money now?"

"It's in a safe at my office, and I have to get to an estates lawyer to put it in a bank, for Iris's estate." Judy had already emailed her friend and she'd get to his office after her deposition. She held on to the greasy leather strap as the cab braked in stop-and-go traffic. "Even if you don't believe me, I think you should pass the word to Iris's roommates."

"You think they're in physical danger?"

"Absolutely." Judy reflexively touched the goose egg, which

had looked redder than yesterday in the bathroom mirror this morning, like she majorly needed Pro-Activ.

"Judy, you have all this wrong. You're judging Iris without knowing her."

"I don't think so, Father. I got my aunt out of her house until we can figure out what's going on." Judy glanced over her shoulder as the cab turned left onto Pine Street. She wondered if her aunt was being wheeled into the operating room right now, if the plastic mask was being put over her face, or if she was under the knife this very minute. Tears came to Judy's eyes but she blinked them away.

"Judy, are you there? Hello?"

"Father?" Judy said, speaking from the heart. "May I ask you to pray for someone?"

Chapter Twenty-three

Judy hit the office running, her head buzzing with Aunt Barb, Iris, the deposition she had to get ready for, and the fifty grand she had to get rid off. She had almost forgotten about the damages cases, but the cardboard boxes dominated the reception area. She hurried past them to the desk, where their receptionist Marshall Trow was talking with Allegra.

"Hi Judy," Marshall said, with an easy smile. She was in her early thirties and had a wholesome, natural prettiness, with bright blue eyes and light brown hair pulled back into a long braid. "What happened to your forehead?"

Allegra's eyes widened behind her big glasses. "You look like a Cyclops! How did you hurt yourself?"

"It's a long story, ladies, but I don't have time to tell it." Judy looked at Allegra. "Why aren't you in school?"

"It's a teachers' in-service day, so I thought I'd come in. Bennie said you could use me on some new cases."

"Did she?" Judy held her tongue, and Marshall handed her a pink stack of phone messages.

"You got a bunch of calls on Friday, and about those boxes"—Marshall gestured at them—"Bennie asked me to get them out of here. She didn't want them cluttering up reception for the start of business. The building guys are on the way to move them. Where should we put them?"

"There's so many, I'll need two conference rooms. Let's put the bulk of them in B, since it's bigger, and put any leftover in A. A is free, right? I have to take a deposition." Judy checked the modern glass clock on Marshall's desk. "The dep starts at nine o'clock."

"It's free. I'll try to get the boxes put away before then."

"Great. Start with A so we don't get interrupted, okay? Where's Mary?"

"A pretrial conference. She should be in in an hour, she said."

"Thanks. Allegra, come with me." Judy took off with the intern, down the hall. She wasn't as close to Allegra as Mary was, but she wasn't as close to anybody as Mary was. "Let me get you started, then I have to get ready for my dep."

"Okay." Allegra trotted obediently beside her, a slip of a girl with light footfalls, especially in her moccasins. Her long brown hair swung behind her, wavy and unstyled, and she was wearing black tights and a yellow wool sweater dress, which Judy suspected was as close as she could get to dressing like a bee, since the girl was a bee fanatic.

"Here's what I want you to do." Judy slid her laptop from her messenger bag as she reached her open door, went to her messy desk, cleared a spot, opened the lid, and fired up the laptop. "I got an email last night from one of the paralegals at Leighton and Reese in New York, and I'm going to forward it to you."

"Okay."

"Here we go." Judy plunked down in her desk chair, scrolled to find the email, and sent it to Allegra. She couldn't stop thinking of her aunt Barb, who must be on the operating table right now. Father Keegan had promised he'd pray for her, and if her aunt survived her dreaded illness, Judy would rethink her position on the deity.

"Judy? You were saying?"

"I just sent you an email that lists all seventy-five new matters."

"Wow! Seventy-five!" Allegra's pale blue eyes lit up behind her glasses, and Judy wished she could share the intern's enthusiasm.

"Print the email, open the boxes, and use it as a checklist." Judy checked her laptop screen, momentarily distracted by the sight of her other email piling onto her monitor screen by the dozen, making a hill she could never climb. She flashed on Bennie's telling her last night that she didn't have a client base. It was true, but today it seemed beside the point, because she sure had tons of work.

"Then what?"

"Then—" Judy looked up from her laptop to see that Allegra wasn't taking any notes. "How are you going to remember this?"

"I'll remember."

Judy let it go. Allegra was allegedly a Girl Genius, but it was still a little hard to believe. "Make sure we have each of the files."

"Then what do you want me to do, once I see if all the files are there?"

"We'll have to organize them." Judy slid her phone from her purse and placed it on the desk, so she wouldn't miss a call from her mother at the hospital.

"How? Alphabetically by plaintiff? By date of complaint? By trial date?"

"I'm not sure yet." Judy's brain was too busy to deal with Allegra's excellent questions and/or youthful enthusiasm right now. "I've never run litigation this extensive. You'll probably be in college by the time we're finished trying those cases."

"I'm already in college."

"What?"

"I take college courses, at Penn State's branch campus." Allegra grinned. "Anyway, can I come to the deposition? Bennie said it would be good if I did. That's why I dressed up."

"All right," Judy said, though she was getting tired of Bennie running her practice.

"Yay! What do I do?"

"Just sit quietly and take notes, or act like you're taking notes. Be unobtrusive. If they object to your being there, I'll have to ask you to leave. Only parties and counsel are permitted at depositions, but I'm going to pass you off as a paralegal."

"I can act like a paralegal. Hard-working and underpaid. Same as an intern."

Judy smiled, for the first time that day. "Have you ever been to a deposition before?"

"Yes, with Mary, but she was defending it, not taking it."

"It's a very different purpose." Judy got up, went to her credenza, and pulled out the case file while she spoke. "When you take a deposition, the purpose is to find out as much as you can from the witness, so you're prepared for anything he says on the stand at trial. This is going to be boring, I'm afraid."

"That's okay. I like to learn."

"Good. This is just a step in the process, the beginning of the exercise in delayed gratification that's the life of the trial lawyer."

"Okay."

"What that means in practical terms is that I want the witness to relax at the deposition. I'm going to ask open-ended questions. I'm going to let him yap. I'm not going to cross-examine him, like at trial. No pyrotechnics. No *Law & Order*." Judy found the case file in the drawer, slid it out, and let the drawer roll closed. "It'll be like watching someone lay bricks, one by one. I'm building a foundation for a case at trial. You understand?"

"Yes."

"So if I act nice to him, don't be fooled. On the stand, I'm going to make him wish he'd never met me."

"Whoa," Allegra said, her eyes glittering. "It's Dark Judy."

"Right." Judy did feel bile course through her system, but maybe because she had so much on her mind lately, like Aunt Barb, Iris, and her mother. And Frank, who'd left the apartment last night with barely a peck on the cheek. "But not today. Today will be a snoozefest. His lawyer, who's good, will try to stop him from talking. They will have met before the deposition, and his lawyer will have told him not to volunteer, answer only the question asked, and keep his answers to yes or no. This matters a lot in this case, because it hinges entirely on a credibility question."

"What's the credibility question?"

"This is a sex-discrimination case, and our client is Linda Adler, a financial consultant at PennBank, who says she didn't get a promotion to branch manager because she's a woman. The reason she thinks that it was discrimination is that she heard that her boss said to the witness, 'there's no room for women at the top at PennBank.'"

"That's terrible!" Allegra's slim hand flew to her mouth, and Judy noticed her fingernails were bitten down.

"It happens, still." Judy closed the lid of her laptop, to take it with her, like a security blanket for grown-ups. "The witness today is Devi Govinda. He wasn't the one who made the statement, that's his boss Guy Morrell, but I'm saving Morrell for the last deposition."

"Why?"

"I want to get as much information as I can before I meet

Morrell, because he's the person who decided not to promote Linda." Judy slid her notes from the case file and skimmed them quickly while she spoke. "The only fact we have against us is that some of the comments in Linda's employment reviews aren't stellar, so the company is claiming that's the reason they didn't promote her. She doesn't believe that that's the real reason and I don't either, but under the law, I have to prove that it's a pretext."

"Why don't you believe it was her performance?"

"Because Morrell reviews her performance and his view is tainted, and any employee review is subjective in itself." Judy glanced at her phone to make sure her mother wasn't calling from the hospital. "Also, when I look at the personnel files of other women in the department, they tend to be reviewed more harshly than men would be in the same position."

"Oh no."

"Oh yes. That's not easy to prove, but that's what makes it a lawsuit. Conflict. Difference of opinion. Dispute. Understand?"

"Yes."

"Bottom line, I'm going to soften Govinda up and see if I can get him to wobble and give up a little of what Morrell said. It's a long shot because it would cost him his job, and he's not going to admit it. Unless he's drunk, which actually happened to me once." Judy looked over as the buzzer sounded on her desk phone, signaling a call from the reception desk, and she picked up. "Yes, Marshall?"

"Opposing counsel and the witness are getting off the elevator right now. The court reporter's already here. The boxes are in the conference room. What do you want me to do?"

"Please set us up with some coffee and send out for the good Danish, so they feel the love. I'll come out and greet everybody."

"On it."

"Thanks." Judy hung up, rising. She gathered up her file, laptop, and phone, checking the screen for the umpteenth time. "Let's roll, little one."

"Exciting!" Allegra popped to her feet.

"Not hardly," Judy told her, but she was already skipping out the door.

Chapter Twenty-four

Judy tried to pick up the pace after the preliminaries, like name, address, and employment history, even though she already had some of the information from the personnel file. She was getting a feel for Devi Govinda, a somber Indian-American man in his mid-forties, with a stilted air and round, excessively vigilant eyes behind beaded, gold-rimmed glasses. His glossy jet-black hair was neatly trimmed, albeit thinning, and he was slightly overweight, so that his neck spilled over the stiffness of the light blue collar, which he had on with a worn patterned tie and a nondescript dark suit.

"Mr. Govinda, you work at the Narberth branch of Penn-Bank, is that correct?" Judy continued, trying to find a rhythm to her questions. She'd started the way she usually did, with softballs, so she could get a lot of yesses in response and build a nice momentum. It wasn't working so far because she couldn't keep her eyes from straying to her phone or her thoughts from Aunt Barb, lying on the operating table only ten blocks away.

"Yes."

"And what do you do at the branch?"

"Do you mean what is my job?"

"Yes." Judy could see that Govinda had been well-coached and also that the cheese Danish wasn't working its carbohydrate magic. His lawyer, Richard Kelin, was equally silent, a short, squat lawyer from Prendergast Manning, a notoriously jerky firm. He had on a dark suit, an Hermès tie with little orange H's, and horn-rimmed glasses. His face was pudgy, and his gray-eyed gaze fixed outside the window, even though the view was only of the air-conditioning ducts and fans atop the building next door.

"I am a financial consultant at the branch."

"Tell me what that means."

"I'm not sure of your question." Govinda pursed fleshy lips. "I don't understand."

"Sorry, perhaps I could be more clear." Judy couldn't find her groove. "What are your job duties as a financial consultant?"

"I sell various banking products to customers who are interested in instruments or potential investments over $100,000."

"How long have you worked in the branch, in that capacity?"

"Five years."

"And Linda Adler, the plaintiff, was a financial sales consultant in the Narberth branch, for the past three years. Is that correct?"

"Yes."

"Let's talk for a moment about the corporate structure at PennBank, just so I'm clear. The Narberth branch is one of fifteen branch banks in the Philadelphia area. Is that correct?"

"Yes, though we call it the Philadelphia Metro Region."

"Thank you." Judy made a mental note that Govinda was precise. She'd have to step up her game. The clock on the credenza said it was 9:25, so they were into her aunt's operation. "And there are no other financial sales consultants in the branch. Is that also correct?"

"Yes."

"How many licensed financial sales consultants are in the Philadelphia Metro Region?"

"Four others, five total."

"How many are women and how many men?"

"Four men, one woman."

"And what are their names?" Judy looked over as Allegra glanced up from her legal pad, then returned to her note-taking. It reminded her of the days when she'd sit next to Mary and they'd write each other notes on their pads. She wondered if that would ever happen again, but the answer was staring her in the face from the far wall of the conference room, where some boxes from the damages trials had been stacked, a cardboard wall of associatehood.

"Stan Barstal, Jerry Moore, and John Morales."

Judy checked the notes in the file in front of her, but they were on a different subject. "Uh, let me see, the regional manager who oversees fifteen branches in the Philadelphia Metro Region is Mr. Guy Morrell. Is that correct?"

"Yes."

"Where is his office?"

"Center City."

Judy's eyes strayed to her phone, wishing her mother could text, at least. She didn't take notes, so she could help Govinda forget it was a legal proceeding, but she was having a harder time than usual listening. "Mr. Govinda, let's shift gears. As a financial sales consultant, what were Ms. Adler's job responsibilities?"

Kelin interrupted, "If you know."

Govinda nodded. "Linda was supposed to sell investment and traditional banking products to our customers, including checking accounts, savings accounts, credit cards, and loans."

Judy made a mental note that he used her client's first name. "Are you aware that as a financial sales consultant, Ms. Adler had a quota of minimum monthly production goals to meet?"

"Yes."

"Her monthly investment production goal was $1,000 and her minimum revenue requirements were sixty thousand minimum revenue credits. Is that correct?"

"Yes."

"And she received incentive pay as well, did she not, for meeting those quotas?"

"Yes."

Kelin sighed, still gazing out the window. "I'm not bothering to object, but is this line of questioning necessary, Judy? You can confirm it from her personnel file."

Judy knew it wasn't objectionable. "I'm trying to understand how much about Ms. Adler's performance Mr. Govinda knows, and the only way to do that is to ask him." Judy turned to Govinda. "To the best of your knowledge, did Ms. Adler meet those minimums every month of this year?"

"Yes."

"How about the two previous years she's been employed by Penn Bank?"

"Yes."

"To whom does Ms. Adler report?"

"To the regional manager, Mr. Morrell."

"To whom do you report?"

"I also report to Mr. Morrell."

"How is it that you have information regarding whether she meets her minimum revenue goals or not?"

"She told me, uh, us, at lunch."

"And was it part of Linda Adler's job to refer clients to you?"

"Yes. She wasn't licensed to sell investments over $100,000 and she referred those clients to me."

"How many such clients has she referred to you this year, to date?"

"Sixteen."

"How many of those resulted in closed sales?"

"Sixteen."

"And the year before that?"

"Fifteen."

"How many of those resulted in closed sales?"

"Fourteen."

Judy skipped ahead, growing impatient and edgy. "Mr. Govinda, does the fact that you were able to close the sales reflect on Ms. Adler in any way?"

"Yes. She cultivated high-quality targets."

"Do you know how she did that?"

"Yes, through cold calls and a network in the community."

"What was Ms. Adler's network, to which you just referred?"

"She belongs to Curves and she's in a few book clubs. One of our customers came from her book club and another from church. They were high-net-worth individuals and I was able to close the sale with them."

"Do the four other financial sales consultants in the Philadelphia Metro Region refer clients to you?"

"Yes."

"Did any of them send you as many referrals as Ms. Adler did?"

"No."

Judy knew she should ask for the details to lay her brick foundation, but she couldn't fight her anger at him, at the injustice to Linda Adler, at Bennie, at the hidden money, and even at breast cancer. "Do you believe that Ms. Adler deserved the promotion to branch manager?"

"Objection!" Kelin swiveled his neat head around, with a new frown. "It's irrelevant whether or not the witness believed Ms. Adler was entitled to the promotion."

Judy felt herself losing her temper. "No it isn't, and we both know that relevance isn't a proper objection at deposition. Mr. Govinda, you may answer the question."

Kelin snorted. "Don't answer, Devi. I'm instructing you not to answer."

Judy reached into the middle of the table and snatched the telephone receiver from its cradle. "Rick, shall I call the judge right now and get a ruling? You tell me."

"Fine, that won't be necessary." Kelin rolled his eyes. "Mr. Govinda, you may answer the question. I'll note for the record that this is Mr. Govinda's opinion only."

Judy faced Govinda, trying to get in control. "Mr. Govinda, did you think Ms. Adler deserved that promotion?"

"It's not for me to say," Govinda answered, his expression impassive.

"It is now," Judy shot back, and Allegra looked over, her fair skin flushing. "Mr. Govinda, I'm asking you a question, and you are compelled to answer. In your opinion, didn't Ms. Adler deserve that promotion?"

"Again, I cannot say. I'm not her superior. I don't have the complete facts."

"But you know that she referred you more customers than any of the other financial sales consultants, and that she made her quota for all three years." Judy leaned forward, urgent. "What other facts do you need, Mr. Govinda?"

Kelin shook his head. "Objection, arguing with the witness."

Govinda's head swiveled to Judy. "I would need to know more facts concerning the employee who received the promotion. He was a new hire from PNC, and we didn't know him."

Judy threw up her hands. "It's not a relative question. I'm not asking you to make a comparison. I'm asking you, simply upon the facts you have, did Ms. Adler deserve that promotion?"

Kelin interjected, "Objection, calls for speculation."

Govinda blinked. "I cannot speculate."

Judy cut to the chase. "Mr. Govinda, isn't it true that Mr. Morrell told you that there was 'no room for women at the top of PennBank'?"

"No."

Judy wasn't about to stop. "Mr. Govinda, I remind you that you're under oath here, and I'm going to ask you again, isn't it true that Mr. Morrell said that to you?"

Kelin scowled. "Objection, asked and answered!"

"Rick, I'm allowed to press him. Mr. Govinda, answer the question."

"No, that's not true," Govinda answered, but he averted his eyes.

Judy tried a lateral attack. "Mr. Govinda, did Mr. Morrell hire you?"

"Yes."

"Does he have the power to fire you?"

"Yes."

"Does Mr. Morrell review your performance?"

"Yes."

"Does he decide whether you receive raises or incentive pay?"

"Yes."

"Have you received incentive pay?"

"Yes," Govinda answered, then he volunteered, "every quarter since I've been at PennBank."

"How about raises?"

"Yes, same thing."

"Mr. Govinda, when I get you on the stand at trial, there will be a judge and a jury. Are you going to lie to them? Because we both know that Mr. Morrell said to you there was 'no room for women—' "

"Objection, this is harassment!"

"No, this is *litigation,* and Mr. Govinda better get used to it."

Judy faced Govinda, her emotions bubbling over. "You're lying through your teeth. You won't get away with it, not in court, and neither will Morrell—"

"—Judy, objection! This is argumentative and—"

"—and I want you to worry about it every night until trial, I want you to lose sleep over it." Judy felt her temper give way, which she'd never done in a deposition in her life. "I want you to tell Morrell you can't keep his secret, that you won't perjure yourself to cover his ass or to keep your job—"

"—improper! You have no right to speak to my client this way—"

"—and I am going to hammer you both until I find out the truth and nobody is going to believe you after I get through with you—"

"We're leaving!" Kelin jumped to his wingtips, yanking Govinda out of his seat by his jacket sleeve. "This deposition is over!"

"—and anybody can see that you're protecting your boss, and they're going to know you're covering up the truth!" Judy jumped up, as Govinda hustled to the door behind Kelin. "You better tell Morrell, too! You're not going to get away with this! I'm coming for you!"

Kelin and Govinda left the conference room, the door slammed closed behind them, and the air went abruptly still.

"Wow, Judy!" Allegra shot up like a rocket, her cheeks flushed with excitement. "That wasn't boring at all!"

The court reporter looked up, her hooded eyes confused and fingers poised over the stenography machine. "Counsel, I'm not sure I understood that last exchange."

Me neither, Judy thought, but didn't say. She picked up her laptop, case files, and papers. She was trying to figure out what just happened, but Allegra was bouncing around the conference room like an overexcited puppy.

"Judy, that was amazing!" Allegra's eyes went wide behind her glasses. "I totally want to be a lawyer when I grow up! It's so exciting!"

"It's not always that exciting," Judy said, dismayed. Aunt Barb's operation, Iris's death, the secret cash, the damages cases, it had all gotten to her. She checked her phone, but her mother still hadn't called. She clutched her stuff to her chest and went to the door, with Allegra bopping along behind her.

"That was the coolest thing ever! You went right at them! They ran away!"

"But, listen, that's not the best thing." Judy held the door for Allegra, only to see Bennie standing in the hallway, holding a boxy trial bag and talking to Mary. Judy touched Allegra's arm. "Allegra, don't tell them about—"

"Guys!" Allegra called out, and before Judy could finish her sentence, the intern was off and running. "Guess what Judy just did!"

Chapter Twenty-five

"Guys, you're not going to believe what happened in our deposition!" Allegra raced off to meet Bennie and Mary, who turned to her.

"What?" Mary asked with an interested smile.

"Judy scared that lawyer away, and the witness too! They were lying, and she called them out on it, and they *bounced*!" Allegra's words poured out in a rush, and as Judy came up from behind her, she could see Mary's smile freeze in place.

Bennie stiffened. "Carrier, they ended the deposition?" she asked, checking her watch. "It's ten o'clock. You weren't even in there an hour. How could—"

"Bennie, it was amazing!" Allegra interrupted. "It was Dark Judy! I so want to be a lawyer! I can't even wait!"

Mary said, "Dark Judy?"

Bennie frowned. "Carrier, what happened?"

"Nothing, really," Judy answered, not wanting to justify herself to Bennie. She could see that Mary was already worried for her. "Aren't you going to court?"

"Fill me in. We're starting late today, and I have time." Bennie set down her trial bag. "This was in *Adler,* wasn't it? Whom did you depose today, Morrell or Govinda?"

"Govinda."

Allegra chirped up, "Every question Judy asked the witness, he didn't want to answer, so she told him she was going to get him at trial—"

Bennie's eyes flared an incredulous blue. "Carrier, you told him *what*?"

Allegra answered, "And she told him—"

"Allegra," Bennie snapped. "Let Judy tell the story."

"But she's too modest," Allegra insisted. "She doesn't want to brag about herself. You know how she is—"

Judy put a hand on Allegra's shoulder, moving her out of the crossfire. "Bennie, if you remember the details of the case, the statement was made that 'there's no room—' "

"I remember the statement. So what happened? You asked him if Morrell made the statement and he denied it?"

"Of course." Judy felt a renewed flicker of anger. "So I pressed him, as I should."

"You had to do more than press him for them to get up and walk out."

"I pressed him hard." Judy bristled. "I challenged him."

"How much did you challenge him?" Bennie recoiled. "You can't challenge him so much they walk out. You crossed the line."

"No I didn't." Judy knew she had crossed the line, but she shouldn't be called on the carpet for it, on her own case. She couldn't bear to look at Mary. It was just like what had happened last night, only worse.

"You had to have crossed the line, and it's a dumb thing to do with Rick Kelin. I've known him for twenty years, and he's one of the biggest jerks around. What did you do?"

"My job."

"How do you figure that?"

"It's strategy." Judy thought on her feet. "Govinda is the weak link, and I want him to worry, tell Morrell that he won't lie for him or at least that they won't get away with it, and that will provoke a settlement."

"That's quite a gamble." Bennie pursed her lips. "You need to know what Govinda will say at trial and you won't get a second bite at the apple. That was your shot."

"I know what he'll say at trial. I intend to beat him before we get there. He's wound too tight, and the anticipation of being embarrassed and humiliated will eat away at him, I can tell."

"So you intimidated him."

"I destabilized him."

Bennie blinked. "Dark Judy, indeed."

Judy held her tongue. "Even if we don't settle, he'll be a wreck on the stand. I won't have to break him down at trial, he'll break himself down before then."

"Still there's other things you could've explored."

"I didn't need anything else from him. The case is the statement. I got what I needed for the case. Bennie, whatever the strategy is, it's my strategy."

"But it's my case. Linda Adler is my client."

"And you assigned the case to me as soon as the complaint came in."

"I'm the billing partner."

"But I interviewed her on intake, sent out interrogatories and document requests, and defended her deposition. I'm working the case."

"If you're working the case, I don't expect a call from the client. She called me because you didn't return her call."

Judy felt herself redden. "I told you, the call fell through the cracks this weekend, but I'm working the case like I always do."

"You're *not* working it like you always do." Bennie picked up the trial bag. "All of a sudden, you're not getting along with anyone. Fighting in depositions, giving me pushback on *Benda-flex*. And now, this? It's not like you. What's gotten into you?"

Everything, Judy wanted to say. But what she answered was: "I'm fine."

"And what's up with the fifty grand? Please tell me you're getting it out of my safe."

"It will be gone by the end of the day." Judy would have to deal with it before she went to the hospital.

"Good, talk to Marshall when you're ready to remove it. She has the combination. I have to go. Take care."

"Good luck," Judy said, catching Mary's eye, then she noticed Allegra's lower lip puckering.

"Judy," Allegra said, "I didn't mean to get you in trouble."

"You didn't." Judy patted her shoulder. "Don't worry, cheer up. You didn't do anything wrong, and I'm a big girl."

"I never saw Bennie get that mad."

"You haven't been here that long," Judy said, forcing a chuckle.

"Judy," Mary said, frowning. "Can I talk with you a minute, alone?" She smiled at Allegra. "It's not personal, but you can't be there when I slap her around."

"Okay," Allegra said, with a shaky smile, but Judy was already in motion, heading for her office, plopping her files and laptop down on the desk, with Mary following her inside and closing the door behind them.

"So, are you okay?" she asked, when they were alone.

"I'm just so, arg." Judy set her phone face-up on her desk, where she could see if a call was coming in. "Meanwhile, what is my mother's problem? I've texted twice. She can't return a text?"

"Come on, why don't you tell Bennie about your aunt?"

"It's not her business." Judy started pacing, too agitated to sit down. Unfortunately she had a small office, so there wasn't far to walk, plus the floor was a mess, which only bothered her more.

"Bennie asked you directly, and it explains what's bugging you."

"No it doesn't. What's bugging me—" Judy stopped pacing to try to figure out how to finish this sentence, but threw her hands up. "It doesn't matter."

"Yes it does."

"I don't agree with her, how about that?"

"Okay," Mary said slowly. She cocked her head the way she always did when she listened carefully, and she folded her arms, in a dark charcoal pantsuit.

"And the fact that my aunt has cancer doesn't have anything to do with my not agreeing with Bennie." Judy couldn't tell if she was thinking clearly or emotionally, or both.

"So tell her anyway. What's the harm? She'll understand. She's another woman."

"I don't want to be cut slack because my aunt is ill."

"Why not? Everybody needs a break sometime."

"I don't need a break, that's not the problem." Judy stopped pacing, caught up short with the realization. "The problem is that I'm starting to be really unhappy here, because the lines of authority are not clear."

"What are you talking about?" Mary asked, her expression bewildered. "I didn't know you were unhappy."

"I didn't know it, either. Not until recently." Judy shrugged, pained. She was thinking aloud, which she had done with Mary for as long as they'd known each other. "I recognize that I'm only an associate, but don't I have any autonomy at all?"

"Of course you do."

"No I don't. I'm not allowed to decide which cases I take. I'm not even allowed to make the decisions in cases I'm assigned to. Am I even a lawyer?"

"Aw, honey." Mary moaned. "She didn't mean it that way."

"Yes she did. Since when is that the way we work, take it and shut up?" The more Judy thought about it, the more right she felt, which was something that happened to her often. "What about female empowerment and all that? Or does it only apply when men are bossing us around, not women?"

Suddenly Judy's phone rang on her desk, and she leapt for it, her heart beginning to hammer. The iPhone screen showed it was Rick Kelin calling. "Oh crap, I should take this, it's Rick. Give me a minute."

"Go ahead, and make nice."

Judy picked up the call. "Rick, hi."

"Judy?" Rick said, in a huff. "What the hell was *that* about?"

"Come on, Rick, since when did you turn into such a baby?"

"You think I'm going to sit there while you *harass* my witness?"

"Oh will you stop using that word? There's no jury around. The case turns on credibility, and I'm entitled to press him. How long have you been practicing law? You've never had a rough deposition? You've never thrown an elbow?"

"You tore into the guy!"

"The hell I did!" Judy raised her voice, though Mary was flashing her the peace sign.

"I'm calling because I expected you to apologize."

"Don't hold your breath."

"I'm warning you, I'm not going to let you treat Morrell that way tomorrow. I'm not."

"He's a liar, and I'll do what I have to do." Judy heard a click on the phone, which told her that another call was coming through. She checked the screen, and it was her mother calling from the hospital. She couldn't let it go to voicemail. "Rick, hold on, I have to take this call."

"We're in the middle of a conversation!"

"It's that emergency you couldn't let me postpone for. I'm sorry, please hold, and I'll be right back." Judy pressed the screen to hold his call, then picked up on her mother. "Mom, how is she?"

"Judy, this is your mother."

Judy felt like her head was going to explode. "Yes I know, I can tell from the phone screen. How's Aunt Barb?"

"The nurse just came out to say she's still in surgery, but that everything is going well."

"Thank God." Judy exhaled with relief. "Okay, Mom, let me call you right back, I'm on the other line."

"The nurse said it's going to take longer, but not to worry."

"Why longer?" Judy was about to swap calls but stopped herself.

"I don't know, dear."

"Does it mean something went wrong?" Judy felt a tremor of fear for her aunt.

"She told me not to worry."

"Did you ask what she meant?" Judy asked, her tone sharper than she intended.

"Don't be so critical."

"I wasn't being critical. I just asked a question."

"It's your tone, dear. Your tone is very critical."

"Mom, really?"

"What, 'Mom, really?'" Her mother imitated her, which was something Judy hated, but she let it go. She glanced at the phone screen, but Rick had hung up.

"I'm sorry, I'm trying to get as much information as I possibly can, because if the surgery takes longer—"

"Please stop. You're giving me a headache. This has been such a difficult morning. I've been updating your aunt's friends. Colleen keeps calling. They mean well, but it's a chore." Her mother sighed. "Between you and your aunt, I'm caught in the middle, pulled in both directions."

"No you're not, Mom." Judy exchanged a look with Mary, who got the message and let herself out of her office, which showed excellent judgment. "Look, I'm going to leave for the hospital. My deposition is over, so I'm going to pack some work and—"

"Why? There's no reason for you to come yet. She's still in surgery."

"I want to be there. I can work from there."

"Why go to the trouble?"

"It's no trouble, and I can be there when she gets out of surgery." Judy tried not to notice that her mother didn't say they could keep each other company.

"By the way, your aunt keeps talking about Iris. She even started crying about her, right before she left for the operating room."

"That's understandable, isn't it? They were friends." Judy remembered it was a touchy subject, so she dialed it back. "And any loss is traumatic, especially coming after Uncle Steve."

"Anyway, she wanted me to remind you to find out about the autopsy. She said the results were supposed to be in today."

"Okay, I'll follow up." Judy realized that her mother wasn't up to speed on Iris news. "Also I found out that Iris's apartment was broken into last night and searched. Her roommates weren't home, so nobody was hurt, but this confirms that the guy who hit me last night wasn't random."

"You keep saying that, dear, but I'm not sure you're right. There's a lot of crime in their neighborhoods."

Judy shuddered. "Mom, that sounds racist."

"No it's not. It's the truth. You told me that yourself. The police said robbery is rampant with the illegals."

Judy let that go, too. She didn't want to get into a political discussion. "Mom, I should hang up, okay? I'll make a call about the autopsy and pack up."

"Judy, there's one last thing. I don't think we should tell your aunt about this robbery business."

"You mean the fact that Iris's apartment was broken into?"

"Yes. I don't think there's any reason for her to know that right now."

"Why not?"

"She has much too much going on. I'd like her to focus on herself. Why stress her more?"

Judy hesitated. "I don't like keeping things from her."

"It's for her own good. I want her to take her mind off these morbid subjects, take care of herself, and get well. Trust me on this."

"Okay," Judy said, hearing the finality in her mother's tone. "We can tell her another time."

"That's right, when she's feeling better. Timing is everything."

"See you soon."

"Fine."

"And text me if there's anything—" Judy said, but her mother had already hung up.

Chapter Twenty-six

Judy hustled around her office, grabbing case files and packing her messenger bag, worried about her aunt. She wanted to get to the hospital right away, though she'd have to stop to drop off the fifty grand with the estates lawyer. Meanwhile, she was also on her cell phone, her white earwire jumping around as she moved, waiting for the call to Rick Kelin to connect.

"Richard Kelin's office," said a female voice, picking up.

"Hi, is he in?" Judy asked, then introduced herself because she didn't recognize the voice as Terry's, Kelin's secretary.

"No, he's out for the rest of the day. I can tell him you called."

"May I have his cell number?" Judy stuffed the *Adler* file into her messenger bag. She wanted to get on a better footing with Kelin before Morrell's deposition, but she'd be damned if she'd apologize. On the contrary, the way he'd overacted made her think that she was on the right track. She knew that Govinda would tell Morrell and that both men would have a few sleepless nights, which was the desired effect.

"I'm not permitted to give out his cell number. Sorry."

"He knows me, I'm opposing counsel, at Rosato and Di-Nunzio." Judy wedged her laptop into the messenger bag next to the *Adler* file.

"I'm sorry, I'm just not permitted to do that."

"Is Terry in? She knows me."

"She's on vacation this week."

"Okay, could you just tell him I called and he can return my call at my cell number?" Judy gave the secretary her number while she hoisted her messenger bag on her shoulder, then went into her desk and grabbed her purse.

"Will do, thank you."

"Thanks." Judy hung up, went online, and Googled the Chester County Coroner as she left her office. She pressed in the phone number and hurried down the hallway while the call connected, wondering if she could ever do just one thing at a time.

"Coroner's Office of Chester County, may I help you? This is the assistant coroner."

"Yes, thanks, I'm Judy Carrier and I'm calling about the autopsy of Iris Juarez. I think the results were supposed to be in today."

"Are you next of kin?"

"No, there's no next of kin in the country. I'm calling for my aunt, who will be taking care of the burial." Judy caught sight of Allegra in the library, opening cardboard boxes of the damages cases, and she took a quick turn to check in with her. Allegra looked up expectantly, and Judy flashed her the one-minute signal.

The assistant coroner continued, "In that case, there will be a fee for the report. Let me check if it's available. Please stay on the line."

"Thank you." Judy put the phone on mute and peeked in the cardboard box, which groaned with thick red accordions. She said to Allegra, "Are you checking to make sure we have the right files?"

"Yes." Allegra nodded, holding the list of case captions that Judy had emailed her.

"Good. Set them up for new matter reports, too."

"I will, but there are so many boxes, like three hundred."

"Why so many?"

"The medical files take up so much room. Some were scanned onto discs, but some of the cases are so old, it's mostly hard copy."

"Good job." Judy gave her a quick pat on the back, then turned to go. "Call me if you have any questions. I'll be at the hospital."

"I hope everything is okay," Allegra called after her.

"Hello, Ms. Carrier?" said the assistant coroner, returning. "I'm sorry, but that report has not been completed."

"Has the autopsy been performed?" Judy headed for the reception area, where Marshall stood beside her desk with the duffel bag of cash. There were two clients in the waiting room, and Marshall handed the bag over discreetly, then they nodded good-bye to each other.

The assistant coroner was saying, "Yes, the autopsy has been performed, but the report will not be complete until the close of business today. You'll have to call back then."

"Okay, I will. By the way, is there a toxicology report?" Judy hit the DOWN button for the elevator, hoisting the heavy bag to her shoulder.

"Yes, there is an initial toxicology report and it screens for the presence of illegal drugs."

"What about legal drugs? Does it test for that, too?" Judy wondered if Iris was abusing prescription medication, even counterfeit prescription medication.

"No. Further testing would be required to determine the presence of legal drugs, but there's a fee for that and we don't do it unless the coroner determines that it would be necessary."

The elevator arrived, the stainless steel doors rattled open, and Judy stepped inside the cab.

"Where is the body now?"

"In the hospital morgue. We should be releasing it tomorrow, so you may want to contact your funeral director. He will call us to coordinate the release on your behalf, rather, on your aunt's behalf."

"Thank you. I'll call later for the report."

"Good-bye now."

"Bye." Judy got off the elevator cab on the bottom floor and hurried through the crowded lobby with the duffel, trying not to be nervous that she was carrying so much cash. She acted normal, checking her email on the fly like everybody else. She scrolled through the first ten incoming and ascertained nothing needed immediate attention as she hurried through the exit doors, hit the pavement, strode to the curb, and spotted a Yellow cab almost instantly.

"Yo!" she called, flagging it down. She jogged to meet the cab at the curb, jumped inside, and closed the door behind her. The cabbie was a young African-American man, and he turned to her.

"Looks like you're in a hurry," he said with a friendly smile.

"I am. Can you take me to Fifteenth and Locust, then I'm going to run inside and ask you to wait?"

"Sure, no problem." The cabbie hit the gas, and Judy faced the window of the cab as they took off. The traffic wasn't bad, and the city whizzed past her, but she didn't see anything. She was worried sick about Aunt Barb. They reached the office quickly, and Judy flew out the cab door, into the mirrored building, up the shiny elevator, and finally into the old-school reception room of Eastwood & Respondi, where her classmate worked. He was one of the smartest kids on Law Review with her, but she hadn't seen him in ages. She hurried to the front desk with the duffel bag, where a dark-haired receptionist smiled up at her.

"Hello, how may I help you?"

"I'm Judy Carrier, here to see John Foxman, he's expecting me."

"Please have a seat," the receptionist said, picking up the receiver of the desk phone.

"But I'm in a hurry—"

"Judy?" said a voice that Judy recognized, and she looked over. It sounded like John, but it didn't look like John. She remembered him as super tall and super skinny, with thick glasses and an insanely studious manner, but he had changed, to say the least.

"John?" Judy asked, trying to keep the shock from her voice, and if John noticed that she was drooling, he didn't let it show. Either he had been working out or he was on steroids, but he looked tall and cut, filling out a sharply tailored dark suit with style. His formerly frizzy red hair had been tamed into short layers, and his blue eyes sparkled with amusement, which she guessed came with his new contact lenses.

"Judy, if you're in a hurry, come with me. We'll get this done quickly." John crossed the carpet to meet her and reached for the duffel. "Let me take the bag."

"Thanks." Judy handed it over and fell into step beside him, though his strides were big as they hustled down the hall. "Nice of you to see me on such short notice."

"I wanted to. You look great."

"You, too."

"I remember the way you used to dress." John smiled. "So . . . fun."

"I still dress fun, if not funny. I had a dep."

"You don't go to the reunions."

"No."

"You should. You're missed."

"Aw, thanks," Judy said, surprised at his warmth. They had been fellow Comment Editors, working together plenty of late nights, but hadn't dated. She couldn't even remember if he had a girlfriend in law school, just that he was one of the scruffy guys in hoodies that hung out in the Law Review office. "It's been a long time."

"Too long."

Well. "We grew up."

"It can't be avoided, can it?" John grinned crookedly, gesturing her into his office with a long arm.

"Thanks." Judy glanced around. His office was small but immaculate, with files organized on the credenza, labeled looseleaf binders on the shelves, and diplomas and certificates of admission on the walls. It was the décor of the geeky boy she remembered, but he had grown into a very different sort of man.

"If you could just sign these forms, I'll put this money in the bank next door, right away." John set the duffel down and reached for some blank forms on his desk, which had a polished maplewood top that was clear except for a laptop.

"It's not a PennBank, is it? I'm suing them."

"No, it's not, but I'm glad to see you're still the firebrand I remember." John slid the forms to Judy, then handed her a black enamel pen from his breast pocket. "Here, use my show-off pen. My father gave it to me when I passed the bar, back when pens still mattered."

"I will, thanks." Judy accepted the pen, and scribbled her name on the first form, noticing that John wasn't wearing a wedding ring and there was no masonry dust under his fingernail. Then she realized with a start that she hadn't thought of Frank today until this very moment, and not in a good way.

"You're signing a form that will permit me to set up an IOLTA account."

"What does that mean anyway?" Judy signed the second form.

"An Interest Only Lawyers' Trust Account. It's a clunky acronym for holding account, that's all. Any fund generates interest, and the question is where the interest goes and who owns it."

"Why didn't they just say that?"

"Because they're politicians."

"Ha." Judy finished signing the forms and handed him back the pen, which he returned to his breast pocket.

"Under the statute, the interest flows into a general fund used to improve access to the civil legal system."

"That's nice."

"Isn't it? We need the money in a safe place while we set up the estate, which will take some time to do. If we could open an estate in a day, then we wouldn't need the IOLTA account."

"I understand." Judy liked that John said *we,* as if her problem was his problem, too.

"If the money is put in an IOLTA account, there is no need to identify the owner to the bank. That works well in this situation, since we don't know who the rightful owner is."

"Right."

"Just so we're clear, the decedent was a Pennsylvania resident, correct?"

"Yes, but she was undocumented."

"That doesn't matter, for present purposes. As a Pennsylvania resident, her estate administration is governed by the Pennsylvania Estate and Fiduciary Code. You remember the basics from law school? The jurisdiction was different, but the legal fundamentals remain the same."

"No, I sucked at trusts and estates."

"I know you did. I remember." John chuckled, and so did Judy. "Anyway, the PEF Code gives a priority list of persons entitled to administer an estate. There is no will, I presume?"

"Not as far as I know."

"We can talk later about the larger questions regarding the administration of the estate, when you have more time. I wanted to make sure we were on the same page." John extended his hand, palm up. "May I have your driver's license, please? I need ID to set up the account, then I can let you go on your way."

"Thanks." Judy went into her purse, extracted her driver's license from her wallet, and handed it to him.

"Great." John slid out his iPhone, took a picture of her driver's license, and handed it back to her.

"So now the money's in your hands."

"It's more complicated than that, but I can explain it to you later. These funds are considered qualified funds under the Code of Professional Responsibility."

"Okay," Judy said, and she could tell from the authoritative tone in his voice that he knew what he was talking about, and she didn't have time to find out. "I should be getting to the hospital. My aunt's pretty sick."

"I'm sorry to hear that." John frowned slightly, with genuine sympathy in his eyes. "It would be gentlemanly of me to walk you to the elevator, but there are fifty thousand reasons I should stay right here."

"I agree." Judy smiled, and John smiled back, meeting her eye more directly than was professional.

"Why don't you call me tonight or tomorrow, and we can set up a time to talk about the next steps? It's a fairly involved process, getting you or your aunt appointed as the administrator of the estate."

"Really, why?" Judy asked, going to the threshold of his office.

"The world isn't set up for $50,000 that nobody wants to keep."

"It's not easy to do the right thing."

"No, it's not easy to do the *legal* thing." John titled his chin up, smiling. "I admire your aunt."

"So do I," Judy said, feeling her emotions well up. "Well, I'd better go. Thanks so much."

"Bye now. Call me."

"I will, thanks." Judy left the office and hustled down the hall through the reception room, down the elevator and out the lobby to the street, where the cabdriver was still waiting. She climbed in the cab and slammed the door behind her. "Thanks for hanging in."

"No problem. Where to?"

"The hospital, please."

"You got it." They took off, switching lanes in traffic, and Judy's head was swimming. She slid out her phone and checked to see if her mother had called or texted, but she hadn't. She checked her email reflexively, and noticed that new email had popped onto the screen. It was an official filing from the United States District Court, which permitted electronic filing in motions and cases, so it had to be something important.

She opened the email, concerned. **MOTION FOR SANCTIONS AGAINST PLAINTIFF'S COUNSEL JUDY CARRIER, ESQ., PURSUANT TO FEDERAL RULE OF CIVIL PROCEDURE 37**, read the title of the motion, and the caption of the action was *Linda Adler v. PennBank*. The motion had been filed on behalf of PennBank by Rick Kelin.

"What?" Judy gasped, aghast. Her heart sank as she skimmed the first few lines: **Movant PennBank asks this Court to sanction Plaintiff's Counsel Judy Carrier, Esq., for failure to cooperate in discovery, i.e., for inappropriate and abusive misconduct during the deposition of witness Mr. Devi Govinda . . .**

Judy couldn't believe what she was reading. Rule 37 was an extreme remedy, a last resort for when the discovery process was being obstructed, blocked, or the like. She had never seen it used the way Kelin was using it, against her. She read on: **Plaintiff's Counsel badgered and harassed the witness . . . Plaintiff's Counsel threatened that she would 'get' the witness at trial . . . Plaintiff's Counsel left Defense Counsel no alternative but to flee the deposition, in order to protect the shaken witness from further distress . . .**

The cab veered around the corner, and Judy scrolled through the motion, which was short, only two pages long. That must've been how Kelin had gotten it written and filed so quickly; either that or he had it ready, on a form. She turned to the last page, which was a certification signed by counsel that he had attempted to confer, in an effort to settle the dispute. At the bottom of the page was Richard Kelin's signature, after: **Defense Counsel called Plaintiff's Counsel and attempted to discuss this matter with her today, to no avail. Plaintiff's Counsel rudely cut off the conversation, then hung up on Defense Counsel . . . Defense Counsel cannot subject Witness Phillip Morrell to Plaintiff's Counsel, until this Court has ruled . . .**

Judy shook her head, disgusted. She understood what Kelin was up to and she kicked herself for leaving herself vulnerable. He wouldn't win the motion, but he'd bring her conduct to the attention of the Court, prejudicing the judge against her. She'd have to file a reply explaining herself, but the judge's first impression of her would be as a hothead. She had to hope it wouldn't prejudice him against Linda's case, or she'd never forgive herself.

Judy gritted her teeth, jostling in the moving cab. She had misjudged Kelin as a spoiled baby, but he was a sharp and aggressive litigator. His motion was typical of the behind-the-scenes gamesmanship that she hated, but she had no one but herself to blame. Her thoughts raced ahead, and the implications fell like dominoes, in a cause-and-effect chain of collapse. She'd have to write, research, and file a response to the motion right away, to mitigate the damage with the judge. She'd have to get the Morrell deposition rescheduled. She'd have to explain it to Linda, and worse, to Bennie.

The cab raced toward the hospital, and Judy looked to the window, realizing that as bad as it was, it paled in comparison to what Aunt Barb was going through.

This very minute.

Chapter Twenty-seven

"So what did the nurse say?" Judy asked, dumping her messenger bag and purse on the chair next to her mother, in the quiet waiting room. A young receptionist sat at the front desk, tapping on the computer keyboard, and the only other people were an older couple sitting together at the far end of the row, watching the news on a TV mounted in the corner, with closed captioning.

"She hasn't said anything new, since what I told you on the phone."

"What about why it was taking longer?" Judy slid out of her coat and put it on top of her stuff. "Did you ask why?"

"Yes, and she said she didn't know, but she'd keep us posted." Her mother pursed her lips, lipsticked a tasteful pink, which told Judy that she had just been in the bathroom, freshening her makeup.

"So that conversation was at about ten thirty, correct?"

"Yes, I suppose so, if I'm to be cross-examined." Her mother gestured at the empty chair beside her. "Please, have a seat."

Judy checked her watch, which showed 12:01. "So that was an hour and a half ago."

"I can subtract, dear. Sit down."

"Hold on." Judy hovered over her chair and glanced back at the receptionist. "I'm saying because it's been an hour and a half, so it seems reasonable to ask how things are going."

"Don't ask any more questions. If there's something we need to know, they'll tell us."

Judy almost laughed out loud. "Mom, I'm a lawyer. If I ran my life that way, I'd be out of a job."

"Do you have to be a lawyer, every minute?"

"Honestly, yes."

"You're not in a courtroom. You're in a hospital."

"So what? I don't think it's a bad thing, to be a lawyer in a hospital."

"I do."

"I don't," Judy shot back, defensive. "It's good to be an advocate when you're in a hospital. Aunt Barb can't do it herself, so she needs us to be her advocate."

"Oh for goodness' sake, sit down."

Judy glanced back at the receptionist, who was now on the phone. "What's the big deal? I can't go ask a question?"

"She's just a receptionist. She's not a nurse. She doesn't know anything." Her mother inhaled slowly, which Judy recognized as her long-suffering martyr sound.

"She can find it out, Mom."

"That's not how it works. The doctor comes out and talks to you, or the nurse. The receptionist doesn't tell you anything." Her mother brushed a hair back into its silky blonde topknot, a reflexive gesture, since every strand was in place.

"That doesn't mean you can't ask."

"But what's the point?" her mother asked sharply.

"The point is that I'm worried something happened!" Judy raised her voice, not bothering to check herself. She couldn't shake the stress of the morning, the botched deposition, or the

Rule 37 motion. "Don't you want to know what's going on in there? She's your sister!"

"No, I don't want to know." Her mother rolled her eyes. "She's my own sister but I don't care. You're the only one who cares. Thank God you've arrived."

"Mom, really?"

"That must be it. You love her more than I do. To prove it, you'll go running around willy-nilly, asking questions that nobody will answer."

Judy felt her temper give way. "Mom, what's your problem? That's not what I'm going to do at all, and you can't know if somebody won't answer a question until you ask."

"Then *go ask!*" her mother hissed, her blue eyes flashing with anger. Her fair skin flushed under her foundation. "Why are you bothering me? You're a big girl. You're a lawyer, twenty-four/seven. If there isn't a fight, you'll pick one. You'll find one. You're not happy unless you're unhappy!" Her mother threw a hand toward the reception desk, then turned away. "Go ask whatever questions you want! You don't need my permission. God knows you never listened to me anyway."

Stung, Judy pivoted on her heel and charged toward the front desk, where the receptionist was hanging up the phone. "Excuse me, I was wondering—"

"Yes, I just got word that your aunt is out of surgery. She is being taken to the recovery room now and you'll be able to see her when she wakes up."

"Great." Judy felt tears of relief, or maybe frustration, come to her eyes, but she blinked them away. "When will that be?"

"It's usually an hour or more."

"Do you know why it took longer?"

"No, I don't."

"Is that typical or atypical?" Judy asked, without knowing exactly why. Maybe she wanted to know what to expect when she saw her aunt. Maybe she didn't trust the hospital to be forth-coming about anything that had gone wrong. Or maybe her mother was right, that if there wasn't a fight, she'd pick one.

"I don't know. I'm just a receptionist, not a nurse." The receptionist's dark eyes shifted toward Judy's mother and back again, and Judy felt embarrassed that the receptionist had over-heard her mother's comment.

"Sorry about that."

"No apologies are necessary." The receptionist looked away. "Unfortunately, the doctor was called in on another operation and so he won't be able to speak with you yet. The schedule is running behind, and he'll meet you in the recovery room just as soon as he can. He'll be able to answer your questions at that time. I can have a nurse come out and give you an update mo-mentarily."

"I would like that, thank you very much. Thank you." Judy walked stiffly back to the row of chairs against the wall and sat down next to her mother, who turned away, fake-reading an old copy of *People*. "She's fine and the nurse will see us—"

"I heard," her mother said, without looking up from the mag-azine, and Judy turned in the opposite direction and reached for her laptop to get started on a response to the Rule 37 motion. Mother and daughter sat stiffly side-by-side for the next fifteen minutes, until a cheery nurse in a blue scrub cap and patterned scrubs emerged from the door behind the reception desk and made a beeline for them.

"Ms. Carrier?" asked the nurse, and as she approached, a blue lanyard bearing her hospital ID bounced on her ample bosom.

"Yes?" her mother answered, looking up.

"That's us." Judy took her laptop off her lap and stood up to meet the nurse, who touched her arm with a friendly, reassuring smile.

"I have good news, ladies."

"Thank God." Judy eased back down in her chair, awash in a warm wave of gratitude as the nurse explained that Aunt Barb's surgery had been successful, but they were still waiting on further pathology tests of her tissue. The nurse said that she didn't know why it took longer, but that wasn't atypical, and she promised that the doctor would fill them in in the recovery room once Aunt Barb woke up. Judy's mother asked about the pain medication, which was Vicodin, and the drains, which seemed to preoccupy her, but Judy felt increasingly too emotional to bother with the medical details. She barely listened to her mother and the nurse, talking about the emptying and stripping of drains. She was just happy Aunt Barb had come through her surgery.

"Well, that's a relief," her mother said after the nurse had left, then returned to her magazine.

"I know." Judy felt the urge to hug her mother, who was evidently memorizing the magazine. "I'm sorry if I was short with you, Mom. I was just upset—"

"We both were," her mother answered without looking up, then lapsed into silence.

Judy didn't know whether her mother officially wasn't speaking to her and let it go. She picked up her laptop, turned her attention to the Rule 37 motion, and tried to draft coherent sentences, writing that she hadn't been abusive during Govinda's deposition, hadn't forced the witness or his lawyer to leave, and hadn't intentionally hung up on Kelin, but that the conversation had been accidentally terminated by an incoming call, which she explained only as a family emergency. She'd be damned if she'd trade Aunt Barb's privacy to win the motion, or for any other reason.

One hour stretched into two as Judy worked, keeping an eye on her laptop clock and wondering why Aunt Barb was taking so long to wake up. She finalized the motion, filed it electronically with the Court, then checked her email, which was piling up, and her phone messages, which would have to wait. Frank had texted **How's Aunt Barb?** And she texted back, **still waiting to hear the details, but it went okay, thx xoxo**. She thought briefly of John and felt reassured that the money was safe, even if its ownership caused problems they'd have to resolve down the line.

Finally, the nurse reappeared and escorted Judy and her mother to the recovery room, where Aunt Barb lay sleeping in a hospital bed, her head to the side, still in her plastic cap. Layers of cotton blankets covered her to her shoulders, and oddly, an IV port was stuck in the side of her neck as well as the top of her hand. Her skin had a gravely ashy hue, and her eyelids barely fluttered open when Judy and her mother took their places on opposite sides of her bed.

"Is she okay?" Judy asked the nurse, alarmed, as she set her stuff down on a chair. "She looks so pale."

"She's fine." The nurse closed the patterned curtain around them, giving them some privacy. "She's had something to drink, but she's sleepy. We gave her something for nausea, and you can expect her to have a dry throat from the intubation. She'll be in and out of sleep for the next hour or two, until she's up for good."

Judy took her aunt's hand, which felt chilly. "Aunt Barb, we're here. We love you."

Her mother frowned. "Don't wake her. She needs to sleep."

The nurse walked to the bed and picked up a white cylinder with a bright green light on one end, which was attached to a covered dispenser on a stalk. "Ladies, this is her pain medication. All she has to do is press this green light. It will dispense morphine every fifteen minutes, but not more frequently than that." She crossed back to an opening in the privacy curtain. "I'm here if you need anything. I'll be back to check on her."

"Thank you," Judy and her mother said in unison, then when they were alone, silence descended again, for a moment.

"Judy," her mother said, her tone weary. She sank into an institutional chair on the other side of the bed. Her makeup had worn off and her features finally relaxed, as if she had kicked out the emotional jambs. "Let go of her hand and sit down. It's going to be a while."

"I guess you're right." Judy was hoping to make peace, so she released her aunt's hand, rolled over a stool on wheels, and perched on it uncomfortably.

"She doesn't look that good, does she?" Her mother gazed down at Aunt Barb, with a slight frown. "She is pale, but it's probably the stress of the procedure. The trauma of it."

"I'm sure but they got all the cancer, so that's wonderful." Judy felt her heart lift, but her mother seemed not to hear her.

"I watched a video of it on YouTube. It's not a pretty operation."

Judy recoiled. "I'm just glad it was a success."

"They have everything on the Internet nowadays." Her mother's gaze remained on Aunt Barb. "You can see medical videos of a breast reconstruction, of mastectomies with the flap or without one, same with expanders. Everything you can imagine. Women make their own video blogs, too. Survivors, that is. I found it very helpful. You should take a look."

Judy couldn't imagine taking a look.

"It's a wealth of information."

Judy didn't reply, realizing that when she and her mother were talking, it was never real conversation, wherein one person replied to the other. It was more like they both took turns filling up the air with words, in a series of familial non sequiturs.

"We should be quiet so she can sleep," her mother added,

though she was the only one talking, so Judy conceded the obvious, that she might as well work while her aunt was asleep. She leaned over, grabbed her bag, unpacked her laptop, and lost herself in her email for another hour.

"Iris?" her aunt whispered, out of the blue.

"Huh?" Judy placed the laptop on the floor and rolled her stool over to the bed and clutched the bed rail, and her mother did the same thing on the other side of the bed.

"It's Delia. Barb? Are you awake?"

"Iris?" her aunt whispered again, her eyelids fluttering.

"Not Iris, Delia," her mother answered, pursing her lips.

"Aunt Barb, it's Judy and Mom." Judy reached for her aunt's hand, which felt warmer. "We're here, and you're fine. Your operation was fine."

"Iris," her aunt said, more distinctly, and opened her eyes. Her gaze was an unfocused blue, shifting from Judy to her mother, taking them in only vaguely. "Oh, hello . . . I was thinking of . . . Iris."

Judy squeezed her hand. "We love you, Aunt Barb. We're here for you."

"Iris was with me . . . she helped me . . ." Her aunt's voice trailed off. "She was there with me . . . in the beginning, before they put the mask on . . . I could feel her presence . . ."

"Really?" Judy asked, surprised, but her mother shot her a look.

"Judy, please don't encourage this. You'll have her seeing ghosts, for God's sake." Her mother picked up a small bottle of water from the bed table and twisted off the cap. "Barb, are you thirsty? Does your throat hurt?"

"Judy?" Aunt Barb turned her head toward Judy and squeezed her hand, though her grip was weak. "Do you . . . hear me . . . about Iris? I mean, I know she's . . . gone . . . but she was *there* . . . she told me everything was going to be okay . . . I felt so *comforted* . . ."

"Aw," Judy said, touched. "I bet that was very comforting."

"It was and I . . . I . . . want to know what happened to her . . . I want to know . . . what time is it . . . today is Monday, right? Is it?"

"Yes, it's Monday." Judy checked her watch. "It's about five thirty."

"Today was the day . . . you were going to find out . . . you're going to call somebody . . . about Iris . . ."

Judy's mother interjected, "Barb, have some water, will you? The nurse told us your throat would be dry. Are you in any pain?"

Aunt Barb shook her head, agitated. "It hurts, my chest . . ."

Judy's mother reached for the white morphine dispenser. "Here. You have pain meds, dear."

Aunt Barb ignored her, turning to Judy. "Judy, did you . . . call? What did they . . . say?"

Judy patted her aunt's hand. "You mean about Iris's autopsy? I called earlier today, but they said to call back later and I didn't get a chance."

"Call them . . . I want you to call them . . . I want to know . . . I want to know what happened to Iris . . . I owe that to her . . ."

"Now?" Judy asked, off-balance. "You really want to know that now?"

"Barb, I can't stand to see you in pain." Her mother thrust the morphine cylinder toward Aunt Barb. "Please press the button. You'll feel better. This isn't the time to be worrying about Iris. This is the time to be worrying about yourself."

Judy added, "Aunt Barb, I wonder if they're even there. It's after business hours."

Judy's mother pressed the green button for the morphine. "Here, let me help. This will make you feel better. Calmer."

Judy looked over, as the clear morphine ran down the tube. "Mom, she should do that, not you. Don't you think?"

Her mother raised an eyebrow. "Why? I want her to be comfortable."

"Call them . . . Call them . . . they have to be there . . ." Her aunt shook her head in confusion, and whether it was the effect of the drugs or she was really concerned, Judy wanted to placate her.

"Okay, Aunt Barb. I'll go call them and be right back." Judy released her aunt's hand, dug in her blazer pocket for her phone, and passed through the opening in the privacy curtain. Signs were posted prohibiting the use of cell phones, so she hurried from the recovery room, through a swinging door past the reception desk, and into the waiting area. Most of the seats were filled with people on phones and e-readers, plus reading some actual books, so she scrolled through her recent phone calls, located the number, and pressed CALL.

"Chester County Coroner's Office," answered a young woman's voice.

"I'm Judy Carrier, and I spoke earlier to the assistant deputy coroner. I'm wondering about the results on the autopsy of Iris Juarez. Would you happen to know if those results are in?"

"I'll try to find out, bear with me," the woman answered, and in the background came the clacking of computer keystrokes. "This isn't usually my job. I'm filling in because we're shorthanded."

"I understand."

"I see a notation that you called earlier and that you're an attorney with Rosato and DiNunzio, representing the family."

"Yes, that's me." Judy wasn't about to bother with technicalities. "Do you have the results?"

"No, sorry, I don't know how to open the file from the pathologist. I don't have the password. Like I say, this isn't my job."

"When can I get the results?"

"It will have to wait till tomorrow. Call or come by. Are you local?"

"Kind of."

"Sorry about the inconvenience. Everybody's out at a job tonight, a high-profile case. It's very sad, you'll probably see it on the news. One of our local priests, Father Keegan, was killed tonight in a hit-and-run."

Chapter Twenty-eight

Judy walked down the glistening hallway, her mind reeling. Hospital staff and families with get-well flowers and Mylar balloons passed her, but she avoided eye contact. Father Keegan had been killed, when she had just talked to him this morning. She didn't know how to react, or what to do, or whether to tell her aunt. She spotted a restroom down the hall and hustled there.

She pressed open the door, crossed to the sink, and splashed cold water on her face, trying to recover. The ladies' room was empty and small, only three sinks and stalls. The chill of the water woke her up, but she couldn't deny the growing realization that something was really wrong. She reached for a paper towel and dried her face, but her thoughts kept churning. Father Keegan's death struck her as too coincidental. The coroner's office had said it was a hit-and-run, but maybe it wasn't an accident. Maybe it was connected to Iris's death. And Daniella's disappearance.

Judy tossed the paper towel in the bin and tried to gather her thoughts. She knew she was speculating, but she couldn't help herself. She replayed her conversation with Father Keegan in her mind and couldn't fight an increasing sense of guilt for what happened to him. She leaned against the white tile wall, closing her eyes in pain. She had told the priest that Iris was involved in wrongdoing. He hadn't believed her; he'd found it inconceivable. What if he had started to dig and one of the conspirators had found out? Would they kill him to stop him from digging further? Was it the same people who had attacked her last night? What was going on?

Judy slid her phone from her pocket and pressed FAVORITES. The call rang twice, and she said, "Mary, do you have a minute?"

"What's the matter?" Mary asked, alarmed. "Is Aunt Barb okay?"

"She's fine, but I just found out that Father Keegan is dead, in a hit-and-run."

"The priest? Oh no." Mary moaned.

"I feel so terrible." Tears came to Judy's eyes. "It's my fault. I didn't know, I didn't think—"

"What are you talking about? How can it be your fault?"

"I told him about the money today and that I thought Iris was dealing drugs. He didn't think it was true. What if he started digging and they killed him?"

"That's possible, but that doesn't mean it's your fault."

"Why not?" Judy asked miserably. "I told him about it. If he wanted to get to the bottom of it, it was because of our conversation."

"No, you're not responsible for that. Whoever hit him was responsible for that, whether it was an accident or not. Why do you think it's not an accident? Have you spoken to the police?"

"No, the coroner, but it just seems too coincidental. Think of the chain of events. Iris's death, finding the money, my getting attacked, and Iris's apartment was ransacked last night, too."

"It was?"

"Yes, right before we were attacked. That's what Father

Keegan called to tell me about. Somebody is looking for that money."

"You think?"

"Yes, I think that Father Keegan started asking around after he spoke to me, and somehow at the end of the day, he ended up . . ." Judy couldn't bring herself to say the words. "Oh my God. This is terrible. It could've been murder."

"You don't know that yet. You don't have any real evidence or facts."

"Agree, it's circumstantial, but it's compelling."

"I have to admit, it is, and we know that every hit-and-run isn't necessarily an accident." Mary's tone turned grave, and Judy remembered that Mary's first husband was murdered almost the same way, struck by a car years ago, while he was riding his bicycle on West River Drive.

"I'm sorry, I didn't mean to bring that up."

"No, honey, it's okay," Mary added quickly. "So where are you now? What are you going to do?"

"I'm at the hospital. Should I tell my aunt? I didn't tell her about Iris's apartment being broken into. My mother didn't want me to."

"I get that, and I'd hold off for now. Is she okay? She has to be going through hell."

"The surgery went fine, and she's coming around." Judy made a gut decision. "I don't think I'll tell her, yet. But she's going to want to know the autopsy results on Iris and I don't have those yet."

"So tell her that, but not about the priest."

"Agree." Judy felt reassured that she and Mary were on the same page.

"She'll be stronger tomorrow, and you'll know more."

"I hope so." Judy straightened up, with a final sniffle. "I better go back now."

"You need anything? I can come down there. I'm home, or-dering takeout."

Judy hadn't eaten but didn't feel hungry. "No thanks, I'm fine, and by the way, the money's safe in a bank."

"Good. Keep me posted. Love you."

"Love you too, bye." Judy pressed END to hang up, slipped the phone back into her jacket, and checked her reflection on the way out. The strain showed on her face, and her blue dressed-up-for-deposition suit was rumpled, but she tried to get it together as she left the bathroom. She hit the hallway and hurried back to the recovery room, where she pushed the pri-vacy curtain aside to find her mother helping her aunt sip some water from a bottle.

"What did you find out?" her aunt asked, after her mother moved the bottle.

"So far, not much." Judy managed a smile, crossing to her aunt's bedside. "I . . . couldn't find the right person to talk to. How do you feel?"

"Better," her aunt answered, though the corners of her mouth turned down. "There's pain, but I'm thinking more clearly. What do you mean, you couldn't find the right person?"

"I mean, the deputy assistant coroner wasn't there and the young woman I spoke with didn't know how to open the re-port." Judy went with a half-truth, since she was the worst liar in the Bar Association.

"So there's a report, but they couldn't open it?"

"Evidently. I'll try again tomorrow."

"Isn't there someone else you can call? I won't sleep until I know what happened to her."

Judy's mother snorted, easing back into her chair. "After that morphine, you'll be asleep in ten minutes."

Judy started to get another idea. "I suppose I could make a few more calls, but it would be easier to do from the office.

They're not big fans of cell phones here. The sign says it interferes with the machines."

Aunt Barb blinked. "So go to the office. I'd love it if you can find out those results and I know you have work to do. Feel free to go, really."

Judy's mother nodded. "Honestly, honey, I can handle everything here. The nurse was just in and said they're going to move her to a room. I'll stay and get her situated, and by then visiting hours will be over. They end at eight o'clock."

Judy looked from her aunt to her mother, her heart beginning to beat with anticipation. "You sure you don't need me here to help?"

Aunt Barb smiled wanly. "You can help me the most by getting the coroner's report."

Her mother flashed a smile that looked oddly relieved. "You can help me the most by getting out of my hair."

"Very funny," Judy said, faking a smile. She had better things to do than fight with her mother.

An hour and a half later, Judy was getting out of her car, having found a parking space in the municipal lot across from the Kennett Square Police Station. She felt bad about lying to her mother and aunt, but she'd had no intention of going into the office. She was burning to find out what happened to Father Keegan, having driven here with her brain on fire, convincing herself of a connection between Iris's and the priest's deaths. She hoped that she could convince the police that she was right, or at least to consider the possibility and investigate her theory. Detective Boone had given her his business card, and she'd tried to call him on the way over, but there had been no answer and the message had gone to voicemail.

Judy walked through the parking lot, heading for the police station, which was completely unassuming. It bore no sign except for a small navy-blue keystone, which was unlighted and therefore unreadable in the darkness. Only a single light over its paneled front door illuminated the small, red brick building that could have passed for a modest single-story house, situated between a low-rise Tudor apartment building and a stop-time laundromat, with a misspelled sign that read LAUNDERMAT. A small parking lot around the right side of the station house held five police cruisers, white with a black stripe, and one all-black car, unmarked.

Judy approached the paved entrance in front of the station, which buzzed with activity. Men in suits and brown-uniformed police stood outside, talking or smoking in groups, and neighbors filled the sidewalk, gawking at TV reporters who were positioning themselves in calcium-white circles of klieglights. Boxy newsvans with local TV logos lined the curb, their black rubbery wires making tripping hazards on the sidewalk and their mobile microwave towers dwarfing the colonial rowhouses on the quaint side streets.

Judy made her way through the crowd to the front door, then opened it onto a small, square waiting room full of personnel, reporters, and men in suits. To her left was a closed door with a sign that read MAYOR'S OFFICE, and to her right were blue-padded chairs where reporters and cameramen sat drinking covered cups of coffee, cameras on their lap.

She walked past them, doing a double-take when she spotted on the wall a signed lithograph from one of the Wyeths, the famed painting family who lived in nearby Brandywine. The art alone qualified Kennett Square's as one of the nicest station houses she'd ever seen, but it also had a thick lapis-blue rug, eggshell-white walls, and one of exposed brick, in which was embedded a rectangular window of glass.

Judy went to the window and introduced herself to a middle-aged woman with bright blue eyes and a warm, professional smile, then said, "I'd like to speak with Detective Boone, in connection with the death tonight of Father Keegan."

"Is he expecting you?" the woman asked, brightly. She wore her light brown hair in a bun and had on an orange T-shirt with KENNETT SQUARE POLICE printed onto the breast pocket, with khaki pants.

"No, but I left a phone message."

"Is this a tip? Because he's very busy tonight." The woman shook her head sadly. "It's a terrible loss."

"I do have information that I believe can help him. He knows me because he's been working on a case involving my aunt, Barb Moyer."

"Oh, my, I know who you are." The woman's eyes registered recognition. "You're the woman who was assaulted last night, aren't you?"

"Yes," Judy answered, moving her hair aside to show her goose egg. "This is me, the real thing."

"Go to your left, and I'll buzz you in the door," the woman said, hurrying off.

Chapter Twenty-nine

"We're meeting in here?" Judy asked, following Detective Boone, who was unlocking the door to the Mayor's Office. "Won't the mayor mind?"

"This is Kennett Square, not New York City." Detective Boone led her inside a small, completely empty office lined with tasteful walnut bookshelves full of leather-bound volumes of law books and black plastic binders. A clean mahogany desk and old-school courtroom chair sat in the far corner next to the American flag, and nearest the door was a modern round conference table, also of walnut, with three matching chairs.

"Where's the mayor?"

"It's after hours." Detective Boone tugged out one of the chairs and gestured to Judy to sit down. "Please."

"Thanks." Judy sat down, getting her bearings. "I thought we'd meet in the squad room, like they do in Philadelphia."

"Technically, it's not my squad room." Detective Boone sat down in the chair opposite her. "The county detectives' office is in West Chester. When we're out on a job, like tonight, we're squatters. How's that noggin of yours?"

"Fine, but I'm so sorry to hear about Father Keegan."

"Me, too. He was a great guy. It's a real blow to the community." Detective Boone slid a ballpoint pen from his pocket, along with his skinny spiral notebook. He looked the same as he had last night; his close-set blue eyes intense and concerned behind his wire-rimmed glasses, his sandy brown hair in its short, professional cut, and he had on another boxy dark suit with a patterned tie. "Do you have something for me, on Keegan? They said you had a tip."

"I spoke to him this morning, on the phone. He called me because he'd read that I was assaulted and he wanted to tell me that Iris's apartment had been broken into and ransacked. Did you know about that?"

"No." Detective Boone flipped open the cardboard top to his notebook. "Anybody assaulted or injured?"

"No. Nobody was home."

"Anything taken?" Detective Boone started taking notes.

"Nothing of value. I think they were looking for the money that Iris had stashed in my aunt's house." Judy wanted to get to the point. "Detective, I believe that Father Keegan's death is linked to Iris Juarez's. I think they were both murdered."

"What are you talking about?" Detective Boone frowned, looking up from his note-taking. "Father Keegan was a hit-and-run accident."

"Can you explain to me how it happened?"

Detective Boone hesitated. "I'll tell you what's public record. He was struck from behind, along the curve, walking to his car. It's very dangerous there, there's no sidewalk. It happened at about five fifteen, and it was dark. The car was driving north, so it couldn't have seen him when it turned the corner."

Judy tried to visualize the scene, though she had never been there, and it tugged at her heart to imagine the priest in the last minutes of his life, not knowing that a deadly car was bearing down on him. Still she reminded herself not to be emotional. If she really wanted to convince the detective of anything, she had to keep her wits about her. She asked, "What was he doing there, by the side of the road?"

"There's a little restaurant, called Jamie's. He was walking from the restaurant to his car, which was parked in the side lot."

"Where's the restaurant?"

"On Warm Spring Road, number 870, I believe. It's at the curve."

Judy made a mental note. "What's the cross street?"

"Closest one is Buck and Doe."

"That's a street name?"

"Yes, city girl." Detective Boone almost smiled.

"Did anybody see anything, like in any of the surrounding stores or houses?"

"There aren't any. It's on the outskirts of town."

"Another remote stretch? Why am I not surprised?" Judy felt more convinced than ever, now that she was getting the facts. "Was he alone?"

"Yes. He eats there every night, the early-bird special, soup and sandwich."

Judy thought a minute. "How do you know that? From asking around?"

"Of course, yes."

"So it was generally known?"

"Everybody knew about it, in the parish. He even used to meet with parishioners there. They would seek him out. I heard that from more than one person."

"It was that well-established a routine?"

"Most of us are creatures of habit. That doesn't mean anything." Detective Boone cocked his head. "We figure it was a drunk driver. We get a lot of that out here. Country life can be boring, for kids and the like. And if they're undocumented, they're going to keep driving. Either way, they won't get away with it. We're all over it." He gestured toward the waiting room. "But let's go back a moment. When was Iris's apartment burglarized?"

"Last night at about six o'clock, right before I was attacked at my aunt's house. I think the bad guys, whoever they are, are looking for the money. They went to her apartment, then they went to my aunt's."

"The address we have? On Point Breeze?"

"Yes."

"Were there any witnesses?"

"Not that I know of, but you have to follow up with that."

"We will, but it's going through the motions. They're not going to tell us anything, just like they didn't report it."

"But you will try anyway, won't you?"

"Of course."

"What about Iris's phone? Did you follow up with that, about that call she got?"

"Yes, but we can't find a phone. The police at the scene didn't bag one, neither did the coroner."

Judy blinked. "She had one, I saw it."

"Do you know for a fact that she had it on her?"

"No, but why wouldn't she?" Judy thought about it. "Whoever killed her took it."

"I'll keep investigating." Detective Boone returned to his note-taking. "What about the money? What did you decide to do with it?"

"It's safely in a bank right now." Judy had to get back on track. "I called the coroner to find out the autopsy results on Iris, but I couldn't because they were all working on the Father Keegan case. But if it turns out that she died of unnatural causes—"

"Excuse me, I'm not following." Detective Boone held up a hammy hand, with the pen. "What does Father Keegan have to do with Iris? I'm assuming she was a parishioner, but what of it? Most of the Mexicans in the county belong to that church, or St. Agnes."

"When I spoke to him this morning, I told him about the cash in my aunt's house and that I thought that Iris was in a drug ring. He knew her very well, and he refused to believe that she would be involved with anything illegal." Judy felt her chest tighten, and another wave of guilt washed over her, but she tried to stay on point. "I'm betting that after he hung up, he tried to get to the bottom of it. Maybe he started asking questions about her death, or about drug dealing in the community, and whoever is selling the drugs, or whatever, got wind of it and killed him to silence him."

"This is speculation," Detective Boone said, but his wrinkled forehead showed that he was mulling it over.

"It's not speculation, it's circumstantial, and there's a difference." Judy found her bearings, now that she'd learned the facts about how the priest had died. "If Father Keegan had a routine of going to this restaurant and the bad guys heard that he was digging around, then they could very easily predict where he'd be, right?"

Detective Boone didn't reply, but met her eye and ceased his note-taking.

"It gets dark early, this time of year. If they know generally what time he leaves the restaurant, they could plan for it and run him over. It would look like a hit-and-run, but it could really be murder." Judy leaned forward, encouraged by his interest. "What do you think?"

"That's a possibility," Detective Boone answered, after a moment.

"It certainly is. Between what I know and what you know, if we work together, we can figure this thing out."

Detective Boone lifted an eyebrow. "Don't get the wrong idea here. I'm listening to you, but I am *not* working with you."

"Okay, I understand." Judy dialed back her enthusiasm.

"The other possibility is that Father Keegan's death was an accident and Iris Juarez died of natural causes. You call this circumstantial, but I think it's speculation, and either way, none of it is supported by any evidence or facts." Detective Boone picked up his notepad and abruptly rose to his feet. "Excuse me for five minutes."

"Sure," Judy answered, surprised. "Where are you going?"

"Be right back," Detective Boone answered, heading for the door. He opened it, letting in noise and chatter from the waiting room, then closed it behind him.

Judy sat back in her chair, feeling her heart begin to thump. The more she thought about it, the more her theory made sense, though she had no idea how to go about proving it. She felt driven to find out what had really happened to Father Keegan, not only to bring his killers to justice, but to help her redeem herself for his death. She felt her throat tighten with emotion but swallowed hard to keep it at bay.

Judy reflexively pulled out her phone to check her text and email, on lawyer autopilot. There were no new texts from Frank and she read through her incoming email, but there was nothing important from any of her clients or from opposing counsel, like Rick Kelin. She'd have to catch up with their other cases at some point, but she couldn't begin to think about that now. She scrolled to the phone function to call her mother and check on Aunt Barb. The call went to voicemail after one ring, but she didn't leave a message.

Suddenly, the door to the office opened, letting in a burst of crowd noise as Detective Boone entered the room carrying a sheaf of papers, but his demeanor had changed. His expression had snapped back into its official mask, his blue-eyed gaze had cooled and his thin lips formed an unsmiling, if professional, line. "You want facts? I have facts."

"What?" Judy asked, intrigued.

"Iris Juarez died of natural causes. She had a heart attack. This is the pathologist's report." Detective Boone set down the sheaf of papers on the conference table. "I spoke with him and he emailed me a copy of his findings."

Judy felt dumbfounded as she slid the papers over. Her eyes shot to the top line, which had a blank for **Cause of Death** and stated **MYOCARDIAL INFARCTION**. "Oh no."

"In law enforcement, we consider this good news. A natural death is better than murder, correct?" Detective Boone walked around the table, returned to his chair, and sat down, crossing his legs.

"I can't believe this." Judy skimmed the report, which seemed like a thorough autopsy report, typical in every way.

"I think this should put your theory to rest, on Father Keegan as well."

"I don't get it," Judy said, stumped. She flipped through the report until she reached the section for **Internal Examination of Organs**, and the description of Iris's heart read that its **arteries showed evidence of atherosclerotic cardiovascular disease, A.S.C.V.D.**

"He said that there's a real problem in the undocumented community because they don't get the medical care they need to control heart disease and hypertension."

"Did they find any drugs in her system?" Judy flipped to the back of the report, where the toxicological screens were usually attached as an appendix, but there wasn't one.

"The tox screen takes two to three weeks to come in and it will show if there was alcohol or drugs in her system."

"What about legal drugs?"

"The basic covers only illegal drugs, not legal ones."

Judy looked up. "Can we test her now for legal drugs? Do they keep the blood? How does that work?"

"An expanded takes longer, and it doesn't happen unless a detective or the pathologist believes it's in order. He didn't request it."

"Would you request it?"

"No." Detective Boone shook his head. "Iris Juarez died a natural death. She wasn't the victim of a homicide. You're a lawyer, you know that police departments are subject to budget constraints. If I authorize expenditures on Juarez, then I won't have it in a case where I have evidence of a suspicious death."

"How much does it cost?"

"Basic is $120, expanded is $160."

"Listen, if it's just a question of cost, I'll pay for it myself. I'd like to request the coroner to do a screen of her blood for legal or prescription drugs, an expanded. How do I do that?"

"You have to get in touch with the coroner's office tomorrow. They may or may not do it." Detective Boone shook his head. "But what is it *exactly* you're hoping to find?"

"Detective, I admit, I don't know what I'm looking for. If I did, I wouldn't be looking for it. Maybe abuse of prescription medication, counterfeit medication, something like that."

"Point of information, what comes in from Mexico isn't prescription meds or counterfeits. It's heroin. And it doesn't originate in Mexico but comes through it, because it's easier to smuggle heroin into Mexico than the States. Generally, the dealers pay mules to carry it up north, for distribution and sale."

Judy couldn't picture Iris as a heroin smuggler or dealer, but something still stunk to high heaven. "Do you have a heroin problem in the county?"

"No more than elsewhere in the state, to my knowledge."

Detective Boone paused. "If the pathologist had found trace evidence of heroin on her hands or fingers, it'd be different. But he didn't."

Judy checked the report, flipping to the external examination of Iris's hands, which read, **broken fingernails on right index and right middle finger with superficial scrapes on fingerpads**. "Look at this, the broken fingernails. How did she get those?"

"She could have done that a number of ways, none of which is suspicious at all."

"In a struggle?"

"There weren't any signs of any struggle or defensive wounds of any kind."

Judy tried another tack. "What about heroin on the money? How do I get the money tested?"

"I believe there are private labs that do that. Check online."

Judy gathered the autopsy report in case her aunt wanted to see it. "What about the fifty grand, the assault on me, and Father Keegan? How do you explain it?"

"Rest assured, we're investigating the hit-and-run and will continue to do so. Father Keegan meant a great deal to us, and we will give him a hundred percent of our efforts. As for the money"—Detective Boone shrugged mildly—"granted, I can't explain it, but there's no crime that has been committed and even if there were, it's a matter for the Kennett Square police. They have only twelve officers full time, so they work closely together. They're all aware of what happened at your aunt's house. That's how you got past the front desk to me tonight, isn't it?"

"Yes," Judy had to concede.

"Trust me, it's the talk of the squad room. Leave it to them. They're small-town, but they're professional. Don't underestimate them just because they're not big-city." Detective Boone rose, brushing down his slacks. "If you observe anything further or, God forbid, are a victim of another attack, you need to call them."

"I appreciate your time, but I just can't accept this, not yet anyway." Judy rose, feeling as if she had failed Father Keegan, Iris, and her aunt. Even herself. "Maybe if the only thing that happened was that Iris had a heart attack, I would believe it, but taken as a whole, I'm just not buying that it's all innocent."

"Good night." Detective Boone walked to the doorway, put his hand on the doorknob, and opened the door. "If there's anything you need to know, we will contact you."

"Thank you," Judy said miserably, but she was already thinking of her next move.

Chapter Thirty

Judy pulled over and let the engine idle across the street from Jamie's Restaurant, unable to get closer because the area had been cordoned off with parked cruisers, flares, and sawhorses. Uniformed police and other personnel gathered in groups inside the perimeter, and reporters clustered on the outside. A chubby traffic cop stood with an orange flashlight, ready to direct traffic around the scene, though the only car was Judy's.

The coroner's van must have already gone, and a police truck was towing away an old blue minivan, presumably Father Keegan's. Judy felt a pang at the sight, thinking how awful it must have been for the priest to die this way, by the side of the road, in shock and pain. She felt a new wave of guilt and grief, and being there felt like an awful replay of Saturday night, when Iris had been found in her car.

Judy cut the ignition, and got out of the car to look around. The air was cold, and Warm Springs Road would have been pitch black except for the lights from the police vehicles. She surveyed the street, which was just as she had pictured it, completely deserted and lined by tangled underbrush and thick dark woods on both sides, with no houses or shops. It was barely wide enough to accommodate two lanes, which ran in different directions and curved dramatically around the restaurant, a small converted house of white clapboard that couldn't have held more than eight tables. Light came from inside the restaurant, and she could see police personnel milling at the counter.

Judy walked along the road toward the restaurant, and now that she could see the lay of the land, it was easy to reconstruct how Father Keegan could have been killed. The restaurant was situated at the elbow of the curve, and a car driving past could have targeted someone walking toward its parking lot, with their back turned. There was neither a curb nor a shoulder, just some gravel, and nothing would have protected the priest from a driver cutting the corner, intentionally or not.

Judy hurried across the street to the perimeter, but noticed she had drawn the attention of the traffic cop, who lumbered toward her, waving his orange flashlight. She pretended not to see him, turned away, and hustled in the opposite direction along the perimeter. When she got closer to the opposite side of the street, she could see in the flickering of the flares that several bouquets of flowers had been left there, a sight that broke her heart.

"Miss, Miss, please don't go back there!" the traffic cop called, catching up with her. "Miss, excuse me!"

"Officer, I just wanted to see." Judy gestured at the flowers, and the chubby face of the traffic cop softened under his cap.

"Condolences, but you can't be leaving your car where you did, Miss." The traffic cop waved his flashlight toward her car. "Please, move it out."

"Can't I just take a minute and look around?"

"No, you may not. You're creating a traffic hazard." The traffic cop waved her off again. "You want to pay your respects, you'd be better advised to do that in the daytime, when it's safer, or to head on over to the church tonight. I hear there's plenty of folks there, doing the same thing."

"Good idea. Thanks, Officer," Judy said, meaning it. She turned around and jogged toward her car, wondering why she hadn't thought of it herself.

Half an hour later, she was slipping into the back pew of the beautiful Madre de Dios Church, near where she had sat just yesterday morning, when she had come to Mass with her aunt. The lovely altar, with its simple crucifix and graceful marble statuary, was vacant now. It seemed impossible to fathom that Father Keegan had conducted that very Mass and shown such kindness to her and her aunt, as well as comfort to his congregation, and now, he was no longer here.

Tears came to Judy's eyes, but she didn't bother to blink them away, because she felt as if she belonged here, for the first time. It was emotion that connected her to the congregation, and it was her heart that connected her to all of the other hearts in the church. Grieving families filled the pews, their expressions stricken and their heads bowed, sniffling as they knelt with rosary beads hanging between their fingers, some praying silently and others whispering their prayers in Spanish or English. Women lit candles in front of a statue of the Virgin of Guadalupe near the altar, and a young priest went from one parishioner to the next, putting an arm around them and engaging them in quiet conversation.

Judy watched him, wishing again that she had some sort of religion, because she could see before her eyes the power that the priest had to comfort people and to ease their pain. The only thing she believed in was love, and that came close to a spiritual belief, maybe as close as she would ever get. The second thing she knew that she believed in was the law, and she felt her emotions slip into default mode, anger at the injustice of a crime as heinous as murder, especially of Father Keegan, a man of goodwill and open heart. She couldn't stay out of it, no matter what Detective Boone had said. She wouldn't rest until she learned the truth.

Judy kept an eye on the young priest and wondered if he could have information about what Father Keegan had been up to today, or know something else that could help her. She worried briefly that this wasn't the time or the place, but decided that there was no better time or place. She stood up, made her way out of the pew, and walked down the wide, tiled aisle of the church toward the priest.

He was speaking with an older woman near the altar and appeared to be finishing up, because he caught Judy's eye with a sad smile. He was short and stocky, and the shine in his round brown eyes betrayed the grief he was undoubtedly keeping inside. He looked in his thirties, with a head of thick black hair and no wrinkles in his wide face, just a smattering of pitting in his cheeks. He was dressed in a simple black uniform with a collar, not the vestments of a formal Mass.

"Hello, welcome to our church," the priest said, when he turned to Judy. His voice sounded soft with pain, and his English was perfect. "I'm Father Oscar Vega."

"Thank you, I'm Judy Carrier, and please accept my deepest sympathies on the loss of Father Keegan. I didn't know him well, but I can see that he was a remarkable man."

"He was, he was, truly." Father Vega winced, evidence of his grief. "I came to this parish two years ago, and he took me under his wing. He was old-school, but at the same time such an innovator, working hard with the outreach groups with parenting education, literacy education, and substance-abuse counseling. We won't see another one like him."

"I'm sure that's right. I came just yesterday, for the first time. It's so hard to believe that Father Keegan is gone, that quickly."

"I understand how you feel." Father Vega nodded, buckling

his lower lip. "I feel the same way, and he mentioned to me that he had met you, Ms. Carrier."

"Please, call me Judy. He did?"

"Yes, and your aunt Barb is a very kind person. My sympathies to you both on the loss of Iris. Your aunt must be very upset."

"Thank you, she is." Judy had to find a way to get to the point, because the women in line behind them kept glancing over, wanting their turn.

"We will have to endure these tragedies with prayer and supporting each other. We have to remember times like this that God doesn't send us more than we can bear. He knows our strength more than we do ourselves."

"That's right." Judy saw her opening in the conversation. "Did Father Keegan mention to you that he spoke with me about Iris?"

"No, he didn't."

"Did you see him today, at all?"

"Yes, in the morning."

"Where was that?"

"At the rectory." Father Vega blinked, and Judy could see he didn't understand why she was asking, so she lowered her voice, not to be heard by the women in the line to light candles.

"I know this seems inappropriate, but I wanted to take this chance to explore with you anything you know about Iris. I feel that her death was suspicious and even Father Keegan's death, as well."

"What?" Father Vega's dark eyes flared with alarm. "Are you serious?"

"Yes." Judy almost regretted bringing it up, but she didn't want to wait. "Do you know what Father Keegan did today? If he met with anyone, visited anyone? Even called anyone?"

"As far as I know, he conducted a funeral mass in the morning."

"Why do you say, 'as far as I know'?"

"I wasn't here. On Mondays I travel to another church in Octorara. There's a shortage of priests, as you may know, and we're spread thin."

"So you wouldn't know firsthand what he did today? For example, if he made any phone calls or had any visits with anyone?"

"No, I wouldn't."

"You didn't see him or talk with him before he went to dinner?"

"No, I haven't seen him since this morning."

"And it's true that he eats dinner at Jamie's, in the early evening?" Judy found herself lapsing into deposition mode.

"Yes, I told the police that, too. They came by earlier this evening. They're the ones who notified me of his death."

Judy could see that the women behind him were waiting to talk to him, so she didn't mince words. "Father, I feel that Iris might have been involved with some kind of drug ring or some other illegal business that generated a lot of money. She hid cash in my aunt's house, and her death seems very suspicious."

"Drugs? Iris? No, not possible." Father Vega shook his head. "I understood she had a heart attack."

"I just don't believe it, and it seems too coincidental, now that Father Keegan was killed. It's also very strange that Iris's best friend Daniella suddenly decided to go back to Mexico—"

"What did you say?" Father Vega interrupted, a frown creasing his short forehead.

"Daniella went back to Mexico."

"She did? How do you know that?"

"That's what they told me at the mission yesterday. That's why she wasn't working there yesterday."

"She didn't tell me. Neither did anyone else." Father Vega shook his head again. "You must be mistaken, Judy."

"That's what they said. How do you know so much about her? I had the impression she wasn't a regular churchgoer."

"She wasn't but I was helping her, with counseling. Daniella is from my town at home. I heard about her from my mother and my sisters." Father Vega permitted himself a tight smile. "There's no Internet like Mexican family."

"Would she have gone back?"

"No. I haven't heard from her lately, but I'll call her at my first opportunity. I can't do it now, I'm busy." Father Vega gestured behind him at the line, where an older woman behind him kept looking over, impatient to speak with him.

"Do you have her number? May I have it?"

"I wouldn't do that without her permission. You understand."

Judy let it go. "Father Vega, I'm surprised that Father Keegan didn't tell me this when he found out that Daniella was gone, because I told him."

"He wouldn't know. I would."

"Is Daniella's family here? Do you think I could go speak with them?"

"The only ones in the country are in Newark, New Jersey."

"Is she married?"

"No longer, but there's a man she's been seeing." Father Vega's lips flattened in a way that suggested he wasn't a fan. "She met him at work."

"At Mike's Exotics?"

"Yes. I don't know much about him, but Daniella brought him to Mass one time and introduced me."

"What's his name?"

"Carlos Ramiro," Father Vega answered, and the older woman behind him stepped closer to him, hovering at his elbow.

"Where does he live?"

"In the barracks."

"What do you mean?"

"Some of the mushroom growers house their workers in barracks. His are on Mallard Road, where it meets Ravine."

"Thanks." Judy made a mental note, beginning to feel like a GPS map of Chester County.

"*Padre Vega?*" said the old woman, teary-eyed. She placed a hand on the priest's arm.

Father Vega turned to her, caught betwixt and between. "*Sí, Guadalupe, uno momento, por favor.*"

Judy knew it was time to go. "Father, I didn't mean to monopolize you. Thank you so much."

"*Padre Vega,*" the woman said again.

"Good night, Father." Judy turned away, hurried down the aisle, and out of the church.

Chapter Thirty-one

Judy braked, hesitating before she turned onto the makeshift driveway, two dirt ruts that divided a black tangle of underbrush tall enough to obscure whatever lay on the other side. The only reason she knew it had to be the barracks was that she was at the intersection on Ravine Road, a single-lane backroad with neither houses, stores, nor streetlights, in a rural pocket of East Grove, about six miles from Kennett Square and civilization.

Judy was brave, but not crazy, so she put the car in neutral, reached for her phone, and pressed in the number for Detective Boone. She wanted to see if she could convince him to meet her. The phone rang, but her call went to voicemail and she left a message: "Detective, this is Judy, I'm at the barracks at Mallard and Ravine. I want to find Carlos Ramiro, Daniella's boyfriend, and ask him a few questions about Iris's death. Call me when you get this message please. Thanks so much."

Judy hung up, only temporarily defeated. She listened to the efficient rumble of her VW engine and gazed through her windshield into the blackness and the thorny tangle of bramblebushes under her headlights. She didn't love the idea of going to the barracks alone, but she didn't see any option. She couldn't justify calling 911 and she didn't want to worry Mary. It struck her that she didn't even consider calling Frank, but she didn't have time now to ponder the reason. She couldn't let it go and come back tomorrow, because she had to work.

She eyed the bramblebushes, which oddly reminded her of *The Bramblebush,* an old book about the philosophy of law that every law student hears about first year, which Judy had actually loved. The gist was that the law itself was a bramblebush, and that reminded Judy of her purpose at the barracks. Justice for Iris and Father Keegan. She couldn't turn away, not when she'd come this far. She was here and she wanted to get it done now. She was strong and not completely unprepared, and if she kept her wits about her, she told herself she'd be fine.

She steered the wheel to the right, turned onto the driveway, and flicked on the high beams, traveling slowly. The driveway was unpaved and lined with more bramble and multiflora, and her headlights flashed on the blood-red eyes of something darting across her path. Spooked, she braked the car, her heart hammering until she realized it was just a fox, his bushy tail flying behind him as he disappeared into the underbrush.

She willed herself not to be afraid and cruised forward. Her headlights illuminated the dark outline of a building that lay ahead. There were no light fixtures to delineate its outline from the blackness of the night sky, but as she got closer, she could see that it was about fifty feet long, made of unpainted cinderblock, a flat roof, and a single front door, with only three small windows, each a lighted square, for its entire length. She thought she heard some sort of mechanical noise coming from the barracks, but wasn't sure, so she lowered her window and confirmed it, hearing a loud thrumming from a machine she couldn't identify.

Suddenly the engine noise cut out and the lights in the

doorway and windows flickered off, plunging them all into darkness except for her headlights. Judy swallowed hard. She put the car in reverse, ready to get the hell out of there. In the stillness, she heard dogs barking and men laughing and shouting to each other in Spanish, with peppy music playing from a radio.

She told herself to stay calm. The stench of compost wafted through her open window. She didn't know where the mushroom growers were, but they couldn't be far. In the next moment, the engine noise started up again and the lights went back on abruptly.

She put the car in forward gear and cruised ahead. Her eyes adjusted to the darkness, and in the headlights she could see that a group of men were hanging out in front of the barracks, their white PVC chairs an unnaturally bright white. The engine noise was coming from a portable generator. The only illumination came from the open doorway, which was wide, like a barn door, and threw a warped square of light onto the hard ground, casting harsh shadows on the men. Their beer bottles glinted brown, and the ends of their cigarettes burned red.

They all stopped laughing and talking, and turned toward her, some getting out of chairs and others walking over. Judy's mouth went dry. She realized there were probably ten or twelve of them, more than she'd reckoned for. She didn't know what to do. She didn't want to reverse, but she was in no hurry to get out of the car. Two little mutts came running toward her, barking and jumping up on her door, their toenails clacking.

"Settle down, guys," Judy said, though she wasn't sure if she was talking to the dogs or the men. She told herself to remain calm as the first man approached her car, cocking his head to peer at her. His body made a short and wiry silhouette in the light coming from the doorway, and she could see he was wearing a grimy white tank top and floppy work pants, but she couldn't tell what he looked like, or even if he was smiling or hostile, because he was backlighted. His odor reached her before he did, a strong mix of cigarettes, aftershave, and compost.

"Miss, are you lost?" he asked, with a light Spanish accent, coming over to her car door and shooing the barking dogs away.

"Uh, no." Judy could see in the reflected light from her dashboard that he couldn't have been more than seventeen years old, with handsome features and a friendly smile, so she relaxed. "My name is Judy Carrier and I'm looking for Carlos Ramiro. I was told he lives here, by Father Vega."

The young man frowned. "Are you from the church? Or Mike's? I never saw you there."

"No, I'm just a lawyer from the city."

"You look like you're from a D.A. or federal, like."

"No, not at all. I'm in general practice."

"Is anybody with you? You came alone?"

"Yes, I don't have anything to do with immigration or anything like that, I promise you. Hold on, I'll show you." Judy reached into her purse, grabbed her wallet, and pulled out a business card, handing it to him. "This is me. I work at a law firm."

"This looks nice, very nice." The young man squinted at the card, though Judy doubted he had enough light to read it properly, and it gave her a moment to look at his face. He had fine features, with a small mouth, narrow nose, and brown eyes, with eyelashes to die for. His hair was a shaved fade that looked oiled, his long neck bore a tattooed crucifix, and his eyebrows were plucked.

"I'm not here in any official way. I just wanted to talk to Carlos about his girlfriend, Daniella. I'm a friend of her best friend, Iris."

"Okay." The young man smiled. "Wait here. You can get out if you want. The dogs don't bite."

"Sure, thanks." Judy watched the young man jog back to the group, the dogs running to greet him, yapping at his heels. The men clustered around him, and there was more talking and a new wave of laughter, but Judy was beginning to find her bearings. She cut the engine, told herself not to be a chicken, and got out of the car.

The dogs raced back, barking and wagging their tails. She offered her hand, which they started licking, so she petted them. From her new vantage point, she could see inside the barracks, and as appalling as the sight was, it didn't completely surprise her. The building had only a dirt floor, cinderblock walls, and a row of wooden bunk beds that looked almost exactly like the mushroom bed she'd seen in the growing house. There didn't appear to be any other furniture. A soft orange glow suggested that there were space heaters inside, probably powered by the generator. She caught a whiff of cooking chicken coming from the doorway, but she didn't know what they were making it on, maybe a hot plate. At the far end of the building stood a battered blue PortaJohn.

"Miss Judy!" the young man called out, motioning to her to come over to the group. "Carlos wants to see you!"

"Great." Judy ignored her jitters, held her head high, and walked over to the men, who gathered around, a group of short and stocky silhouettes whose faces she couldn't see. She had no way of knowing which man was Carlos, but she wasn't going any closer.

"My name is Domingo," the young man said, touching his chest. "I speak English, so I can translate if you want to talk to Carlos."

"Thank you," Judy said, forcing a smile. The dogs danced around her ankles. "Hi, everybody."

"*Hola, gringa!*" a man called out, and there was general laughter.

"This is Carlos," Domingo said, gesturing to a thickly muscled man who emerged from the crowd, smoking a cigarette. His shoulders were broad and strong, and he stood with his barrel chest puffed out, straining his grimy T-shirt, a stance so exaggerated it would have been comical if it weren't genuinely menacing.

Judy found herself stepping back, without knowing why. Then she realized it wasn't a reaction to him, but rather an unconscious imitation of the crowd, who also edged away, according him a certain status or just giving him a wide berth. She couldn't see his features in detail, but his eyes were slits in a wide face, his hair was thick and oiled, and his arms were covered with tattoos. The man had the kind of presence that made her instantly sorry she'd come.

"Miss Judy, what did you want from Carlos?" Domingo asked, but Judy noticed a new tension in his tone.

"Can you ask him if he knows where Daniella is? I'm trying to find her so I can ask about Iris."

Domingo turned to Carlos and spoke to him in rapid Spanish, and Judy didn't recognize any words except for the names Daniella and Iris. Carlos replied in equally rapid Spanish, speaking without even looking at Domingo, and Judy felt her gut tighten when she recognized one of the words, *puta,* which meant whore.

Domingo said to Judy, "He says Daniella is home in Mexico."

Judy hesitated. "Can you ask him if he's sure? Also didn't she care that she was going to miss Iris's funeral?"

Domingo turned to Carlos and translated, and Carlos replied, again without looking at Domingo. Judy sensed that Carlos didn't like Domingo, realizing why when she recognized another word, *maricon,* or, gay. Judy heard a quiet descend and sensed a growing fear in the crowd.

Domingo said to Judy, "He said he's sure she's there. He drove her to the bus himself. She went home again because she was sad about Iris. She wanted to be with her family."

Judy hesitated. "Father Vega told me she wouldn't miss Iris's funeral."

Domingo turned to translate, but before he could say a word, Carlos exploded in anger, shoving him in his chest and shouting in Spanish. Domingo reeled, staggering off-balance, but didn't lose his footing.

Judy gasped, edging away. She had to go. Trouble was breaking out. The dogs started barking and running around.

Carlos advanced on Judy, shouting in Spanish, his dark eyes glittering with malice. Her heart jumped through her chest.

Domingo came over, shaken. "Miss Judy, leave right away. Go. Now. Run."

Suddenly Carlos lunged at Judy and grabbed her by the shoulders. He reeked of beer and body odor.

"No, no!" Judy struggled in his grasp, terrified. She couldn't get away. Carlos dug his nails into her, yanked her off her feet toward him, and pressed his body against hers.

"No!" Judy tried to get away but Carlos overpowered her. He thrust his hips into her, his crotch hard.

Judy couldn't get her hands free. Carlos was shoving her backwards to the ground. Fear electrified her, jolting all of her senses to high alert. Adrenaline poured into her system. She was going to be raped or killed. She had to save herself.

Carlos pulled her close, pressed his wet lips to her, and bit her hard on the lips, leaving spittle on her lips, the revolting kiss of a sadist.

Judy exploded in disgust, kneeing him with all her might. Carlos crumpled in pain and shock.

Judy reeled but kept her wits about her. She broke free,

whipped her can of Mace from her blazer pocket, and aimed it directly at his eyes.

"No, no, NO!" Judy roared, scrambling backwards toward her car. "Stay away from me! Stay *back*!"

She jumped into the car, locked the doors, started the engine, and reversed at speed, almost veering off the driveway.

Her heart didn't stop hammering until she reached the city.

Chapter Thirty-two

"Penny, down!" Judy petted the dog's fluffy head, set her purse on the floor, and closed her apartment door behind her, dismayed to find her mother coming from the living room. The eleven o'clock news was on TV, and she'd thought her mother would have already gone to bed. Judy tilted her head down, because she didn't want her mother to see the bite mark from Carlos, on her mouth.

"Honey, what kept you?"

"Sorry, I had a lot of work. Is Aunt Barb okay?" Judy kept her head down, making much of petting the dog, who was sniffing her shoes and legs, undoubtedly getting the scent of the dogs from the barracks.

"She's fine and says hi. Her room is private until she gets a roommate, and there were lots of flowers waiting for her, one from that estates lawyer you know. Foxman, his name is?"

"How nice." Judy kept her head turned away from her mother as she straightened up and headed for the staircase. "Be right down, I need to go to the bathroom."

"What?"

"I have to pee!" Judy called after her, taking the stairs two by two, with Penny bounding after her.

"Honey?"

Judy hustled into the small bathroom, switching on the light and letting Penny in, because the dog would not be denied. She closed the door, checked her reflection in the mirror over the sink, and grimaced, which hurt. The bite mark looked worse than it had in the rearview mirror, splitting her lower lip on the side, leaving it bloody and swollen. A tremor of fear rippled through her body, an aftershock of the trauma and the very thought of what could have happened.

Judy heard her mother's footsteps on the stairs and got busy. She twisted on the faucet, pumped some cleanser into her hand, and washed her face and mouth with warm water. The wound stung, so she switched to cold, snatched a washrag from the rack, ran it under the water, and pressed it to her lips, trying to control the swelling.

"Judy, what's going on?"

"I'm in the bathroom, Mom." Judy checked the washrag, and a pinkish stain blotted the terrycloth, but the bleeding had stopped.

"What are you doing?"

"What do you think?" Judy kept her tone impatient to back her mother off. "I'm washing up and going to the bathroom."

"With the dog?"

"If I leave her outside, she'll scratch the door."

"I took her out, but you know, I think you might have a flea problem."

"Really." Judy cringed. It was the last thing she wanted for her aunt, to worry about fleas.

"You'll have to get her dipped. Stop that before it starts. You have no idea what a headache that can be, washing the sheets and everything."

"Good to know, thanks." Judy held the cold compress on her lip and reached over to flush the toilet. Penny kept smelling her legs and shoes, sniffing excitedly. "Mom, can I have some privacy?"

"Since when do you want privacy in the bathroom? When you were growing up, you left the bathroom door open all the time." Judy's mother wiggled the doorknob. "Honey, let me in. I thought I saw something on your face."

"I . . . hurt myself a little." Suddenly Judy's cell phone started ringing, and she pulled it from her pocket, checking the screen. It was Detective Boone, and she couldn't miss the call.

"Judy?"

"Mom, I'll be right out. Frank's on the phone and I want to talk to him. Can you please give me a minute?"

"Judy, what's going on? Something is going on."

The phone rang again, and Judy had no choice but to answer, but she couldn't very well fill Detective Boone in without being overheard by her mother. She pressed ANSWER and said, "Hi, thanks for calling back."

"Judy?" Detective Boone asked, concerned. "Are you okay? What were you doing at the barracks?"

"I'm fine, and I'm home now. Can I call you tomorrow morning and fill you in?"

"Sure," Detective Boone answered, sounding puzzled. "But I got a call late tonight from Father Vega at the church."

"Oh, really." Judy tried to keep her tone casual for her mother's benefit.

"Judy, we would appreciate it if you would refrain from stirring up speculation—"

"We'll talk about this tomorrow morning. I have to go, okay?"

"You're doing a great deal of harm, fomenting trouble, and if the press gets wind of it—"

"They won't, I have to go. Bye!"

Detective Boone paused. "Fine, good night."

"Good night." Judy hung up, slipped the phone back into her pocket, and opened the door, holding the compress to her mouth. Penny scooted out of the bathroom, going to Judy's mother. "Mom, I'm fine."

"Oh really." Her mother cocked her head and folded her arms over her chest, managing to look concerned and chic at the same time. "Let me see your face."

"I hurt my mouth but it's not a big deal. See?" Judy moved the washrag, and her mother recoiled.

"Oh my, how did you do that? Did somebody *hit* you?"

"No, of course not." Judy tried to think of a good lie, fast. "I stopped short in the car because I thought something ran across my path, and I hit my mouth on the steering wheel."

"Didn't you have your seat belt on?" Her mother scrutinized the wound. "You're going to need to put some Neosporin on that."

"No, I had just started the car, so I didn't have it on yet." Judy set the wet rag on the sink, went into the medicine cabinet, and found a tube of Neosporin.

"You should put your seat belt on *before* you start the car. You know that. Here, let me help." Suddenly her mother stepped forward to grab the tube of Neosporin, startling Judy, who cringed reflexively, her body remembering what her brain wanted to forget. Her mother's mouth dropped open and her forehead wrinkled with confusion. "Honey, what's the matter with you? I'm not going to hurt you."

"I know, let me do it." Judy took back the tube, but her hand shook, and she and her mother saw it at the same time.

"Judy, somebody hit you."

"No they didn't."

"Yes, they did. I wasn't born yesterday." Her mother pursed her lips, blinking. "Why can't you tell me?"

"There's nothing to tell."

"Why can't you be honest with me?" her mother asked, wounded. Her blue eyes filmed with tears that seemed to come out of nowhere, and her gaze held Judy's for a moment of naked pain, unlike any Judy had ever seen in her.

"Mom," Judy started to say, but her mother turned away and walked down the hall. Judy went after her, following her into the bedroom to find her mother slumping at the edge of the bed, wiping tears away. She looked so out of place, a forlorn figure against the sunny yellow walls of the bedroom, filled with Judy's vivid, colorful oils. "I'm sorry, Mom. Please don't be upset."

Her mother stifled a sob, covering her mouth with her hand, and Judy felt surprised and guilty at making her mother cry. She didn't know where it had come from, and the only time she'd ever seen her mother cry was at Judy's grandfather's funeral.

"I'm really sorry, Mom." Judy sat down beside her and put an arm around her mother's shoulders, while Penny jumped onto the bed and flopped down on the comforter behind them.

"It's just hard, that's all. It's very hard." Her mother shook her head, but didn't look over.

"I know, there's a lot going on right now, with Aunt Barb and everything. It's just all catching up with you." Judy hugged her shoulders gently. "Why don't I make us some tea, some chamomile, and then we can go to bed?"

Her mother kept shaking her head. "It's not that. It's not Barb. It's us. It's me. We're not close, we can't even talk about anything."

"What do you mean, Mom?" Judy felt terrible that her

mother was so upset, but there was no way she could tell her about the barracks.

"It's just so hard, to be a mother, there's so many things I didn't understand." Her mother's tone softened, pained. "It's like you have a window of time, and it's a small window. It's not much time, really. They say life is short, but the truth is, motherhood is short."

Judy didn't understand. "Motherhood is forever, Mom. A girl always needs her mom."

"No, it's like you have one shot to be a good mother. The window is until your child's twelve or thirteen, and by then, I knew I had blown it with you. I just had blown it. What I did with the boys didn't work with you."

"You didn't blow it, Mom." Judy had never seen her mother like this, so vulnerable, and they'd never talked about their relationship, so directly. "You were a great mother, and you still are. You're a great mother."

"No, honestly, I'm not, I'm a terrible mother to you. I don't know what I did wrong. I failed." Her mother's shoulders shuddered with a new sob, and Judy held her tighter.

"That's not true, I love you. We love each other."

"No, I love you, but I've done a terrible job. I've made a mess of it. I failed *you*." Her mother heaved another sob, trying to strangle it in her throat but not succeeding, and Judy's heart broke at the sound.

"Mom, now, this isn't true. You've always been there for me, I know that."

"How do you know that?" Her mother looked up at her abruptly, her eyes brimming and bloodshot. "I'm asking you a question. How do you know that? How do you know I'm there for you, if you never tell me anything? Never call upon me? Never even *call me*?"

Judy thought a minute, seeing from her mother's questioning

gaze that she wouldn't get away with less than the absolute truth. "You know how I know, Mom? You really want to know how I know?"

"Yes." Her mother nodded, sniffling.

"Wait." Judy put her hand in her blazer pocket and withdrew the palm-size canister of Mace, which happened to be hot pink. "Do you recognize this? This looks like something Barbie would have, but this is the Mace you gave me last Christmas, which replaced the Mace that you gave me the year before that, in case it expired. I carry it with me in my purse, all the time, because you have drilled that propaganda into my head. Every time I see it in my purse, I think to myself, my mother loves me. This is Exhibit A." Judy felt her own chest tighten, but didn't want to cry now, because she needed her mother to hear her. "And the same thing happens every time I see that dopey red fire extinguisher that you bought me for the kitchen, in case there's a grease fire. I think to myself, my mother loves me. My mother cares about me. My mother is always there for me, no matter what, in any emergency."

"Really?" Her mother half-smiled, though her lips trembled.

"*Really.*" Judy sniffled, feeling her heart ache, which she hadn't even known was possible. "And I'm not going to get into it, because I don't want to upset you more than I already have, but tonight, this Mace saved my ass. Even though you weren't there and you're *never* going to find out what happened, you saved me. You saved me from harm. You might have even saved my life. That's how there for me you are. It doesn't get better than that, Mom. It just doesn't." Judy felt her mouth twist with sobs she was holding back, perhaps a lifetime's worth of them. "I love you, Mom. I really do."

"I love you, too, sweetie." Her mother seemed to collapse into her arms, and Judy held her tight.

"And we'll make things better, starting now. I'll be a better daughter, I promise. I'll call you more, I will."

"It's not you, it was me. I held back, I guess. I see that now. But now it's too late." Her mother burst into tears in her embrace. "It's too . . . late."

"No, it isn't," Judy said, meaning it. "You'll see, you won't even be able to get me off the phone. As long as we're both alive, it's not too late. It's never too late."

"Yes . . . it is." Her mother began to cry in earnest, hiccupping sobs racking her frame. "You're all . . . grown-up. I'm . . . out of . . . time."

"No, you're not." Judy felt so much love for her then, though she couldn't understand why her mother wasn't coming around, but seemed to be hurting even more. "Mom, it's okay. Everything's going to be all right. I'm not grown-up yet, God knows. As long as we're mother and daughter, we're all right."

"No, no . . . no. That's . . . the . . . problem."

"What is?"

Her mother looked up from her arms, her bloodshot eyes agonized and her expression stricken. "Honey, I'm . . . not your . . . mother."

Chapter Thirty-three

"What did you say?" Judy asked, thinking she must've heard wrong.

"I'm not . . . your mother." Her mother looked at her directly, focusing on Judy through pooling tears.

"Is this a joke?"

"No, it's the truth, the absolute truth." Her mother wiped her eyes, leaving a pinkish streak, then heaved a final sob, trying to stop crying. "I'm not your mother. I'm not your real mother."

Judy recoiled, not understanding. "What are you talking about? Are you saying I'm adopted?"

"In a way, yes." Her mother nodded, wiping her runny nose on her sleeve.

"What the hell?" Judy's mouth went dry. "What's going on? Is this for real?"

"Yes, it is."

"I'm *adopted*?"

"Not exactly. Your mother is Aunt Barb."

"*What?*" Judy felt thunderstruck. "What are you talking about?"

"I can explain—"

"Are you *serious*?"

"Yes, we were going to tell you later in the week, when she came home from the hospital and felt better—"

"Are you *kidding me right now*?" Judy jumped to her feet without knowing why. "What are you talking about, you were going to tell me?"

"Please, sit down, honey." Her mother gestured her back, but Judy wasn't having any.

"I don't want to sit down. Tell me what's going on. What are you talking about?"

"Please don't be angry. I can explain—"

"I'm not angry," Judy said, though she had no idea what emotion she was feeling, because she was feeling so many at once. Disbelief, shock, complete and utter bewilderment. "I don't understand. I'm just trying to understand. If this is real, then explain it to me."

"Okay, well, Aunt Barb had you, she's the one who gave birth to you, when she was sixteen—"

"Are you *kidding me*?" Judy interrupted, knowing she was repeating herself but not being able to help it.

"This is the truth. The way it happened was that she was in high school and she fell in love, puppy love, and got pregnant by one of the enlisted men on the base. In Pensacola."

"Aunt Barb's really my mother?" Judy asked, like a nightmare echo chamber.

"Yes. Our father, your grandfather, you know the general, he was not about to have any of that. Neither was my mother. Appearances mattered to them, too much."

Judy tried to listen, but all of the words got tangled up, a bewildering bolus of father, mother, grandfather, grandmother.

"I was twenty-four years old and already married, and your brother Tom was only one . . ."

Judy lost track when she thought about Tom, her older brother who was no longer her real brother.

". . . and my parents, your grandparents, decided that the only way to solve the problem was to have me take the baby and raise her as my own. It worked out because we were doing so well and we were about to move to another base, Frankfurt, so nobody knew . . ."

Judy kept trying to follow, realizing that the baby her mother was talking about was Judy herself.

". . . Barb took a year off from high school, then she gave birth and went back to school." Her mother paused, pursing her lips. "Barb didn't want to give you up, but our parents gave her no options, except have you adopted by strangers, so she went along with it. She always loved you, even from the beginning, and we all agreed that when you got older, when the time was right, we would tell you."

Judy couldn't believe her ears, but she knew from her mother's anguished words that it was all true. "This is unreal."

"I know, I'm sorry."

"You're telling me this, *now*?"

"Yes."

"So what makes this time right? Why didn't you tell me before?"

"We were going to, but we just couldn't find the right time, and to be fair, we avoided it. We knew how hurt you would be, and I knew that I would lose you then, and that when we told you, that would be . . . the end of my time with you." Her mother's voice broke, but she didn't stop talking, as if the words were coming out with a force of their own. "We were going to tell you after college, but then you were so busy, and in law school you were working so hard, then when you moved to Philadelphia, you were on one coast and I was on the other. That's why Barb moved here to be near you."

Judy thought back, remembering. "She said it was because there were better doctors here, for Uncle Steve."

"That wasn't the real reason. He was sick a long time, but she moved to be where you were. She wanted to be close to you, to watch out for you. She loves you with all her heart, as do I."

Judy felt tears come to her eyes, but she shook them off. She hadn't seen this coming, in a million years, but things began to fall into place, like the way her mother seemed jealous of Aunt Barb. "So why didn't you tell me then, after I came here?"

"We both thought you were having so many ups and downs in your new job. It just didn't seem like the right time, and we didn't want to add to your load, and Uncle Steve got sicker."

"Did he know?"

"Yes, he did."

Judy felt struck by a revelation she should've had before. "Then who's my father? You mean Dad isn't—"

"He's not your father."

Judy didn't know what to say for a moment, rocked to her foundations. "He knows about this, too?"

"Yes, of course."

Judy gasped. She'd never been close to her father, but she never doubted that he was her father. In a weird way, finally learning the truth explained a lot about her childhood. Her mind raced to consider the implications. "What's the guy's name, the enlisted guy? My father."

"John Ward."

"Where is he?"

"He was killed in action in Bosnia."

"*Bosnia?*" Judy's mouth fell open. She had written a paper about the Bosnian conflict for her American history class, never thinking that her own father died there. "Did he know, like, what happened to me?"

"Yes." Her mother sighed heavily. "Honey, this is a lot to digest—"

"Ya *think*?" Judy shot back, with an abrupt, mirthless laugh. Her mother sat crestfallen on the bed, her strong shoulders collapsed and her head tilted down, and behind her, Judy caught a glimpse of the framed photographs on her dresser, smiling happy pictures of herself with people who weren't who she'd thought they were—Aunt Barb, her brothers, her mother and father, all of them skiing, climbing rock faces, and celebrating each other's birthdays. She looked away, because it killed her to think that none of it was true, or real, not from day one.

"I'm sorry, I'm so very sorry. We tried to solve the problem the best way we could—"

"Mom"—Judy caught herself—"or whatever I'm supposed to call you, please stop saying *the problem. I was* the problem. The problem was a person. The problem is standing right in front of you, trying to figure out what the hell is going on."

"I know, I'm sorry." Her mother put up a gentle hand. "We agreed that we were going to tell you this spring, when your dad could get the time off and we could both make the trip east. We wanted to sit down and tell you, the three of us, together."

"Not Dad. He's not my dad. My dad is dead." Judy heard the awful ring of the words and felt a loss she couldn't begin to understand.

Her mother nodded, tacitly accepting the correction. "But the thing is, we're all so proud of you, the way you've grown up, a lawyer making a wonderful living, you and Frank on your way to getting married. Barb has even been saving up all these years for your wedding, she wants to pay for everything—"

"I'm not marrying Frank," Judy blurted out, surprising even herself.

Her mother blinked, her tears gone, though her eyes were

red and puffy. "Well, whatever you choose to do, Barb and I thought it was getting on time to tell you, but then her illness shifted everything forward."

Judy tried to follow the timeline. "Did you know she had breast cancer before this weekend? Did you know about the chemo?"

"No, that came as a surprise to me, too. Barb thought she could beat it and she didn't want to worry me, but when she needed the surgery, she decided not to wait any longer, to tell you."

Judy swallowed hard, thinking of how awful Aunt Barb must be feeling, looking down the barrel at a dreaded diagnosis, and on top of that, knowing that she was keeping a terrible secret.

"Needless to say, if anything happens to her, she wants you to know the truth, while she's still alive. She wants to be able to explain her actions and she wants you to be able to hear it from her."

"What do you want?" Judy said, speaking from the heart. She suddenly knew how her mother must be feeling and even why she'd put off telling the truth for so long. Because suddenly, Judy was losing the only mother she had ever known.

"I wanted you," her mother said, leaning forward urgently, her hands clasped together on her lap. "I wanted you from the minute I saw you, an adorable, blue-eyed baby girl. We were so happy, very happy, all of us together. You fit right in, and then we had Billy and John, and we became a family, a real family."

"Not a real family. It wasn't real." Judy tried to process it, thinking of her brothers. "Do they know, too? Billy and John? And Tommy? Do they all know?"

"No. They thought we were a family, and I thought we were, too. But we weren't, I see that now." Her mother frowned deeply, agonized. "That's why I know the problems in our relationship were my fault, my responsibility, and now you know that's true. You've been a good daughter to me, a wonderful daughter. You reached out to me time after time, until you finally gave up."

Judy cringed inwardly, because it struck such a chord. She could remember trying to connect with her mother, but after a while, she had simply stopped.

"I was holding back inside, knowing you weren't mine forever, not like the boys. I was protecting myself, but I hurt you in the process." Her mother shook her head, looking down for a moment. "I'm so sorry. It was a bad and selfish decision, made in a different time, for the wrong reasons. I realize now that we actually picked the worst possible choice. I was afraid to love you fully, and Barb was afraid to love you fully. You never had either of us completely. Our beautiful, blue-eyed baby girl fell between the cracks."

Judy understood her mother and Barb, and she even understood why they'd done what they'd done, but it didn't make it any less sad. Somehow she ended up betwixt and between, hollow and hurting, her hands empty. She felt her eyes well up.

"The amazing thing to me is the natural affinity you and Barb have for each other. You just fit together." Her mother's eyes welled up, too. "You two are a wonderful pair, a true mother and daughter, even though you didn't even know she was your mother. Nothing defeats nature, not even words."

Judy realized it was true, that she had always felt closer to her aunt, and she wondered if her heart had known something she hadn't been willing to acknowledge. She found herself edging backwards toward the threshold, aware of her actions only because Penny bounded off the bed, her tail wagging,

"Are you going somewhere?" her mother asked, rising slowly.

"Uh, yes." Judy didn't know where she was going, but she

knew that she didn't want to stay here. "Just out, I think. I think I'll just go out."

"Don't go." Her mother frowned, plainly worried. "It's late, and it's not a good idea to drive when you're upset."

"I'll drive safe, Mom," Judy said reflexively, then turned away and walked stiffly down the hall, with the dog trotting happily behind her.

Chapter Thirty-four

Judy found herself parked in the dark in front of Frank's grand-father's rowhouse, without remembering having driven here. She wiped her tears with her sleeve, then went into the console and found some napkins, which she used to dry her eyes and blow her juicy nose, hard and noisily. She knew Frank was still awake because the light was on in the front window, and through the old-school sheer curtains, she could see the bright colors of the TV, undoubtedly tuned to *Monday Night Football*. She looked around the skinny side street and spotted Cartman's Jeep parked under a streetlight up ahead, so that meant the boys were over, watching the game again.

She tossed the napkin aside, eased back into the driver's seat, and tried to decide what to do. She must have wanted to see Frank because she'd driven here, but she hadn't realized the game would be on and she didn't know how it would go down if she went inside. The last thing she wanted was an instant re-play, no pun intended, and she knew she must look a mess. She shifted up in her seat and checked the rearview mirror, taken aback at her reflection, even in the dim light. It wasn't only that her eyes, nose, and lips were red and puffy, but for the first time in her life, she looked at her own face through new eyes, as if she had never seen herself before.

She frowned at her eye color, which she had always thought were a china blue like her father's, but now she realized she had no idea what her father looked like. Everyone always said that her mouth was clearly from her mother, but Judy would have to start clarifying the term *mother*, because she was still thinking of her *mother* as her mother, when her *aunt* was really her mother.

She scrutinized her face, pondering her features as if each one were a cardboard piece from a jigsaw puzzle, trying to match her turned-up nose to her Aunt Barb's nose and wondering where her cheekbones fit, because they could have come from a total stranger, who also happened to be dead. Judy felt tears well up again, but she pressed them away. She couldn't sit out here forever and she couldn't overthink it.

She grabbed her purse, got out of the car, and chirped it locked while she walked up to the front door, with its three steps of worn grayish marble. Like the other rowhouses on the street, they were of red brick, with one front window on the first floor, and two above that, then a flat tar roof with a satellite dish aimed for maximum sports reception. South Philly was Mary DiNunzio territory, and Judy didn't fit in here, but she wasn't sure she fit in anywhere, after her conversation with her mother. Then she reminded herself that her mother wasn't her mother anymore, and her real mother had breast cancer, which made her sick at heart. She'd already lost one mother and she didn't know if she could lose another.

Judy set aside her emotions and knocked on the front door, remembering the first time she had been here, when she represented Frank's grandfather Pigeon Tony, on a case. She'd been delighted to meet her new client's hunky grandson, who had swept her off her feet, and while she waited for Frank to answer the door, she wondered if those old feelings were still there, or if they weren't, if she could get them back.

"Babe!" Frank said, opening the door. "Come in!"

"Hi, sure." Judy tried to get her bearings, knowing that it was still dark enough on the stoop for him not to be able to see her clearly. She could hear the noise of the football game and the boys talking inside. "Do you think we can get a minute alone? I just want to talk to you."

"Totally, sure!" Frank was already reaching for her, giving her a hug, and sweeping her inside the little entrance hall, which was divided from the living room by a panel of ridged glass. But when he let her go, he did a double-take, his eyes widening in surprise, then anger. "What happened? Who hit you?"

"WHAT DO YOU MEAN?" Cartman called out. "WHO HIT WHO?"

"Cartman, shut up!" Frank shouted over his shoulder, then put a strong arm around Judy.

"Frank," Judy whispered, "nobody hit me, but can we go somewhere and talk?"

"Come with me, out back."

"Good." Judy kept her head turned, letting Frank run interference for her with the boys and lead her through the tiny dining room and kitchen, then he flicked on the outside light and opened the back door.

"Thanks." Judy stepped into the backyard, a small, rectangular plot of grass, surrounded by whitewashed cinderblock, with two plastic lattice beach chairs in front of a loft that Frank's grandfather had made for his homing pigeons. The loft was about thirty feet long, with a white framed-wire cage on all four sides, containing forty-odd snow-white doves, and reddish-brown Meulemanns and Janssens.

"What happened, baby?" Frank asked, aghast. He touched

her arm, tilting her toward him as he looked at her face. "What the hell? Were you mugged? I'll kill him!"

"I didn't get mugged," Judy began, but she wasn't sure what to say next. She slipped from his grasp, drawn to the loft. Inside the pigeons fluttered this way and that, disturbed by the sudden light and the presence of people, so late. They cooed and called to each other, their wings beating against the wire walls, shedding fuzzy underfeathers that flew around in the quiet night air, sailing on invisible currents. "God, I love these birds."

"What happened, hon?" Frank followed her to the loft, linking his fingers through the cage wire.

"I'm fine, but it's a long story. It's been a long day and night, starting with Aunt Barb's operation." Judy watched as the birds began to find their mates, because homing pigeons were bonded pairs, mated for life. They settled down together, two by two, tucking their white wings neatly at their sides, puffing out their chests, their eyes red and perfectly round, complementing their dark pink, scaly legs. Judy used to let them perch on her fingers, surprised at the warmth of their feet.

"Judy, who hit you? Was it the guys who attacked you at your aunt's? Are they stalking you? Because if the police won't do anything about it, I will."

"The police are all over it, but thanks."

"You don't want to tell me about it?"

"Honestly, I don't want to talk about it." Judy felt that what had happened at the barracks was old news compared with the conversation with her mother, which she needed to hash out with somebody. She watched the birds without seeing them anymore, losing focus. "I had a weird discussion with my mother, though."

"Tell me what happened to your lip, then tell me about your mom."

"My lip doesn't matter, my mom does."

"Your lip matters to me." Frank frowned. "I can't let people take shots at you and get away with it."

"Listen, I appreciate it, but that's not what's on my mind right now. My mother's the thing that's on my mind. My mother is important."

"What's important is that people are attacking you, physically."

"Can't I identify what's important, to me? Can't I decide what I want to talk about?" Judy couldn't tell if she was picking on him or if she was right, but it bugged her just the same. "It's about my need to talk, isn't it? It's not about your need to know. It's not about you."

"Where's this coming from, babe?" Frank was taken aback, looking at her like she was crazy. "I ask how you are and you are pissed at me?"

"I answered how I am, but I told you that I wanted to talk about my mom."

"If you're in danger, I want to know about that." Frank threw up his hands. "What's the point of keeping me in suspense?"

"I'm not keeping you in suspense." Judy didn't want to fight, but she wanted to be heard. "I told you I'm fine."

"Okay, have it your way." Frank folded his arms, his expression newly tense. "Tell me about your mom. You fought over nothing again, right? Because you two always fight. You're oil and water. Am I right or am I right?"

"No, not exactly," Judy said, dismayed. "It wasn't about nothing, and we didn't fight. We talked."

"Okay, tell me what and your mother fought about, or sorry, *talked* about." Frank sat down in one of the beach chairs in front of the loft, next to a round wooden table.

"Oh, jeez." Judy sank into the other chair. "What are we fighting about? Do we have to fight?"

"Lately we do, that's what it seems like. You're unhappy all the time, and I think I know why." Frank unfolded his arms and leaned forward, a familiar warmth returning to his rich brown eyes. "It's not your mom, and it's not even your aunt, getting sick. You've been upset from before that, since Mary and Anthony decided to get married."

"No I haven't," Judy said reflexively. She didn't want to talk about it now, but she was surprised that he'd noticed.

"Yes you have, and I know how women are." Frank's features softened. "It's like when one goes to the ladies' room, you all go to the ladies' room."

"No, I'm not that girl, the one who needs to go to the bathroom just because everybody else is."

"I think you've been worrying about why we're not married, and when I'm going to ask you to marry me." Frank smiled gently, and Judy started to panic inside.

"No, that's not it. I swear, it's not."

"Yes, it is. I'm not dumb." Frank buckled his lower lip, regretful. "We never really talked about it because we both assumed it would happen. But that's not good enough for you anymore. It's not good enough for me anymore, either."

"No, it's fine," Judy rushed to say. "We don't have to get married just because somebody else is getting married. What's right for one couple isn't right for another."

"That's not what I'm saying. I'm saying that it's just a matter of time that we're going to get married, and I want you to know, right now, that I'd marry you in a minute." Frank caressed her arm and smiled crookedly, his trademark loving grin. "I sensed that you weren't ready, and I was waiting for you to come around, but if you're ready, I'm ready. Hell, I'm more than ready. I've got five years on you. I can't wait to make babies and buy a house of our own. In fact, Judy—"

"No, stop." Judy felt a bolt of alarm, realizing from the look in his eyes that he was about to propose. "Frank, listen to me. I don't think I'm ready. I'm not ready."

"I don't believe you," Frank said softly, stroking her arm. "I think you are."

"No, I'm not."

"I think you're scared of taking it to the next level, which is natural, or you're waiting to make partner, which I get, but I say enough is enough. It's time I made an honest woman of you." Frank took her hands in his and began to lower himself off the chair, as if he were going to kneel on bended knee, but Judy yanked her hands away.

"No, Frank, I"—Judy felt pain knife her heart, but realized what she had to do, to be fair to him—"I know what I feel, and I don't want us to get married."

Frank's lips parted, and he eased back onto the chair. "You mean now, right?"

Judy's mouth went dry. "No. I mean ever."

Frank recoiled slowly, his dark eyebrows lifting in astonishment. "I don't get it. You love me, right?"

"Yes, I love you. But I don't think we should get married."

"Ever?"

"Ever."

Frank blinked a few times, then his eyes filmed, but he masked his emotions with a rueful smile. "Oh, man, this sucks. I'm trying to propose, and you're trying to break up."

"I'm really sorry," Judy told him, from her very soul. She met his eye, even though she was responsible for the hurt that was plain in them. "I wish it were otherwise because you're wonderful, you really are."

"Not wonderful enough," Frank said, pursing his lips, but without rancor in his tone.

"Wonderful enough, but that's not the point." Judy flashed unaccountably on what her mother had told her, about how nature couldn't be denied. "We're just not a good pair. We don't fit together so well, when it comes down to it."

"But we love each other."

"We do, but we're not right for each other."

"That sounds like something a lawyer would say," Frank said, with a shaky smile.

"There's a reason for that." Judy felt her eyes film. She'd come here for comfort, not to end their relationship, but it looked like it was happening and she knew it was the right thing.

"Well. Okay." Frank exhaled, angry. "I certainly don't want to be with someone who doesn't appreciate me. I don't have to."

"I agree, you don't, and you shouldn't."

"You're making a huge mistake."

"I could be, I know," Judy told him, meaning it.

"But you're doing it anyway."

"I have to." Judy meant that, too, somehow.

Frank met her eye, wounded but still proud. "So that's that?"

"Yes."

"You're something, Carrier," Frank said, shaking his head, pained.

"I'm sorry."

"Gimme a hug, woman." Frank raised his arms for a final embrace, and Judy almost melted.

"I'd love to," she said, with feeling.

Chapter Thirty-five

Judy got off the elevator and walked through an empty reception area, barely glancing at the gleamy ROSATO & DINUNZIO plaque, feeling lost and rudderless. She hadn't known where else to go except to work, because she didn't want to go home and deal with her mother, or rather, her aunt. The lights were on in the office, but she doubted that Bennie or anybody else was in, because the only sound was a vacuum cleaner and the cleaning staff never started until the lawyers had gone.

She took a right down the hallway and spotted the black electrical wire running into her office, so she ducked her head in and waved to the cleaner, an older woman who looked up, startled, then waved back with a reassured smile. Judy turned around and walked down the hall to her new war room, where she paused in the threshold, taking in the scene. Allegra must have worked her little buns off because the cardboard boxes were gone, evidently broken down and whisked away. Instead, red accordion files, each one representing a separate case, were lined up on the conference table in three rows, like so many legal dominoes. Next to them sat a stapled list.

Judy walked over, set her purse on the table, and picked up

the list. **New Matters**, it read at the top, and she skimmed the list of case captions, organized in alphabetical order: *Morris Abellmen v. Bendaflex industries, Inc., Sam Atwater v. Bendaflex industries, Inc., Melissa Baxter v. Bendaflex industries, Inc.* She flipped the pages idly, coming to the end, which was case number 76, *Jennifer Zwitz v. Bendaflex industries, Inc.*

Judy set the sheet down, reached for the first accordion file, and pulled out the pleading index, a long binder that held all of the papers filed with the Court during the case. She sank into a chair at the head of the conference table and flipped through the cleaning index, skimming the Complaint, the defendant company's Answer, and an endless series of interrogatories, losing focus as she read on. She kept thinking of Frank, hugging her one last time. Then her mother, talking about *the problem*. And Aunt Barb, lying alone in a hospital bed, afraid that she would die before she could answer the questions of her only daughter. And poor Iris, whose death could be mourned, if not completely understood. And a priest, a man of God, dead.

Judy let the pleadings of index flop closed, and her thoughts finally came to rest on Domingo, the young man who had translated for her at the barracks. Her heart went out to him, and Iris, Frank, her mother, Aunt Barb, and Father Keegan as she eased back in her padded chair and faced her damages cases. She realized that she was surrounded on all sides, by all sorts of damage. In her work, in her family, in the man she loved, and in the world entire.

She closed her eyes, feeling a wave of exhaustion and profound sadness wash over her, not for herself, but for everyone. And when she felt herself drifting into sleep, she let slumber come, surrendering.

She woke up to the sound of her cell phone ringing and opened her eyes, trying to orient herself. She was still in the conference room, and the windows were still dark, so it was before dawn. Her cell phone rang again, the sound emanating from her purse, and she reached for it, worried. The call could have something to do with Aunt Barb.

Judy opened the flap to her purse and quickly pulled out the phone, and the screen said 5:06, with an UNKNOWN NUMBER in the 999 area code. "Hello?" she said, rubbing her face to wake up.

"Miss Judy, is that you?" asked a man with a thick Spanish accent, and Judy recognized the voice, though he was slurring his words as if he had been drinking.

"Domingo?"

"Yes, Miss Judy, it's me. I need to see you. I need to see you right away."

"What about?" Judy wondered where he had gotten her cell number, then remembered it was on her business card, which she had given him.

"I need money, Miss Judy. I need money to get out of here. I need to go far away from these men, these bad men."

"Are you okay?" Judy asked, alarmed. "Have you been drinking?"

"A thousand dollars, Miss Judy. You have that much money, you are a lawyer."

"Where are you, at the barracks?"

"No, I left. If you bring me the money, I will tell you what you want to know."

"What do you mean?"

"Bring the money. I know a place to meet. Don't tell anyone. No police, no one else. Just you. Now."

"Now? I'm in the city. I don't understand. What'll you tell me?"

"Pay me, and I will tell you what they did to Iris."

Chapter Thirty-six

Judy raced west, as the sun rose behind her in a clear sky, spilling brightness into the back window of her VW Beetle. She'd hit the highway before rush-hour traffic, having made great time to Chester County. The dashboard clock read 6:15, and she zoomed through East Grove, a small town consisting of an off-brand gas station and a Turkey Hill convenience store. The farther from the city Judy got, the more she left behind what was going on in her personal life and turned her attention to Iris's death. She'd been right that it had been a murder, and that fueled her. She'd tried to convince Domingo on the phone to let her go to the police, but he'd insisted that he wouldn't tell her anything if she did. She'd complied so far, but intended to convince him to notify the authorities, though she had plans even if he didn't.

She accelerated onto a paved country road, then turned left and right, following the GPS directions past fenced pastures with grazing horses in muddy blankets, then long stretches of cornfield, and acres of open space, covered with underbrush. She was heading for a sandwich shop in East Grove, which Domingo had said was hidden enough for their meeting, and her heart began to hammer from a half a mile away. She took another right, then left, in light traffic, mostly pickup trucks, one full of baled hay, and a rusty red Farmall tractor, which pulled over to let her pass.

She spotted an Agway feed store up ahead, then the coffee shop came into view, a white shack with a faded sign that read HALTMAN'S HOAGIES. The two stores sat together alongside the road, and beyond them stretched yet another open field thick with underbrush, then in the distance, a large bluish building with a corrugated roof. Birds flew over the building, seeming to congregate, and Judy didn't know why until she pulled into the side parking lot next to the sandwich shop, turned off the engine, braked, and stepped out of her car. The air reeked of compost, and she assumed that the building out back was a large mushroom grower, which could explain why Domingo had said that nobody ate at the sandwich shop.

Judy could barely take the stench, trying not to breathe as she hurried past a white Ford pickup, went around the building, and entered the sandwich shop, which was practically empty. Domingo had told her that he'd meet her at six thirty, and she was early, so she didn't worry that he'd be a no-show. There were two rows of small white tables on the right, and on the left was a stop-time soda fountain with an older man behind the counter, wearing a white apron over his T-shirt and pants. He was filling up a line of plastic catsup bottles, balancing one upside down on top of another, and he looked up when Judy came in.

"What can I do you for?" he asked, with a smile.

"Coffee and a doughnut would be great, thanks." Judy crossed to the counter and peered at the doughnuts sitting on a cake dish underneath a cloudy plastic dome. Her stomach was too jumpy to eat, but she wanted to get some for Domingo. "What do you suggest, glazed or plain?"

"I'd suggest you go to McDonald's," the old man answered, with a dry chuckle.

"What makes you say that? The smell outside?"

"Heck no, I'm used to that. None of us smell it anymore. I meant the pastry. It's day-old, and my wife is the baker."

Judy smiled. "I'll take my chances with two glazed and two coffees, please." She checked her watch, but it was only 6:27. "Which mushroom grower is back there?"

"In the back field? That's not a grower. That's the plant where they treat the compost, then it gets trucked to the growers. The growers don't treat their own compost." The old man slid the glass pot from an old Bunn coffeemaker and filled a white mug, the pour making a *glug-glug* sound.

"I didn't know you had to treat compost. I thought it was just horse manure."

"No, it's horse, chicken, and whatever chemicals they put in it, then they wash it and dry it out. They gotta treat it, you know, make it sanitary, to grow mushrooms on it. Big government got its eye out, you know, comes out here to inspect." The old man put the two mugs of coffee on the yellowed counter, picked up a plate, and lifted up the lid of the cake dish. "One down, one to go."

"Thanks."

"You go pick a table and I'll come serve you." The old man retrieved two doughnuts with plastic tongs and put them on the same plate, then reached for a dented stainless steel tray.

"Perfect." Judy turned around, scanned the tables, and made her way to one in the corner, where they wouldn't be seen by anybody who came in. The old man followed her, setting down the coffees and the doughnut plate with a napkin.

"Enjoy your meal," he said, with a wink, then returned to the counter while Judy sat down, taking the seat facing the door. She put her phone on the table and slung her shoulder bag on the back of her chair. She sipped her coffee, which was bitter and predictably did nothing to settle her stomach. She checked her watch again, and it read 6:33, though when she looked up, Domingo was coming through the door.

His young expression looked grave, his handsome mouth an unsmiling line, and his bright dark eyes seemed sunken, as if he had been awake all night, hung over, or both. He flashed her an uncertain smile, and she smiled back as he walked toward her table, removing his hands from the pockets of a black hoodie, which he had on with a T-shirt, low-slung jeans, and flat sneakers.

"Domingo, hi, please, sit down." Judy pushed the coffee mug and plate of doughnuts to his side of the table.

"Thank you, I'm so hungry." Domingo took a chair, gulped some coffee, and set down the mug with a *clunk*. "Did you bring the money?"

"Yes."

"Let me see."

"Okay." Judy reached for her purse, slid out the white envelope, and passed it to him across the table. She'd gotten the cash from the office's petty cash and left a personal check in its place.

"Thank you, Miss Judy." Domingo took the envelope quickly, folded it in half, and stuck it in the pocket of his hoodie. "I am sorry about Carlos, what he did to you."

"It's okay."

"Your mouth, it hurts, from him?" Domingo motioned to his lips.

"No, thanks. How are you? I'm worried about you."

"I will be okay with money." Domingo smiled warmly, seeming to relax. He grabbed a doughnut and took a big bite, then another. "I go away, to New York."

"Why there?"

"My uncle, he washes dishes in a restaurant, a nice restaurant." Domingo took two more bites and finished the doughnut. "He said he can get me a job. He likes New York very much. I see it on the TV, *Saturday Night Live*. It looks fun."

"It is fun," Judy said, touched.

"I have to go away from Carlos and Roberto." Domingo's brief smile vanished. "They are not good man. They are the worst man in the world."

Judy got a sick feeling in the pit of her stomach. "Are they the ones that killed Iris?"

"Yes."

Judy swallowed hard. She wanted to know the truth, and at the same time, it was too awful to hear. "How did they do it?"

"Gas."

"What kind of gas?" Judy asked, her mouth going dry.

"Bug killer, and they have a bottle, a soda bottle. They mix bug killer and acid, you know acid?"

"Acid?"

"Yes, acid, they use to clean plumbing and stones. This is the name. I copy from the bottle." Domingo reached into his other pocket, retrieved a crumpled scrap of white paper, and slipped it to her across the table.

Judy opened it up, her heart pounding. On the sheet of paper at were two penciled words in capitals. BONIDE MURIATIC. "Is this English?"

"Yes, yes." Domingo reached his hand across the table and pointed a dirty fingernail at BONIDE. "This kill bugs." Then he moved his finger to MURIATIC. "Mix this, kill people."

Judy gasped. She couldn't speak, horrified. She couldn't bear to imagine the agony of Iris's murder. She couldn't conceive of such cruelty. Her mind went into denial. Perhaps Domingo had been wrong. She asked him, "How do you know this?"

"I saw."

Judy stifled a moan. "What did you see, exactly?"

"At the barracks, I see them, Carlos and Roberto." Domingo picked up his mug and drained it of coffee.

"Roberto who?"

"Rivera." Domingo picked up the second doughnut and began to wolf it down.

"How did they do it?"

"They take Iris and put her in the shed." Domingo finished the doughnut and leaned over the table, his voice urgent. "She scream, 'no, no.' They throw bottle in pipe on top. Bottle break in the shed. No more screaming."

Judy forced herself to understand the scene. "Why weren't they gassed?"

"They wear—" Domingo raised his hand and covered his face.

"Masks?"

"Yes." Judy thought it seemed oddly elaborate and she still doubted him. "Why did they kill her that way?"

"No, at home, the cartel, they do it."

Judy shuddered. "Do Carlos and Roberto sell heroin?"

Domingo hesitated, his tongue licking dry lips. "I don't know."

Judy could see he was lying. "They work for some cartel, don't they?"

"Miss Judy, I don't know. I don't want to . . . say. I tell about Iris, that is all."

"Could that be why they killed Iris? Was she working with them or did she find out about them?"

"I don't know."

"Was anyone there, when they killed her?"

"No."

"I don't understand, what were you doing there? Did you help them?"

"No." Domingo recoiled, blinking. "I would never. It's a sin."

"Where were you?"

Domingo paused. "Inside."

"In the barracks?"

"Yes."

"What were you doing there? Did they know you were there?"

"No." Domingo hesitated. "I was with Pablo. In bed, you understand? Carlos and Roberto, they don't know."

Judy got the gist. "So Pablo saw them, too?"

"Pablo is married. Nobody know about him, only me. His wife at home, three children."

"What's Pablo's last name?"

"Diaz."

"Why did they kill Iris?"

"I don't know."

"Are you sure?" Judy was trying to piece it together. "They didn't say anything or you didn't hear them talking?"

"We hear screaming, a woman screaming, then we see." Domingo shuddered, flattening his lips in disgust. "We want to stop them, but they will kill us, too. They are *killer*." Domingo slid a silver flip phone from his pocket and checked the clock. "Miss Judy, I have to go. I miss the bus."

"Wait. Did they kill Daniella, too?"

"I don't know."

"Domingo, we should go to the police. Please. We should tell them."

"No, I told you. Never." Domingo's eyes flared with fear. "They will kill me."

"The police would never kill you."

"Carlos and Roberto, they will. The police will send me home, but I will not get there." Domingo rose. "Good-bye, Miss Judy. The bus is far to walk."

"Please can we go to the police?'

"No."

"But it's the right thing to do."

"No."

"The police can protect you."

"They will not. My mother, my brothers. Carlos will kill my family." Domingo shook his head. "No, no, no."

"Okay, all right. I'll take you to the bus stop or wherever you need to go." Judy would use the ride to convince him to go to the cops.

"Only to the bus."

"The bus, got it."

"No police."

"No."

"Okay, thank you. Let's go now." Domingo smiled, grateful.

Judy would have to figure another way to convince him. She stood up, got her purse, slid ten dollars from her wallet, and left it on the table, then slipped her phone in her pocket, and followed Domingo outside. They fell into step as they turned toward the parking lot, where Domingo pointed at Judy's VW with a grin.

"Is your car? Is so cute, like a big tomato!"

"It is, isn't it?" Judy chirped the door open as they walked towards the car. "It's because of the color, like tomato soup."

"Yes, I love it. My mother, she always make it for me. Campbell's."

"Mine, too." Judy opened the car door, climbed into the driver's seat, and slid the key into the ignition as Domingo went around to the back of the car.

"Miss, wait a minute!" someone called out, as Judy was about to close the car door. She spotted the old man from the sandwich shop, making his way slowly toward her, trying to flag her down. He walked with a limp, so she climbed out of the car and walked toward him, to save him the trouble.

"Yes, what is it, sir?"

"You forgot your change."

"You can keep it." Judy met him at the corner of the sandwich shop. "Don't worry about it."

"No, it's too much. The tab is only $3.25." The old man handed her a fistful of dollars and some change, but Judy waved him off.

"Please, keep it."

"No, take it." The old man got distracted a moment, looking past Judy and gesturing at the parking lot. "Ha! I think your friend likes the car."

"What?" Judy turned around to see Domingo sliding into the driver's seat of her VW, flashing her a big grin. She called to him, "Domingo, you look damn good in there!"

"I know that's right!" Domingo beeped the horn, turned on the ignition, and burst into laughter.

Suddenly there was an earsplitting *boom*! The VW exploded into a white-hot fireball. Metal and plastic debris flew into the air. The percussive blast hurled Judy backwards.

And everything went black.

Chapter Thirty-seven

Judy woke up on her back in the parking lot. She felt stunned. She couldn't keep her eyes open. She couldn't think. Her head rang. She didn't know how long she had been lying there. The air reeked of smoke, gasoline, and burning rubber. Chunks of metal, broken glass, and charred debris lay everywhere. She couldn't hear a thing.

She propped herself up on her arm and saw the old man lying on his side, his face blackened. He was moving and didn't look injured. Her thoughts cohered in a terrifying moment.

Oh my God.

She looked around her in horror. Bright orange flames engulfed her car, raging through the interior. The conflagration obscured Domingo in the driver's seat. She scrambled to her feet, reeling.

Oh no no.

"Domingo!" she screamed in anguish. She had to get Domingo out of the car. She staggered to the VW. She didn't know how long the fire had been burning. Black smoke filled the air, fogging everything. She lunged to the car but raging flames drove her back. She reached into her pocket for her phone, scrolled frantically to the phone function, and pressed 911.

"Please hurry, I have an emergency, an explosion, a car fire!" Judy couldn't hear the operator or her own voice but kept shouting. "I need an ambulance right away! There's somebody trapped in the car! We're at Haltman's Hoagies in East Grove! Please hurry! I'm hanging up because I can't hear anyway!"

Judy put her phone away. Her eyes watered. Her throat and nostrils filled with smoke and soot. She gasped for breath. She covered her mouth and tried to get to the car. Flames licked at her, keeping her at bay.

Her cheeks and chest burned. Tears streamed down her cheeks. She coughed and coughed. Heat seared her face. Fiery debris flew like a nightmare blizzard, blocking out the sky.

"Domingo, Domingo!" Judy tried to get to the car one more time. The sleeve of her blazer caught fire. She beat the flames with her hand, smothering them. Agonizing pain exploded in her palm.

She couldn't let Domingo die. Her thoughts raced ahead. The sandwich shop must have a fire extinguisher. She whirled around and ran back to the shop through the smoke. A yellow Mini Cooper had stopped at the curb. Two young girls jumped out of the front doors, surveying the scene with horror.

"Help the old man!" Judy yelled to them. The young girls yelled back to her, something she couldn't hear. One young girl raced to the old man, who was struggling to his feet. The other young girl started talking into a cell phone, probably calling 911.

Judy bolted to the sandwich shop, ran inside, and looked wildly around. A small red extinguisher was affixed to the lower wall by the door. She yanked it off and raced outside with it, frantic. She sprinted past the old man and the young girls.

Cars were slowing on the street and pulling to the curb to help.

Judy ran to her VW. An inferno razed the interior. Flames raged skyward. Smoke billowed everywhere. The heat beat her backwards. Her eyes burned in the smoke. She couldn't accept that Domingo was dead. She tucked the fire extinguisher under her arm and pulled out the steel ring on top. Behind her, a trio of Good Samaritans helped the old man to his feet. She recognized one of them, a priest.

"Father Vega?" Judy's heart leapt with hope. "Thank God! Help!"

"Judy?" Father Vega looked over and ran toward her through the smoke, his black jacket flying open. He reached her, his eyes wide with alarm. "What are you doing here? Is that your car?"

"Yes, my friend's inside!" Judy tugged the rubber hose on the extinguisher from its holder and aimed the nozzle at the fire.

"Hurry! Squeeze the black handle! Spray the car! Sweep it from side to side!"

"On it!" Judy squeezed the handle and aimed the nozzle. Acrid pale yellow powder sprayed at the huge flames, though it looked futile. She didn't know what else to do. She glanced at Father Vega and caught him sliding a hunting knife from his jacket pocket, its jagged blade glinting in the sun. The priest was turning toward her, his eyes blazing darkly as he raised the knife in his hand.

"Father Vega?" Judy gasped, thunderstruck. She couldn't begin to comprehend what she was seeing with her own eyes. A man of God, about to stab her with a lethal knife.

And behind him at the curb, jumping out of a battered white pick-up, were Carlos and another man, presumably Roberto.

Chapter Thirty-eight

Judy couldn't believe what was happening. She had thought Father Vega was so kind, but she'd been horribly wrong. It shocked her, but it was unfolding before her. The priest must've been in cahoots with Carlos and Roberto. Father Vega charged at Judy with the hunting knife.

"No!" Judy aimed the nozzle of the fire extinguisher at him and sprayed his face with powder.

"Ahh!" Father Vega cried in pain. His hands flew to his face. He dropped the knife and staggered backwards.

Judy swung the extinguisher toward his head and slammed it into his temple. The priest fell to the ground, and the old man, girls, and Good Samaritans wheeled around, a confused group. Behind them at the curb, Carlos raised an assault rifle and Roberto a handgun, aimed at Judy and the group. They must've followed Domingo to the sandwich shop and planted the bomb on her car. They'd tried to kill her and Domingo. Now they were going to finish the job.

"Watch out, they have guns!" Judy screamed. Roberto fired his weapon. Suddenly red blood spurted from the cheek of one of the girls, who dropped to her knees and fell over.

Pop pop pop! Carlos fired the assault rifle, but Judy was already running for her life. She raced past the burning car and through the parking lot. The smoke and fire screened her from Carlos's view. There were woods behind the sandwich shop, and she ran into it as fast as she could, struggling not to trip on sticks and underbrush.

Tree trunks and limbs exploded on her right, spraying jagged wood chips where bullets hit. She kept her legs churning, full-tilt. She zigzagged between the trees. Their limbs had grown together everywhere. Vines wound around the branches, blocking her path. She pinwheeled her arms to get through them.

Tree limbs and thorns scratched her face and clothes. She veered around one tree, then the next, not knowing which direction she was heading. Her only thought was to run away. Her chest heaved. Her heart pumped with exertion and terror. She coughed and spit. She caught a flash through the trees of the sloped gray roof of the treatment plant, with steel pipes sticking out of the top.

She crashed through the woods, trying to think. Carlos and Roberto couldn't drive a truck through here. They had to chase her on foot. She had a head start. She was younger and in better shape. She had a fighting chance if she could make it to the treatment plant. There would be help there. She thought of shouting for help but that would give away her position. Police would arrive soon. She had to stay alive until then.

Hope fueled her. She kept going, the idea of salvation powering her anew. She heard her own ragged breaths. Her hearing was fully back. She heard gunshots behind her and put on the afterburners. A herd of deer sprang from the underbrush away from her, their stiff white tails high. She kept running and whacked aside the vines as she went. She stumbled, tripping on the gnarled root of a tree. She kept her balance and staggered forward.

She veered left and caught another glimpse of the treatment plant. She was getting closer. Birds and turkey vultures circled overhead. Her nostrils were too full of soot to smell anything.

Gunshots popped behind her, a lethal series. It was too close for comfort. She bolted ahead in terror. She kept going, running straight. She didn't dare look back. Carlos was running after her. Roberto could be with him. It was two against one. They had weapons.

Judy felt rising panic but fought it. She couldn't give up now. She had to get to the police. She had to put Carlos and Roberto away for Iris and the others. She had to tell the police what Domingo had told her. Then she remembered.

My phone.

Judy had recorded her conversation with Domingo on her phone, unbeknownst to him. She had every word he'd said on tape, in case she couldn't persuade him to go to the police. She never dreamed that he would be murdered. Domingo would help her bring his own killers to justice, even though he was gone.

Her phone bounced around in her pocket. She raced toward the treatment plant with her precious cargo.

She would get to the police or die trying.

Chapter Thirty-nine

Judy ran closer to the treatment plant, soaring with hope. She was almost there. Her lungs felt like they were about to burst. Her stomach cramped. Her legs burned but she kept them churning. She pumped her arms, ignoring the ache in her shoulders.

She kept going, getting closer, catching a clear view of a commotion at the plant. For such a large operation, there seemed to be only a handful of employees, and they were gathering in a parking lot in front of a boxy building, like an office.

Judy almost cried with happiness. They would help her. She was almost there, only three hundred yards away. She veered toward them, changing course. She didn't call out because she didn't want to give away her position to Carlos and Roberto.

She sprinted closer and saw the plant employees quickly dispersing to trucks and cars, then speeding off down a side road, spraying gravel and dust. She realized that the road led back to the sandwich shop. The employees must've seen the car fire or heard the gunshots. They were leaving the treatment plant to go help.

No, no, no!

Judy almost shouted to them, but stopped herself. If she called to them now, she'd draw fire for sure. Carlos had an assault rifle and he would shoot them all. She couldn't cause any more death. She ran harder than she ever thought possible. Tears of fright sprang to her eyes. There had to be somebody left at the plant, didn't there? They wouldn't all leave, would they? Cars and trucks drove off down the road at speed.

She kept a bead on the office. Two cars were left in the lot. There had to be somebody there. Or maybe a weapon. Or maybe she could lock herself in a room until the police arrived.

Judy ran and ran, on her way to the edge of the woods. She could see ahead that the trees ended in a trash area filled with Dumpsters, the parking lot, and the door to the office. She would be exposed as soon as she got out of the woods. Her only hope was that Carlos wasn't looking to the right. She prayed he was running straight for the treatment plant, the way she had been before she changed course.

Judy burst out of the woods and raced over the blacktop and past the Dumpsters. She flung open the office door and flew inside. She found herself in a bright entrance hall that was quiet and empty. She ran through it to the next door, which led to a short hallway with an office on either side.

"Help me!" she called out, barely able to catch her breath, running past the empty offices, but there was no response. She looked around frantic for a place to hide but didn't see any. She tested the door to the last office but it didn't lock. She flew back down the hall into a coffee room with brown cabinets, stopping at a wall phone. She snatched the receiver off the cradle, pressed 911, and couldn't wait for the call to connect.

"Help, help!" she said, her chest heaving. "I'm at the treatment plant in East Grove! I'm being chased by men with guns. They killed people at the sandwich shop. Please hurry!" She left the receiver hanging and took off running. She heard a noise behind her in the office area. She glanced back reflexively at the sound. Nobody was there, but they must've been coming. She almost cried out for help, but she couldn't be sure if it was an employee or Carlos.

She burst through the door at the end of the hall into a cavernous building, as big as a warehouse but completely empty. The concrete floor was wet as if it had just been hosed down. She didn't see any employees or anyplace to hide. The air was warm and wet. A tractor-trailer with an empty container sat parked in the open door. Thick industrial orange-and-yellow hook hoses lay nearby. Her heart leapt at the distant sound of sirens. The police were finally getting here. Help was on the way. All she had to do was stay alive.

She heard another noise behind her in the office area. The distinct slamming of a door, then men speaking Spanish. She didn't recognize the voices. She still didn't know if they were employees or Carlos and Roberto. She raced from the empty room, through another door, and almost plowed into a big white cylinder on a cart. HEAT STAR, it read, but she couldn't use it as a weapon or anything else.

She bolted past it into another huge room with a wet floor, looking around wildly for help. The air was hot and more humid. There was nobody. A twenty-foot-tall green machine that read CHRISTIAENS GROUP sat on a rail close to the wall. She bolted behind it to see if it would hide her, but it wouldn't. She looked up, her heart pounding. Gray piping of all kinds was suspended from the corrugated ceiling. None of it could help her. The police sirens sounded closer. So did the men speaking Spanish, calling to each other. They were angry, their words staccato. It had to be Carlos and Roberto.

Judy's heart thundered with terror. Adrenaline poured into her system. She had to think of something. She had to save herself. She spotted a stairway of stainless steel that went from the floor to ceiling and led to a conveyor belt with a sign **Danger: Pinch Points, Peligro: Puntos de Ajustamiento**. She would have run up it but it didn't lead anywhere except the conveyor belt.

She wheeled around in a panic. She ran to a black tractor-trailer that sat parked underneath the conveyor belt. Heat emanated from its massive engine. The driver must have just abandoned it. He could have left the keys in the ignition. She clambered onto the rubber step to the cab, but there was no key.

Police sirens cut the air outside, closer but not here yet. Carlos and Roberto had fallen silent. Judy didn't know where they were. She had to get out of sight. The hall from the office would lead them directly here. Her panicky gaze found a skinny middle ladder that was part of the truck, going up the side.

She jumped onto the closest rung and scrambled to the roof of the container. There was barely a foot between the top of the truck and the corrugated ceiling of the room. She flattened down just in time to see light spill from the door. The silhouette of a short, muscular man stood in the threshold. In his hand was a handgun.

She bit her lip not to cry out in fear. It had to be Roberto because Carlos had a rifle. She turned her head and pressed it flat against the metal roof of the container, which was covered with grit and dirt from the road. She couldn't risk raising her head or she would be seen. Instead she watched Roberto's shadow, moving on the floor. He entered the room and walked around, raising his gun. He was looking for her. He was going to kill her.

Judy remained perfectly still. She could hear his footsteps faintly, in heavy boots. He was trying to walk quietly. She breathed as shallowly as possible. The heat in the room made it hard to inhale. She pressed her face and cheek against the roof of the container.

Suddenly, a shifting movement caught her eye on the other side of the vast room, by the open rolltop door. It was a man. He walked into view and even at a distance, she could see it was Carlos, raising his rifle.

Terror shot through her. The police siren sounded closer, but Carlos and Roberto were in no hurry. She forced herself to think. She had to do something. She realized that Carlos and Roberto couldn't see each other because the truck was in the middle. She would lose the opportunity if they kept moving.

She swept her hand slowly over the surface of the container, feeling the grit for the biggest rock. She found one, closed her hand around it, and waited for the right moment. She tried to control her breathing and her fear. She blocked out the sound of the police sirens. She cleared her head of any other thought.

She watched silently as Carlos walked farther into the room. Then Roberto's shadow vanished, which meant that he was well out of the doorway and closer into the room, but the two killers still couldn't see each other.

Now.

Judy pitched the rock in Roberto's direction and heard it *ping* off something metal. Carlos responded instantly, swinging the rifle back and forth, spraying gunfire. Shots reverberated at deafening levels throughout the corrugated room. A man cried out in pain, then moaned. The gunfire ended abruptly.

Judy realized her move must have worked. One of the bullets had caught Roberto. She kept her head down and flat. Her ears rung. She didn't dare peek to see what was going on. Smoke hung in the air.

She heard footsteps running across the room. Carlos yelled furiously in Spanish, from right in front of the truck. Roberto groaned and moaned, crying piteously. Suddenly another barrage of gunfire went off, then ended abruptly.

Judy squeezed her eyes shut. Carlos had just killed Roberto. He would kill her if he discovered her. She gritted her teeth to stay in control of her emotions. She couldn't predict whether Carlos would go or stay. Whether she would live or die.

She held her breath.

Chapter Forty

Judy stayed as flat as she could on the top of the container. She heard the sound of heavy footsteps walking away. She spotted Carlos's shadow turning around in the light from the door. He raised his gun as he scanned the space for her. Every muscle in her body clenched with fright.

Police sirens screamed louder and closer. Carlos must have heard them. He was running out of time and he knew it. He edged backwards toward the door. She prayed he kept going. In the next moment he turned around, faced the door, and hustled from the room.

Judy thought about staying but worried he'd come back. She had to keep moving. She had to know where he was. She got up from the container roof so quickly she bumped her head on the ceiling. She was too adrenalized to feel a thing. She got low, scrambled around like a crab, and climbed down the ladder as fast as she could, jumping to the wet concrete floor. She couldn't go to the right because Carlos had gone that way. She turned left and ran to the open door of the vast room.

Massive industrial fans whirred in the ceiling, masking the sound of her footsteps as she raced across the concrete floor.

Her heart pounded, her breath came ragged. She reached the door, squinting from the bright sunlight. The police sirens sounded closer, almost at the sandwich shop. She prayed they had gotten her 911 message from the treatment plant, but she couldn't wait for help to come. She scanned the yard to see where she could hide.

The area was paved almost a city block, and on the left stood massive rectangular bales of hay, twelve feet tall and thirty feet wide. There had to be forty of them in the field, and beyond them rose hill-size mounds of dark brown compost, with smoke trailing from their peaks.

Judy clung to the corrugated inside of the room. The big fans whirred overhead. She had to plan her next move or it would be her last. She could run to the hay bales. She could go from one to the next, hiding from Carlos until the police came. She would be exposed as she sprinted across the concrete. But she was out of options.

She spotted Carlos pop from behind one of the hay bales, his back turned. He had anticipated her move. He was going from one bale to the next, searching them for her. She couldn't go that way. She tucked herself from view, waiting for the right moment, keeping an eye on Carlos.

Carlos disappeared behind the next hay bale, and she made her move. She darted out of the doorway, turning left away from where she'd seen him. She ran as hard as she could across the concrete yard, dangerously exposed. Birds and turkey vultures flew overhead. Police sirens sounded at the sandwich shop.

Judy kept running, almost slipping. Filth and muddy tire tracks covered the yard. Huge trucks and equipment sat parked willy-nilly, stopped where they were when the employees had left. She skidded as she raced past a yellow truck pulling a coiled red hose, then three front-end loaders that had their buckets in the air. They offered her no place to hide, but she veered in front of them so they would block her from Carlos. She bolted to a cinderblock building that looked like an operations office. She flung open the door, but passed up the office because it had four glass windows on the other side that would show her hiding there. She whirled around.

Behind her lay a huge concrete structure as tall as a single-story house, with a heavy green rail system over the top. The structure was open on the side facing her, only a roof over six cinderblock bins. The bins had a foot-high shield at the front bottom. She could see in a flash that the four closest bins were empty, their concrete side walls brown with filth. The fifth bin had a dirty dump truck parked in front, its bed in the inclined position. The sixth bin looked closed, roped off with yellow caution tape and an official-looking safety notice.

She realized that the bins were where raw manure got dumped, but they could save her life. Carlos wouldn't suspect she would go in that direction. The fifth bin had enough manure to bury herself in. She could hide behind the structure or run back in the woods.

Police sirens screamed louder. Carlos would be back any minute. If Roberto had driven their white pick-up truck to the plant, it would be parked in front of the office. Carlos would have to run back this way to get the truck and escape the police.

Judy had to do something fast. She sprinted behind the bin structure. The woods were on her left but too far away. She would be exposed for too long if she ran that way. Carlos would cut her down and take off in the truck. On her right was the back of the concrete structure, and it was her only hope. The back of each bin had a heavy mechanized door that closed across the middle. She ran past the first five bins because their doors were chained and padlocked. She ran to the sixth bin on the end, roped off. A handwritten sign read GEARS BROKEN DO NOT USE. The doors of the roped-off bin were open a crack but there was no chain or padlock.

Judy looked around wildly. She had no other choice. She ducked under the caution tape, wedged her hands between the top and bottom doors, and yanked with all her might, trying to open the door. She moved them six inches apart, then a foot, then a little more until they jammed, immovable. Her heart pounded with fear and exertion. The space between the doors looked almost big enough for her body. She heard Carlos running in the concrete yard, cursing in Spanish, his rage boiling over. She was out of time.

She launched herself into the opening, scrambling inside the bin, scraping the outside of the door with her legs and knees. She squeezed inside, wrenching her arm at the socket. She slid down along the filth of the door, keeping a hard grasp of the lid so she wouldn't make a noise when she hit the bottom. She eased herself onto the floor. Raw manure covered the bin bottom.

Carlos ranted, fifty feet away. She made herself as flat as possible against the back of the bin. Her body was hidden by the foot-high rim at the front of the bin. She squeezed her eyes and lips shut. She stuck her face into the crack between the door and the floor, burrowing down into the manure and the darkness. The stench filled her nose. Her gorge rose with disgust. She had to stay calm.

Carlos was only twenty feet away, cursing in frantic Spanish. The police sirens blared louder and louder. The cruisers were coming down the road to the treatment plant. They must have gotten her 911 call. They were on the way. They were going to rescue her just in time.

Judy had to stay alive for just a few more seconds. Carlos must be looking for her, turning this way and that. She could hear his footsteps on the gritty concrete and hear the scrape of his boots. He would have to leave any second. He was cutting it so close. The police were almost here.

Judy willed herself to keep her wits about her. If she wanted to live, she had to stay still and silent.

Suddenly, in her blazer pocket, her phone started ringing.

Chapter Forty-one

Judy reacted instantly, desperate. She grabbed the phone from her pocket and sent it slipping along the mucky floor, so the ringing came from the far side of the bin. Carlos started firing, but aimed a deafening volley at the bin next to her. Scattered bullets punched holes in the front rim of her bin. She bit her lips not to scream.

Abruptly the gunfire stopped. Smoke drifted into the bin. Her phone rang and rang.

"Freeze right there!" an officer shouted. "Police! Put your weapon on the ground! Put your weapon on the ground!"

Judy could only imagine the standoff outside. The police would train their guns on Carlos, thinking he would give up. She knew better. Carlos wanted her dead even if he was captured alive. He had nothing to lose and everything to gain from her murder. He wanted her silenced for good. Her phone finally went quiet.

"Keep lowering your weapon!" another officer yelled. "Lower it and put it on the ground! Put your weapon on the ground!"

Judy's heart pounded like it was trying to get out of her chest. She knew what Carlos would do next. He would shoot the policemen. It sounded like only two cops. Carlos was waiting for just the right moment, tricking the police by lowering his weapon. She couldn't let that happen.

She squeezed both hands around some manure, closed her fists, and jumped up. Carlos was standing five feet from the bin, facing her direction, his gun slightly lowered. She hurled the manure at Carlos's eyes, then sprang out of the way.

Carlos shouted in surprise. His hands flew up reflexively, firing shots wildly into the air. Judy dove toward the floor for safety, just in time to see Carlos lose his balance, whirl away from her, and recover fast enough to aim his weapon at the police.

Pop pop pop! The police responded with a barrage of firepower.

Judy landed on the bottom of the filthy bin. She heard Carlos cry out, then he went silent. The gunfire stopped.

Judy lay perfectly still, afraid to move. She kept her eyes closed. She was in no hurry to get up and see Carlos's bullet-ridden body, even as much as she hated him. She opened her eyes slowly, but didn't understand what she was seeing, amid the brown manure that lay everywhere.

A bright patch of white-and-green paper stood out in the bottom seam of the bin. She reached for it instinctively and pulled. A twenty-dollar bill came from underneath the floor of the bin, attached to another twenty-dollar bill, like Kleenex out of the box. Astounded, she dug her fingers in the seam and pulled out a five-dollar bill and realized that the manure bin must have had a false bottom.

"Miss, are you okay?" the police officers asked, rushing over.

"Look at this, guys," Judy answered, digging for more money.

Chapter Forty-two

Judy sat at the conference table in the mayor's office at the Kennett Square Police Station, having finished giving her statement to a room packed with law enforcement personnel, including Detective Boone and two other detectives, three assistant district attorneys, and a fleet of FBI, DEA, and ICE agents who sat in the back of the room, taking rapid notes. The press thronged outside the building, their newsvans, reporters, and cameramen visible through the old-fashioned venetian blinds.

Before her statement, Judy had asked the police to contact her mother and her office to let them know where she was, then she had been photographed in her filthy clothes for purposes of the investigation, and finally showered in the locker room for female officers and changed into a KSPD sweatshirt and sweatpants one of them had lent her. Given the stink of manure on Judy's skin, she doubted the female officer would want her sweatclothes back.

Judy's filthy phone sat on the table between her and the law enforcement authorities, next to the silvery recording devices from the various agencies and Domingo's scrap of paper that read BONIDE and MURIATIC. She had explained everything that

302 | Lisa Scottoline

had happened at the barracks last night, then what Domingo had told her this morning, playing the recording for them from her phone. Her eyes had filmed at the sound of Domingo's voice, but she'd kept it together. She consoled herself with the notion that Father Vega was in federal custody and charged with an array of crimes, as well as being investigated for the death of Father Keegan. Carlos and Roberto had met their end, but Judy was enough of a lawyer to wish that they'd rot in jail for the rest of their lives. Luckily, they hadn't succeeded in killing the two young girls from the Mini Cooper, the old man at the sandwich shop, or the Good Samaritans. The one girl had been hospitalized, but was expected to recover.

Judy met Detective Boone's eye. "So how much money was under the manure bin?"

"I'm not sure it's been counted yet." Detective Boone kept his tone official, but not unkind.

"Ballpark it for me, would you?" Judy understood his reluctance, reading the body language of the FBI behind him, a collective stiffening of postures that were already stiff, in suits and ties.

"We are not at liberty to discuss that, Judy."

"I think I've earned the right to know, don't you? Modesty aside, nobody would've found any money but for me, and I almost got killed in the process."

"Chester County appreciates your efforts, and as we've already said, you are to be commended as a private citizen for—"

"Please just answer the question." Judy felt too raw and exhausted to mince words. "We both know what a pain in the ass I can be."

Detective Boone almost smiled. "Fine. It will be in the newspapers, so I'll tell you. Estimates are about $760,000."

"Wow." Judy didn't hide her surprise. "Plus the $50,000 that was in my aunt's house, that's a major drug ring, isn't it? Do you think they were dealing heroin?"

"I cannot give you any further details."

"Did you find any money under the other bins, or elsewhere at the treatment plant? I'll keep it confidential, you have my word."

"Not the point. It's police business, and given that you almost lost your life today, you should understand completely the dangerousness of the criminals we're dealing with."

"Please." Judy thought of Iris and couldn't let it go. "I know how they killed Iris, but I still don't know why. Can't you fill me in on your investigation or your next steps?"

"It's no longer our investigation. We'll keep a hand in, but the federal agencies are asserting primary jurisdiction at this point. They will liaise with us, but they're running the show now." Detective Boone gestured to the men behind him, and Judy could see from the tightness around his mouth that he wasn't any happier than she was about the current state of affairs.

"Well, what do you think is going on here, gentlemen?" Judy raised her voice, addressing the room in general.

"Again, we're not going to discuss that with you," Detective Boone answered, presumably for all of them.

"I'm no expert, like you gentlemen, but it must be some type of heroin ring, right? We found where they stash their money, or at least one of the places they stash their money." Judy figured she could think out loud and watch them for reaction, if they weren't going to tell her anything. She thought of the money stored in her aunt's house, now safely in the bank, and she remembered what John Foxman had said about banking laws. "So they're selling heroin and making lots of cash, but they have nowhere to store it. They can't put it in a bank, so they have to launder it, and I'm betting we found their hamper. Sorry, *I* found their hamper."

"Judy, I'm not about to speculate with you." Detective Boone closed his notebook, but Judy continued talking.

"U.S.D.A. inspections take place at the treatment plant, but the government inspects the treated manure, not the raw manure. Hiding the money under the false bottom was pretty smart." Judy noticed one of the FBI agents frowning, so she knew she was right. "Now, it seems unlikely that so much money was hidden at the treatment plant without some of the higher-ups knowing about it, and maybe they're in on it with Father Vega, Carlos, Roberto, or other employees at Mike's Exotics. Maybe even Mike himself." Judy realized that some East Grove police could be involved, since that was where Mike's, the barracks, and the plant were located, but she didn't say so out loud. She did, however, notice that no police personnel from East Grove were present at the meeting. "In any event, it looks like we have a conspiracy to deal heroin and launder money, right here in lovely Chester County. Boys, you have your work cut out for you."

Detective Boone set his pen down. "I think we're finished here, unless anyone has any further questions."

"Wait, hold on," Judy said, thinking of Aunt Barb. "Can I ask you a question about Iris? I know my aunt will want to know."

"Go right ahead," Detective Boone answered, his voice gentler, and Judy sensed he had a soft spot for Aunt Barb.

"Was Domingo right that if you mix Bonide and muriatic acid, they produce a gas that can kill you?"

"Yes."

"How does that work, exactly?" Judy would Google it later, but she wanted to get the official version.

"Bonide is a brand name of a common pesticide on farms, and muriatic acid is a form of hydrochloric acid. It's used in lots of applications, around the house or a farm. Masons use it to clean flagstone and the like. These are common chemicals that, when mixed together, produce a poison gas."

Judy swallowed hard. "Would Iris have suffered a long time?"

"No, death is almost instantaneous."

"Almost." Judy's stomach turned over. "I bet that's how she broke her nails, trying to get out of the shed. Look on the floor of the shed, I bet you find the nail tips, little rhinestones."

"Will do."

"And the car window. Why do you think it was open? Maybe they thought some gas would cling to her? To her clothes or hair?" Judy didn't pause for an answer, because she could see that she wasn't getting one. Her heart ached for Iris, Domingo, and the others. "What about Daniella?"

"We're investigating."

"Did you look at the barracks? If they killed Iris there, they could have killed Daniella there, too."

"We're looking into it."

"Do you think she's still alive?"

"We don't want to speculate."

Judy felt another pang at so much loss. "You know what I don't get? Why did the pathologist say Iris had a heart attack in the autopsy report?"

"Because she did. Hydrogen sulfide gas causes the organs to shut down, resulting in a heart attack. Unlike carbon monoxide, it doesn't turn the skin cherry-red or any other color."

"So it looks like a natural death, but it isn't?"

"Yes, the only way the gas would be detectable at autopsy is that it sometimes leaves a faint rotten-egg smell in the organs, but the pathologist had a head cold. We think that's how he might have missed it, if he did."

Judy cringed inwardly. "Can they confirm that's how she died?"

"The coroner can confirm it by ordering a special test of her blood for the gas. That takes a month or so to do, but it's easily done." Detective Boone paused, glancing over his shoulder at the FBI, DEA, and ICE types. "I can tell you that it's becoming more common in rural areas like ours as a way to commit suicide. We've had cases where people mix the chemicals in the car, then close themselves inside. We started hearing about it last year and put the word out to first responders. We send in the Hazmat Unit to respond to a suicide like that."

"How sad," Judy blurted out, the horror of the day catching up with her. She sensed that the meeting was over because the FBI men were slipping their notepads inside their breast pockets and even Detective Boone stood, brushing down his slacks again.

"Judy, please don't speak to the press, if they call you or show up at your office."

"Of course not, I know the drill." Judy stood up, gesturing at the table. "I'm assuming you want to keep my stinky phone, for evidence."

"Yes, thank you. Might be time for an upgrade, eh?"

"Ya think?" Judy managed a smile, and Detective Boone guided her to the door.

"I've arranged for a uniformed officer to give you a lift back to the city, considering your service to the county today."

"Thanks." Judy flashed on the horrific explosion in her VW. It gave her a jolt, but she had to put it behind her for now. Detective Boone held open the door, and the other Chester County detectives, A.D.A.'s, uniformed officers, and FBI, DEA, and ICE agents gathered around her, thanking her and handing her a flurry of business cards with gold seals and embossed badges.

"I'll take you out back to avoid the press," Detective Boone said after the good-byes were finished, leading her out the door, through the crowded waiting room, and out a side door down a hallway. Judy let herself be steered past a time clock next to a tray of metal slots filled with punch cards, then a scheduling board covered with wipe-off Magic Marker notations, out the back to a small police parking lot. The sunlight was waning, and without her phone, she had no idea how long she'd been inside.

"What time is it?" Judy asked, disoriented.

"Four thirty." Detective Boone gestured to a uniformed police officer who stood waiting beside a Kennett Square police cruiser, its back door open.

"Thanks for the ride."

"We're happy to do it. Officer Kitt will be your driver. Tell him where to take you." Detective Boone put a paternal hand on her shoulder. "Thanks for everything you did. While we appreciate your efforts, I'm officially informing you that we hope you never do it again."

"I won't. Maybe." Judy smiled. "Will you keep me posted?"

"No."

"Aw, come on," Judy whined, and Detective Boone didn't suppress a wry smile.

"Okay, if there's anything you need to know, I will."

"I wish I understood why they killed Iris or what she was doing with the money."

"We'll keep investigating, you can be assured of that." Detective Boone opened the back door of the cruiser while Officer Kitt went around the front, climbed in the driver's seat, and started the big engine. "Travel safe. Please give my best regards to your aunt."

"Will do, thanks." Judy eased into the cruiser, and Detective Boone shut the door behind her, closing her inside. The cruiser took off, taking a left turn to bypass the media, then wound its way through Kennett Square and hit the highway.

Judy rested her head back on the hard plastic seat, closing

her eyes, but she didn't rest. Awful images flooded her brain, of white-hot explosions and fresh red blood. She could hear the noise of the blast, Roberto moaning, and Carlos cursing. She flashed on Father Vega, feeling shocked all over again that he'd tried to stab her to death. The priest had hidden behind the cloth to win the trust of Iris, Daniella, and an entire congregation, but in the end, Father Vega had betrayed them all, even his own, Father Keegan. Judy thought about Iris, who had been so savagely murdered, and it made her angry and frustrated that she still didn't know why. Judy had believed she wanted justice, but what she really wanted was to understand why, though no explanation of motive could make her truly comprehend the human capacity for evil.

She opened her eyes, gazed out the window, and watched the highway whiz past. Twilight fell, painting the sky black as they headed toward the city, and she wondered what she was going back to, since everything had changed. Her mother. Her aunt. Even Frank was gone. She didn't have a car anymore. She didn't even have a purse or a phone. She thought about stopping at a pay phone to call her mother and the office, but the police already had. The Rule 37 motion had been answered, and the rest of her cases could wait. It was impossible to think about work in the aftermath of so much destruction and death.

"Ms. Carrier, we're approaching the city limits," Officer Kitt said, looking into the rearview mirror. "Where would you like to go?"

"Pennsylvania Hospital, please."

"Gotcha." Officer Kitt hit the gas, rolling into the city, then entered the grid that was Center City, choked with rush-hour traffic. Finally, they ended up in front of the hospital, where he dropped her off and she thanked him.

Judy entered the hospital and crossed to the reception desk to get the information about Aunt Barb's room, then went up the elevator. She got off on a floor busy with visitors, doctors, and nurses bustling back and forth. Dinner service had begun, and an orderly pushed a tall, rolling stack of food trays covered with steamy lids, though she couldn't smell anything for the stink of manure and ashes in her nose. She walked down the glistening hall, reading the room numbers until she had located her aunt's room, which was the first closed door. She paused for a moment, bracing herself to see her aunt and her mother, and vice versa, or whatever. She knocked on the door, then opened it to see Aunt Barb in bed, and her mother sitting by her side with a female visitor.

"Hi, everybody," she said, entering the room uncertainly.

"Judy!" Aunt Barb looked up, her lips parting with happiness. Flowers and cards covered the sidetable. "You're here! Are you okay? The police called, and we've been watching on TV! Were you hurt in the explosion? What happened? Thank God you're okay!"

"Honey!" Her mother jumped up and rushed toward her, arms outstretched, and gathered her up for a real hug. "We were worried sick! Are you okay? What did they do to you?"

"I'm fine, I'm okay." Judy hugged her mother back, surprised at the show of emotion, which felt somehow painful. She let her mother go, avoiding her eyes. "It's all right now, so don't worry."

"But look at your face!" her mother said, aghast. "There's little cuts on your cheeks! Is that from the car bomb? Did you get to a hospital? Didn't they take you to an ER? I knew something was wrong, very wrong, when you didn't call me back. I called you this morning, did you get my message?"

"This morning?" Judy realized that her mother must have been the one who'd phoned when she'd been hiding from Carlos in the manure bin. She decided not to share that part of the story. "Sorry, I didn't hear the phone."

"Judy, come over, please!" Aunt Barb was sitting up in bed

and motioning to her, with a hand attached to an IV and a pressure monitor. "I want to see you! You poor thing, what have you been *through*?"

"I'm fine, really." Judy walked over stiffly, unable to shake the awkwardness she felt in the presence of her mother and aunt, especially in front of the female visitor, whom she assumed was a friend of Aunt Barb's. Judy extended a hand. "Hi, nice to see you, I'm Judy."

"Nice to see you, too," answered the woman, with a Spanish accent. "I'm Daniella Gamboa."

Chapter Forty-three

"You're Daniella, *Iris's friend*?" Judy asked, incredulous, and Daniella clasped Judy's hand, covered it with her other hand, and held it for a moment. She looked younger than Iris, in her late forties, and was tall, about five-seven, and slim. Her large brown eyes stood out in a long face, and her shiny black hair was pulled back in a long ponytail. She had on a jeans jacket over a white sweater, with baggy jeans and black sneakers.

"I'm very sorry about what happened to you, from Carlos. They say on TV that your car, it blew up. He is very crazy man, very crazy. And Father Vega, they say on TV he *was* with them! I can' believe that!" Daniella's dark eyes flared in disbelief. "I *know* him. He know my family. We are from the same town. I tell him everything, is all my fault!"

"I understand," Judy said, though she didn't, not yet. "Daniella, I'm just happy you're alive. I was worried about you, so are the police. Where have you been?"

"I'm sorry, so sorry." Daniella shook her head. "I feel so terrible, so sick in my heart, in my soul. I was hiding. I get on the bus and go out of town, to Wilmington."

"Why were you hiding? From Carlos?"

"Yes, from him, from Father Vega, from everybody." Daniella nodded, agitated. "That why I take the money, to get away from Carlos."

"What money?"

Aunt Barb motioned for attention. "Daniella saw on the TV news that Father Vega had been arrested and Carlos and Roberto killed, so she came out of hiding. Iris had told her about me, so she knew where to find me." Aunt Barb's eyes filmed with new tears, and she held the Kleenex to her nose. "Daniella, tell Judy what you told us. I . . . don't want to tell it. I can't."

"Judy, Carlos and Roberto, they kill Iris. They *murder* her."

"I know," Judy said, sinking onto the bed.

"You *know*?" Aunt Barb asked, shocked. "How did you find out? Did they try to kill you? What happened?"

Judy's mother interjected, "Judy, how do you know? How did you get so involved in this? Why didn't the police handle it? What's going on?"

"Ladies, please." Judy waved them both into silence, focusing on Daniella. "*Why* did they kill Iris, do you know?"

"Yes." Daniella pursed her lips, which were thin.

"Please, tell me." Judy eased down onto a corner of the bed, across from Daniella.

"Iris and me, we mee' Carlos when he and Roberto come to Mike's. He is new and his friend Roberto. I like Carlos and he's liking me, so we date, you know?"

"Yes," Judy answered, trying to be patient.

"Carlos drink, all the time, too much, and he is mean, ugly. I know he sell heroin. I want to get away from him, but I cannot. He hit me, all the time. He say I am sleepin' with everybody, the men, the bosses, everybody. He don' want me to work at my job no more. He say he will marry me, give me money. He say he has so much money. He tell me where his money is."

"Where was it?"

"At Mike's. In the shed. He tell me there is a door in the floor."

Judy realized it must have been a second stash. "I don't understand something. Why did he tell you that?"

"When he drink, he tell me. He is out of his mind. He get so angry, he yell at himself. At me. And God." Daniella shook her head, with a deep frown. "Crazy, he get."

"So then what happened?"

"So then we have a big fight and he hit me, here." Daniella pointed to her lower chest. "He break my rib. He say he will kill me. I know I have to get away. I tell Iris, we should get his money. We can take the money and I can go away. Get away from him. I have to do it."

Judy could visualize the two desperate women, best friends trying to help each other.

"But I tell Father Vega, my priest. My *priest.* He help me all the time, with Carlos. He tell me to pray, but he *lie.*" Daniella shook her head, agonized. "I don' know Father Vega is *with* Carlos. I don' know."

"I'm sure." Judy's heart went out to her.

"Carlos drink one night and he fall asleep, from a pill I put in his rum. Iris bring me the sleeping pill, from Barb's house." Daniella winced, gesturing at Aunt Barb, who listened, dabbing her eyes. "Then we go in her car to the shed at Mike's. We find the money and we take some. Iris hide the money at Barb's house."

"Okay."

"So Friday, they move my shif' at work. The boss call me up. He tell me, no afternoon shif' with Iris. Somebody on mornin' shif' call in sick. The boss tell me to come in."

"What's the boss's name?"

"Roy. I worry, it isn' right.' People get sick, Roy don't care. He don't change shif'. He don' bother. I don' tell Iris, I know she worry too much." Daniella paused, with a pained sigh. "I go early, I hear Roy and Carlos talk, they say Father Vega tell them everything I tell him. They know we take the money. I run away. I don' have no money. I don' need no money. I . . ." Daniella made a hitchhiking motion with her thumb, then her face fell. The lines in her forehead formed fissures of deep grief. "I call Iris, I tell her. I leave a message to call me."

"You called her Saturday? Was it around two?"

"Yes."

Judy realized that Daniella had been the one who'd called Iris, in the rose garden.

"I don' know what happen. I hear she die and I know they kill her. I feel terrible, so terrible about Iris. I pray and pray for God to forgive me. I don' forgive myself. I don' know how they kill her but they do."

"You're right, they did."

"How? How do you know?"

"Before we discuss that, let me ask you something. Why did you come forward now?"

"I don' know what to do. I am safe now Carlos is dead but I no feel safe. Other bosses know we take the money. They wan' the money, so I come to Barb to ask her for it." Daniella's eyes turned pleading, and she faced Aunt Barb in bed. "Please, give me the money so I can give it to them. So they will not kill me or my family at home."

Judy held up a hand, interjecting. "Daniella, I don't think it works that way. If you show yourself, they'll kill you. Whoever else is in the conspiracy, they'll kill you. They can't let you live, even if you give them the money back."

"Wha' can I do?" Daniella's eyes brimmed with tears. "Wha' can I do? They will kill my family!"

Judy's thoughts raced ahead. "Let's go to the police. I'll go with you. We can make a deal."

"No, no, never." Daniella shook her head. "They will kill me. You see how they do."

"Let me try to get you a deal." Judy dug in the pocket of her sweatpants and pulled out the array of business cards from the various government agencies. "Look, I just met with all of these cops. FBI, ICE, too. Let me make some phone calls and talk to them. I'm a lawyer. I won't tell them where you are."

"No, I no go to the police." Daniella shook her head again, frightened.

"You can and you should. You have something to trade for a visa. You know about the other stash. There's probably a lot of things you know."

"No, no, no."

"What else do you know about the cartel? Did Carlos ever talk to you about the cartel or his business, when he was drunk?"

"Yes, okay, he did. He brag, all the time. He wan' to be the boss, the top."

"Did he say who he's in business with?"

"Yes, I know, he tell me."

"Are some of the mushroom growers in on it? Mike's? And the treatment plant?"

"Yes, yes."

"What about the police in East Grove?"

"Yes."

"Great," Judy said, then realized how wrong that sounded. "The point is, the government will trade for that information. They want names. That's how they make their case."

"No, they kill me. They kill my family. The cartel, they do what they want."

"What if I could make a deal to protect your family, Daniella?"

"They will find them. They will kill them."

"Let me call. Let me see if I can get a deal to protect them. I won't tell the government where you are until they agree." Judy spoke from the heart. "Daniella, won't you take a chance, for Iris?"

Chapter Forty-four

It was after midnight when Judy finally left the federal building in downtown Philly, turning left and walking down a chilly Chestnut Street. It had rained again, leaving the asphalt a shiny black and the sidewalk slick. Gutters flowed with rainwater, cigarette butts, and other debris. There was almost no traffic except a white Septa bus that rambled by empty, going her way, but Judy didn't try to catch it. She wanted to walk home, to clear her mind.

She shoved her hands in her pockets, heading home, head down. She and Daniella had met with the top brass at the FBI, DEA, and ICE, and Daniella had given the government plenty of good information. They had succeeded, with the help of an immigration lawyer, in securing an S-visa for Daniella, which was a special visa given to confidential informants, the so-called "snitch visa." They also got a deal to protect Daniella's mother and older sister, still living in Mexico, and the three of them were already on their way to their respective safe houses.

Judy passed the Constitution Center on her left and the Liberty Bell on her right, sights that usually gave her a lift, but not tonight. She supposed, at some level, she had gotten justice for

Iris, with the killers now dead and the government on its way to making a case against the rest of the conspirators. She had even learned the reason they had killed Iris, but she felt an emptiness inside that she hadn't anticipated.

She walked down the dark street and crossed into Old City, where all the stores were closed and the shops dark. She thought of the horrors she had witnessed, the loss of poor Domingo, and she felt a wave of sadness sweep over her. Somehow listening to the litany of names that Daniella had given the authorities made her feel even worse, and she wondered if justice was possible in a world full of profoundly evil and damaged human beings, in a veritable universe of damage.

Judy found herself in her apartment without even realizing it, having let herself in from the key in the lockbox that the landlord required them to keep there, for the fire department. She flicked on the light, closed the door behind her, and set the key on the sidetable, with a little *clink*. She didn't bother to check her mail.

She looked around for her mother, or her aunt or whatever, but nobody was downstairs. Her mother had probably gone upstairs to sleep. Of course Frank wasn't home, and Judy tried not to focus on how empty the apartment seemed without him. Penny bounded over, then plopped her butt on the hardwood and started scratching her ear with her back leg, signaling that the fleas were back.

"Hey, girl," Judy said to the dog, petting her. "Can you wait on that walk? I need a shower."

Penny trotted behind as Judy climbed the stairs quietly, so as not to wake up her mother. But when she got to the second floor, she looked down the hall and noticed the bedroom door was open. Her mother slept with the door closed, so Judy tiptoed to the bedroom, peeked inside the room, and could tell in the streetlight from the windows that the bed was empty. She flicked on the overhead light, and her mother wasn't there.

Judy reached for her pocket to get her cell phone, then re-membered her cell phone was gone. She still had a landline on the nightstand next to her bed, so she went over, picked up the receiver, and heard the telltale signal that she had messages. She barely remembered how to retrieve them, but she hit the right numbers, then deleted a series of junk calls until she got a message from her mother.

"Honey," her mother said, her tone uncharacteristically ten-tative. "I'm going to be staying at the hospital tonight. They said I'm allowed, and Barb and I both thought you might like to see Frank, after the hell you've been through. We feel just terrible about displacing him, and when Barb gets discharged tomorrow, she wants to go home to recuperate, instead of the apartment. We both love you, very much. I hope things went well with Daniella, and I'll keep my cell phone on if you want to talk. Good night."

Judy hung up the phone, shaking her head. She turned away from the bed and started to leave the room, then she did a double-take, realizing what she had just seen. She backed up to her closet and looked at it again, but she had been right the first time. The closet door had been rolled back to expose Frank's side of the closet, but his clothes were gone, including the hang-ers, leaving an empty hole. The sweaters, sweatshirts, and T-shirts that he used to jam into the shelves above his clothes were gone, too. She looked down and she could see the floorboards on his side of the closet, which had been covered for as long as she could remember by his pungent jumble of sneakers, loafers, and slide flip-flops. Frank must've come to the apartment today and moved out.

It was over.

Judy blinked, surprised, though she shouldn't have been. Frank wasn't the kind of man to drag things out, and she knew she had hurt him. Her mouth went dry. Something about his being gone seemed inconceivable, though she had willed it to happen. She found herself shaking her head. She crossed to their dresser and pulled out his drawer, which started with the fourth, but it was empty. She closed it and went to the fifth drawer, opening it even though she knew what she'd find, like a psycho ex on autopilot.

She left the drawer hanging open, straightened up, and looked around, seeing a bedroom she barely recognized, now that she started noticing things. Frank's framed photos and favorite Oakley sunglasses were missing from the top of the dresser, and his series of black kettlebells in graduated weights were no longer lined up against the wall, where she used to trip over them. In place of the Frank-things were her mother's things—a pump bottle of Cetaphil hand lotion, a small green jar of La Mer eye cream, and an old-school folding travel clock by the bed—and her Aunt Barb's things—the compression bras she'd bought at the mastectomy boutique, a large-size Ziploc bag of medication in brown plastic bottles, and a stack of mystery novels.

Judy scanned the room, which struck her as a total mess, strewn with debris, damage of its own kind. She couldn't help but see it as a mirror of her life, in matching disarray, with Frank gone and her mother and aunt jumbled together, the lines between the two women blurred, their respective roles impossible to delineate, much less define. Mother and aunt, aunt and mother, both women seemed to be occupying the same place at the same time, which everyone knew was impossible, most especially Mother Nature.

Judy turned away, left the bedroom, and walked stiffly to the bathroom, with the dog at her heels. She flipped on the light switch and avoided looking in the mirror because she didn't want to play match-the-facial-feature again. She reached inside the shower and turned on the faucet, trying not to think another thought or feel another emotion. She undressed while she waited for the water to warm up, shedding her borrowed sweat-clothes, which Penny came over to sniff avidly.

Judy stepped naked into the shower, letting the warm water run over her cuts and bruises, feeling it wash away the manure and the ashes, cleansing her of the blood and the grime, and she didn't know when she started crying, but she was pretty sure she would never, ever stop.

Chapter Forty-five

Next morning, Judy emerged from her front door, reflexively raising her hand against the press stationed outside the rowhouse that held her apartment. Photographers aimed cameras with wide rubber lenses at Judy's face, and TV reporters rushed forward, extending their black bubble microphones. She'd known they were there, having seen them from her window, so she plowed through them with her head down, ignoring their shouted questions.

"Ms. Carrier, was the car bomb intended for you?" "Why were you in Chester County?" "Did you know Carlos Ramiro and Roberto Rivera?" "How are you involved?" "Who are you representing?" "Is it true that Father Oscar Vega assaulted you?"

"No comment!" Judy called, hustling down the street, looking for a cab. Traffic clogged both lanes, and passersby stared at the scene, stopping on their way to work. It was a sunny day, and she knew she'd look like a freak in this light, with foundation hardly covering the tiny cuts on her face and lip gloss doing nothing to her split lip but making it look slicker. She'd dressed in a boring navy sweater and pants, with a trenchcoat on top, in case she had to go back to the FBI offices. Her trenchcoat flew behind her as she broke into a light run, but the reporters ran after her.

"Come on, Judy!" "Don't you have a comment for us, Judy?" "Are you or Bennie Rosato stepping in for the defense of anyone? Do you know who the targets of the federal investigation will be?" "Can you comment on the murder of Domingo Gutierrez?"

Judy cringed at the sound of Domingo's name. She'd thought of him all last night, hardly sleeping and replaying their meeting over and over in her mind. She spotted a cab and flagged it down, with reporters at her heels.

"Ms. Carrier, did you know the men who died at the treatment facility, Carlos Ramiro and Roberto Rivera? Were they conspirators with Domingo Gutierrez?" "How did you get involved?" "Are there any persons of interest? Any indictments coming down the pipeline?"

Judy ran to meet the cab as it pulled over to the curb, and when it stopped, she jumped inside and turned away from the reporters as camera flashes fired at her, inside the backseat.

"You somebody important?" the cabbie called over his shoulder, as the cab took off. He was young and African-American, in a mesh Sixers cap.

"Not in the least," Judy answered, then told him where she needed to go.

Chapter Forty-six

"Hi, Mom, Aunt Barb." Judy entered the hospital room, trying to suppress the tension she felt inside.

"Good morning, dear," her mother said, looking over with a nervous smile. She'd been packing items from the bed table in a white plastic bag, but she walked over, bag in hand, and gave Judy a quick peck on the cheek. She was freshly made-up, back in her favorite long gray sweater, black knit leggings, and black ballet shoes, but her manner was stilted. "Did it go okay, at the FBI?"

"All fine, as expected. That's why I didn't call. Sorry."

"Sure. We understand. And Daniella?"

"She's fine, and in their hands."

"Wonderful." Her mother smiled, almost politely. "Did you sleep well?"

"I did, thanks."

"Are you feeling better?"

"Yes, thanks."

"You sure you don't need to be seen by a doctor? We're in a hospital, after all."

"No, I'm fine."

"I bet Frank was glad to see you."

"Yes," Judy answered, avoiding her mother's eye. She wasn't about to tell them about Frank. She had known both women her whole life, but felt as if she couldn't trust them anymore.

"You're all over the news." Her mother nodded in the direction of the television, which was playing morning shows on mute.

"I know, right?" Judy found herself hesitating before she went over to Aunt Barb, who was sitting inclined in bed, pale and tired under a multicolored cap and buried by a white blanket, her finger hooked up to a monitor and her hand to an IV. Judy learned over and gave her aunt a quick kiss on the cheek, feeling as if she were going through the motions. All of them were.

"Hi, honey." Aunt Barb managed a shaky smile. "Who knew what a mess I'd get you into, huh? We're so proud of you, for everything you did, and for helping Daniella."

"Thanks. How do you feel?" Judy lingered by the bed, glancing at the array of monitors with their blinking lights. The cottony straps of Aunt Barb's vest, with the drain pockets, were visible because her neckline had slipped to the side.

"Not too bad. It feels like there's pressure on my chest, but it's not that bad. They're weaning me off of morphine and onto Demerol." Aunt Barb gestured at the IV drip that ran to a port in the top of her hand. "It supposedly makes your back itch, so I have my back scratcher. See, look." She patted a bamboo back-scratcher by her side.

"So, everything went okay?"

"Perfect." Aunt Barb smiled. "I'm relieved to have it behind me. The doctor said I might not have to have radiation, but we'll see."

"I'm so happy for you," Judy said, meaning it, but she didn't feel happiness, strangely apart form her own emotions. Before, she and her aunt would have been giggling, laughing, and high-fiving. But that was Before, and this was After. "So you ready to go home today?"

"More than ready."

"When do you think you'll be discharged?" Judy asked, making small talk, filling the air with words to dispel the awkwardness.

"They said the doctor should be here in about an hour, then I have to fill out forms and such. Noon, I hope to be out."

"You sure you want to go back to your house?"

"Yes, thanks for the offer of your place, but I'll be more comfy at home, now that it's safe, thanks to you."

Judy's mother returned to the bed table and slipped a brown jug of Sunsweet prune juice in a bag. "We have everything planned. We'll take my car to your apartment, pack her bags, then get her home. Will you join us or do you have to work?"

"No, I have to work," Judy lied. She didn't know what she was going to do today, and nobody at the office would blame her for taking the day off.

"But you'll come out to the house tonight? Say hi? Have dinner?"

"If I can. We'll see."

"Good. I'll make a nice salmon with parsley. You know how you love that dish. Frank can come, too." Her mother wrapped the top of the plastic bag around the bottom, making a neat roll. "Aunt Barb will rest for the afternoon, then she has to do her range-of-motion and breathing exercises."

"Breathing?" Judy faked a smile. "In, out? In, out?"

"With that gadget, a spirometer." Her mother pointed at a transparent plastic tube by the side of the bed, with graduated numbers up the side and a blue plastic bottom. "You inhale and try to get the ball in the air. She has to do it every day, twice a day."

Aunt Barb patted the bed. "Judy, come sit down and tell us how last night went, with the FBI. I'm so curious about how it works, negotiating deals and such."

"It's very bureaucratic," Judy said, suddenly sick of the small talk, of avoiding the subject. She wished she had gone straight to work.

"I doubt that," Aunt Barb said, gently. "Is it like on TV?"

"Barb, of course it isn't." Her mother came over, setting down the bag. "I bet it is bureaucratic. All those government agencies are the same. Everything is political. Right, Judy?"

"I don't want to talk about that," Judy said, the words slipping out of their own accord. "I want to understand what happened with me and you two."

"Here?" Her mother's eyes flared. "Now?"

"Yes, here and now. Why not here and now?" Judy thought better of it when she spotted a pained look crease Aunt Barb's face. "I mean, forget it. You're right. This isn't the time or place, after the operation and all. That was selfish of me, I wasn't thinking."

"No, it's fine," Aunt Barb said firmly. "It is. We can talk about it right now."

"Please, forget it." Judy felt her face heat with shame. "You've just had a major operation. It's just that it's so fake to be together without talking about it, but we can't not be together, so we have to be fake. I'm . . . sorry, that was . . . wrong," she stammered, feeling her emotions rise to the surface, the anger and the love both at once. "It was so selfish."

"No, it's not. Please, Judy, sit down."

"No forget it. It's not fair to you, right now—"

"Yes, I want to talk. Really talk." Aunt Barb patted the bed again, for Judy to sit down. "I don't like pussyfooting around it, either. That's not how we are, or have ever been. There's an elephant in the room, as they say, and we need to deal with it. Sit. Please? I had a mastectomy, but my mouth works fine, believe me."

"Okay, then." Her mother came over, sinking into the heavy chair. "We'll talk."

Judy perched on the corner of the bed, distant from them both, shifting her attention from one woman to the other, the sisters' resemblance clear in the hue of their deep blue eyes, set far apart. Paradoxically, the difference between them could also be found in their eyes, but in the aspect to them; her mother's eyes were more guarded, her lids closed like a shield against some sudden brightness, while Aunt Barb's anguish showed clearly through her frank blue lenses.

"Honey," Aunt Barb said softly. "How can we help you understand this? I'll do anything, and I'll tell you anything."

"Tell me what happened, from your point of view. Because Mom already told me, I mean, my aunt." Judy swallowed hard, a bitter knot twisting in her chest. "I don't even know what to call you. Aunt? Mom? Aunt Mom?"

Aunt Barb cringed. "I know it's hard to process."

"I want to know what you were thinking." Judy modulated her voice, trying to stay calm. "Not just in the beginning, but all these years, keeping it from me. I mean, I trusted you. You lied to me, every time you saw me."

Aunt Barb nodded, pained. "You feel betrayed—"

"Absolutely, of course I do. How could I not?" Judy looked from Aunt Barb to her mother. "Years of Mother's Days, I'm giving cards and presents to someone not my mother? You did betray me, both of you. You've lied to me as long as I've been alive. I don't know who you are, and it makes me feel like I don't know who I am. I've always defined myself in relation to you, at least in the family. I thought I was Aunt Barb's niece and Delia's daughter, but it turns out it's the other way around."

"We screwed this up, royally," Aunt Barb said gently. "But believe me, we didn't mean to."

"We tried to do the right thing," Judy's mother added, pursing her lips.

"Well, you didn't," Judy shot back, trying to suppress her resentment. "The truth is the right thing. You could've told me the truth, sooner. Even if they made you lie when I was born, you could've told me the truth when I grew up, but you didn't. You avoided it. You put it off. You pretended. It was cowardly."

"I'm so sorry," Aunt Barb said, holding tears back. "I'm very sorry, I truly am. I regret that I didn't tell you sooner, and I should have. It wasn't until my diagnosis that I realized the cliché really was true, that life is short. I should have understood it after Steve died, but I was so preoccupied with his illness, I didn't think of myself. Somehow I thought *I* would never get sick. I was in denial. What are the odds, both of us, getting cancer so close together?" Aunt Barb ran a dry tongue over her lips. "But when I got diagnosed, I thought about putting my affairs in order, so if the worst happened, I didn't want to leave this earth without you hearing from me why everything happened the way it did."

"So tell me then."

"It's true, our parents did make us do it. I don't blame them, either, because they were only doing what they thought was right, too. I try not to judge them. I'm in no position to judge anybody."

Judy listened, trying to adjust mentally to the fact that she knew this woman who was talking, and didn't know her, both at the same time.

"We made this decision, and we carried it out, and your mother stepped in to help and—"

"She's not my mother. You're my mother. Can we please be honest, from here on out?"

"Okay, then let me say what I was going to say, something that even your mother can't say, which is that when you were born and our parents gave us this ultimatum, she was amazing." Aunt Barb gestured at Judy's mother, with an IV port attached. "She responded with grace and generosity. She was thrilled to take you and raise you. She gave me a gift, but above all, she gave *you* a gift."

Judy blinked, letting it sink in, because it rang true.

"Think about the position your mother was in. She had a young child at home, but she fell in love with this baby girl, an *infant*, and she took you in with open arms. She knew the entire time that someday we would tell you the truth and that you would react this way." Aunt Barb paused. "But I'm not talking about you yet, I'm talking about her. She had a sword of Damocles hanging over her head every day of her life, not knowing when this day would come, but knowing inevitably that it would. Can you imagine being in that position?"

Judy let it sink in. She had never seen her mother that way, because she couldn't have, but she understood now.

"Imagine opening your heart to let in a child that you know will be angry at you for the decision you made—when you did it with the best of intentions, to give that child a home? And can you understand her not wanting that day to come? For putting off telling you, as long as she could?"

Judy swallowed hard. She glanced at her mother, who kept her head down, rubbing her linked fingers together in her lap.

"Still think she was a coward? I don't. I think she was a human being. I think she was a woman, with a *heart*." Aunt Barb shook her head sadly. "So let's give your mother some credit, because she was your mother, she did raise you, and she didn't tell you the truth because she wanted things to stay the way they were. She's terrified to lose you."

"Mom, you won't lose me," Judy blurted out, though her mother didn't look up. "You could never lose me, either of you. I just feel angry—"

"Of course you do," Aunt Barb said quickly. "We have lived this way for this long, and you can call it a lie or a betrayal, and

I suppose you're right about that, but to me, what we call each other isn't the thing that matters. Even that I'm your birth mother, and your mother is the one who raised you, that doesn't matter either."

"How can you say that?" Judy asked, bewildered. "What matters then?"

"Judy, to me, those things are just on the surface. We're no different from a woman, or a girl, who puts up a child for adoption and is lucky enough to find that child welcomed with loving arms, by another woman. *Both* women are mothers." Aunt Barb's eyes flashed with new animation, and her tone strengthened. "The only difference here is that I was lucky enough to stay in your life, and if you think back, I've been in your life, for all of your life."

Judy thought back, to the events in her life. To college graduation, and law school. Aunt Barb had organized the luncheons afterward, with her mother. Judy remembered when she was a child, to Brownies, then to Girl Scouts. Aunt Barb had sold cookies in front of the supermarket with Judy. Aunt Barb had been the den mother, not her mother, and she had even chaperoned the field trips. Aunt Barb had woven herself into Judy's life, the two of them there for her, for as far back as Judy could remember.

"We shared you, in a way, you know. We sat down with your schedule for your various activities, your choir recitals and such, and even for your soccer games, home and away. Whatever you were doing, we did as many as we could together." Aunt Barb met her gaze directly. "There were times, too, when we actually took turns. Your mom was kind enough to step aside for some things, to let me have you all to myself."

"Like what?"

"I don't know. I don't remember."

"Like the aquarium?" Judy asked, the memory coming out

of the blue. She remembered that the aquarium trip had always been a sore spot with her, because her mother had simply said she was too busy to go, so Aunt Barb had gone instead. "Did you guys agree that you should be the chaperone, not mom?"

"What grade was that in? Remind me." Aunt Barb frowned in confusion. "It's my chemo brain again, or maybe that's an excuse. I remember the trip, but I don't remember the grade."

"Fifth," Judy answered, beginning to feel a new sympathy for her mother, whom she'd blamed whenever she wasn't there, sending Aunt Barb in her place.

"Yes, I remember now. She went to the zoo trip, because I took you to the aquarium. You loved the puffins. You wouldn't stop watching them."

"Yes."

Her mother looked up, with a sad smile. "You came home with the toy puffin. It's still in your room."

"Yes. You named him Mort."

"Right." The sadness left her mother's smile. "What a name."

"Besides I think he's a girl," Aunt Barb chimed in, with a chuckle.

Judy felt the knot in her chest loosen, relieved that all this time, her awkwardness with her mother wasn't her fault, and that nothing she could have done would have made it better. Somehow the lifting of the secret relieved the burden of guilt she'd felt every minute, until now.

Aunt Barb continued, "Judy, we both love you, like a mother. We have both spent our lives mothering you. I completely understand that you think of my sister as your mother, and I would never dream of asking you to change that, nor do I even want you to." Aunt Barb shook her head, her lips pursed with conviction. "Keep calling her your mother. She deserves that. She has earned that, in spades. And please keep calling me Aunt

Barb. I'm used to it, I don't want that to change. It's only super-ficial. It's form over substance. It's not what I want."

"What do you want then?" Judy's emotions welled up. She realized that Aunt Barb really was the unselfish person she'd always believed her to be.

"I want us to be honest and close, and take our new relation-ship as it comes, bit by bit. That's how I took the chemo, that's how I'm taking this mastectomy, and that's how I'll take the radiation, if I have to."

Judy felt her resentment melt away, and Aunt Barb continued talking.

"We will go forward, getting our test results over time, changing our treatments and protocols, our dosages and our meds, revisiting our prognosis. You have to take it as it comes. That's what I've learned, not from cancer, but from life." Aunt Barb faced Judy's mother, with a crooked smile. "We'll muddle through, the three of us. We'll fuss and bicker, but we'll be fine. Won't we, Delia?"

"We sure will," her mother answered warmly, reaching over and patting Aunt Barb's arm.

Judy watched them both, thinking back to last week, when she'd been sitting at a bridal salon, wishing that she were closer to her mother. In the end, it turned out that she really was close to her mother. She just hadn't known who her mother was, until now. It wasn't quite the ending she expected, but it was a happy one.

Her spirits lifted, and her heart filled with love. She had a feel-ing that from now on, things were going to be different. Even, better.

With both her mothers.

And the truth.

Chapter Forty-seven

Judy stepped off the elevator at work, and Mary, Allegra, and Marshall looked over from the reception desk, then burst into excited grins.

"Judy, thank God!" Mary shouted, rushing over with open arms, followed by Marshall and Allegra.

"Judy!" Allegra squealed, as the three of them swarmed Judy, scooping her up with girl hugs and happy noises.

"You guys are too much!" Judy joined them in laughter, disentangling herself from their joyful embrace, fragrant with fresh perfume and overpriced hair products.

Mary beamed. "You're amazing! Are you okay? I called your cell phone a million times!"

Allegra's eyes flared wide behind her glasses. "Who blew up your car? That's so scary! It's like a movie!"

"It's a long story," Judy told them, which was the understatement of the year.

"Judy." Marshall stepped forward with a flurry of phone messages. "Sorry to be a buzz kill, but you have some things to deal with right away. The press has been calling all morning, and I don't know who you want to respond to, if anybody."

"None of them." Judy took the phone messages without looking at them. There had been a slew of reporters in front of the office building, and she had no-commented her way past them.

Mary touched her arm. "Judy, there's one or two reporters you could talk to. You just made huge news. It wouldn't be the worst idea to promote yourself. Bennie would."

"Well, I wouldn't." Judy snorted. Her only remaining nub of resentment was for Bennie, because now it was time to face the damages cases. "Where is the boss, by the way?"

"At her trial. The jury's coming back."

"She better win or I'll fire her ass."

Everybody laughed, including Mary. "Girl, don't start. When the boss gets back from court, you should kiss and make up. Your stock is up right now and you need to parlay that sucker. Parlay, I tell you!"

"I'll get right on that." Judy looked over, seeing that Marshall had more to say, and it wasn't easy to get a word in edgewise in an all-female law firm. "Marshall, what is it?"

"There's good and bad news."

"Good news first," Judy said, her mood improving. Her heart felt lighter since the talk with her mother and aunt, and being back at the office with the girls felt like terra firma, solid under her clogs.

"You won in *Adler*. The judge denied the Rule 37 motion."

"Yay!" Judy cheered, and so did Mary and Allegra.

Marshall grinned. "The judge's order came in your email this morning, and I printed it. It's here with your mail." She handed Judy a thick packet of correspondence. "The judge really nailed Kelin, saying that he wasted the Court's time and acted like a basketball player, faking that he got fouled."

"Wonderful!" Judy thought ahead, anticipating her conversation with Linda Adler. Conversations with clients always went better when they started with victories, and Kelin would think harder about settling the case, now that his gambit had backfired.

"Here's the bad news. John Foxman called and said you need to call him right away. There's a problem with the money for your aunt. The message is on top."

"Thanks, Marshall," Judy said, concerned. She turned toward her office, but her cheering section followed, led by Mary.

"So fill me in." Mary fell into step beside Judy. "How did you get her the deal from the FBI?"

Allegra tagged along. "Judy, what happened to your mouth? Did somebody *hit* you?"

"Fill you guys in later, okay?" Judy's thoughts were elsewhere, wondering what was the matter with the money. Last night at the FBI, she had been so preoccupied with getting a deal for Daniella that she had left that as a loose end. "After I make this phone call, we can yap endlessly."

"Okay, honey," Mary said, falling behind. "Let me know if you need me."

Allegra called after her, "Did you hit him back? Did he have a gun?"

Judy hurried into her office, shed her coat and purse on the chair, and sorted through her phone messages. She found John Foxman's number, went around the desk, picked up the phone receiver, and plugged in the number, sitting down.

"Foxman here," he answered, after one ring.

"John, this is Judy—"

"Judy!" John said, his tone concerned. "I can't believe what I'm reading about you. You're busting drug rings in Chester County now? I called your cell phone a few times, but there was no answer. I hope you weren't injured."

"I'm fine," Judy answered, touched. "And thanks for the flowers you sent my aunt. That was so thoughtful."

"Are you okay? Was this connected to your aunt's money?"

"Yes, but is there a problem with the money? Is that why you called?"

"Not a problem with the money, *per se*. Believe it or not, my firm is closing, going out of business. They just told us, so I'm calling my clients. This is my last day."

"*What?*" Judy asked, incredulous. "Eastman and Respondi is *closing*? That's not possible."

"I hear you, but it's happening. It just became public. It's pretty grim around here. Everybody's in shock. I feel sorry for the staff."

"How? Why?" Judy couldn't get over the news. "You have, like, three hundred associates and partners. It's one of the biggest firms in Philadelphia."

"So was Wolf, Block. Remember them?"

"What happened? Can you say? Do you know?"

"Between us, the firm expanded too fast. We opened offices where we didn't need them and we acquired too much overhead." John *tsk-tsk*ed. "I saw it coming. I've had my résumé out for six months, but so far, not a nibble."

"You're out of a job?" Judy's heart went out to him. "But you're so able. You edited the Law Review."

"Which guarantees nothing, in this economy." John chuckled, without mirth. "If you hear that anybody needs an associate, think of me. I don't only do trusts and estates, I can do any kind of general litigation. I feel weird asking you, but the truth is, I need a job. I'll send you a résumé and my new contact information, if you don't mind."

"Not at all, please send it. Any firm would be lucky to have you."

"Thanks." John's tone changed, back to business. "Anyway, since the firm is closing, I have to make some changes to the paperwork for your aunt's account, immediately. It doesn't alter the account, but because my firm's name is on the papers, we'll have to redo and refile them. Can you come over to sign the new papers, sooner rather than later? They're ready whenever you are."

"Sure," Judy answered, but she was starting to get an idea. "Did you say you do general litigation?"

"Yes. I was a trial lawyer for five years, at Thomas, Main and Henderson."

"That's a litigation firm. You must've gone to court a lot."

"All the time, for all kinds of civil cases, both defense and plaintiff's side. It's really my forte. Eastman needed me in trusts and estates, so I played ball, but I'm itching to get back in the courtroom."

Judy thought fast. "I know of a job you might be interested in. It's not that great, but you'd be in court every day."

"Fine with me. Where's the job?"

Judy took a flyer. "Here at Rosato, working for me."

John burst into surprised laughter. "Are you serious?"

"Absolutely!" Judy said, feeling a flush of satisfaction. The more she thought about the idea, the more she liked it, which we all know was something that happened with her. If John took the job, she could avoid trying the damages cases herself, get a superb trial lawyer on board, and keep the legal work for the firm. It didn't hurt that he was superhot, and her very next thought violated federal sexual harassment law.

"Really? You want me to come work for you?"

"Why not?" Judy stopped herself, out of fairness to him. "But I don't want to misrepresent anything. I need somebody to try seventy-five cases that I'm hating on, asbestos work referred to me by a New York firm. Damages cases."

"Ugh."

"I know. Would you consider it?"

"You know what, I'll do more than consider it. What's it pay?"

"We can negotiate that, when I come sign the papers."

"Ha!" John chuckled. "Watch out, I'm a great negotiator."

"Not better than I am, dude. You just told me I'm the only buyer."

"Ouch!" John burst into new laughter. "I was bluffing!"

"The hell you were!" Judy told him, smiling. "Get ready for me to lowball you."

"We'll see about that. When are you coming over?"

"Right now. I'll be there in fifteen."

"See you." John chuckled again. "Bring your calculator."

"Very funny. Bye now." Judy smiled as she hung up, popped up from her seat, grabbed her bag and coat from the chair, and hurried out of her office.

She hustled down the hall to the reception area, toward what sounded like a happy commotion. She turned the corner to see Mary, Allegra, and Marshall clustered excitedly around Bennie and Anne, who must've just gotten back from trial. She gathered that they had won, because everybody was beaming, and trial exhibits and boxy trial bags had been abandoned around the reception room.

Judy made a beeline for the happy group, in high spirits herself. "Congratulations, Bennie and Anne!" she called to them, and everybody looked over, flush with victory.

"Thanks, Carrier!" Bennie grinned. "Meanwhile, way to go! You hit *another* one out of the park! There are so many reporters outside, and they're all asking about you!"

Next to her, Anne smiled her dazzling smile. "Judy, what happened to you this weekend? When do I get to hear this story?"

"Hold that thought." Judy crossed to the elevator. "I have an errand to run that will take half an hour, then we can go out to lunch and celebrate, on me."

Mary grinned. "I'm in!"

Anne nodded. "Me, too!"

Allegra hopped up and down. "Me, three!" she said, because she was still young.

Only Bennie looked at Judy like she was crazy. "Carrier, it's too early for lunch. Also, where are you going? Why aren't you setting up a press conference? What errand can be so important?"

Judy hit the button to call the elevator cab. "Actually, I'm off to hire somebody to work the damages cases, from Bendaflex."

"Oh." Bennie lifted her eyebrows, intrigued. "Don't you want to run the candidate by me?"

"No, thanks. You told me I could hire anybody I wanted, and I did."

"Right." Bennie blinked. "So who'd you hire?"

"An experienced litigator I know just freed up, and I hopped on it."

"Great. What's her name?"

"John Foxman."

Everybody froze for a moment, falling silent. *Ping,* went the elevator, signaling the arrival of the cab.

"Carrier, did I hear you right?" Bennie asked, in disbelief. "We're an all-woman law firm, and you hired a *man*?"

"Yep." Judy stepped into the elevator, pressed the DOWN button, and hoped the doors closed fast.

"How's *that* going to work?" Bennie's eyes flew open, an incredulous blue.

"I don't know." Judy shrugged, just as the elevator doors began to slide closed. "But we're going to find out, aren't we?"

Acknowledgments

It's important to understand at the outset that this is a novel, a work of fiction. In other words, though Chester County, Pennsylvania, exists, as does the town of Kennett Square, I made up all of the events and people in the book. Now to the thank-yous, where I thank all of those experts and kind souls who helped me with *Betrayed,* and I make clear that any and all mistakes herein are mine.

Thank you to Deputy Coroner Patricia Emmons of the Chester County Coroner's Office, who helped me so much with the forensics and procedural questions in the novel. I won't say more or I'll give away some spoilers.

Thank you very much to Police Chief Edward Zunnino of Kennett Square, who patiently explained the police procedures in that lovely town. Thanks to the ladies at the front desk, who staff his office with such diligence and kindness.

Thanks to Jim Angelucci, an expert in mushroom growing for some forty years and a pioneer in the business in Chester County, as well as one of the most upstanding members of the grower community. Jim took me on a super-informative tour of the Phillips Mushroom Farm, owned by the wonderful Phillips family, and it's one of the finest in the county. It should go without saying that the independent grower herein is completely fictional. Thanks, too, to Jim for taking me on a tour of the Laurel Valley Farms, the composting cooperative, and for introducing me to Glenn Cote, its general manager, who answered even more questions for me. Finally, an excellent work on mushroom growing in Chester County is Bruce Mowday's *Chester County Mushroom Farming* (2008).

Special thanks to Father Depner of the St. Rocco Church in Avondale who welcomed me into his wonderful church and selflessly provided so much information to inform the book.

Thanks to Rebecca Zerr, a brilliant and wonderful young woman who took so much time to answer all of my questions about the undocumented in Chester County. She referred me to some excellent works on the subject: *Between Two Worlds* (1996) by David Gutiérrez, *The World of Mexican Migrants* (2008) by Judith Hellman, and *Beyond Borders* (2011) by Timothy Henderson. Kudos to Drs. Victor Garcia and Laura Gonzales, who have done excellent research and written so much about the undocumented workers in Chester County.

A special thanks to my friends in the breast cancer community, who helped me with this book. One was Kathy Robbins, and she was so very helpful in detailing her own fight with this disease, as well as her inspiring recovery. Thank you so much, Kathy! I also read so many thoughtful and moving blogs and memoirs, especially Barbara Delinsky's *Uplift*.

I'm a lawyer, but criminal law wasn't my field. My first lawyerly thank-you, as always, goes to a brilliant and dedicated public servant, Chief Deputy District Attorney Nicholas Casenta, Esq., of the Chester County District Attorney's Office. Nick heads the Appeals Unit and was just named Prosecutor of the Year. Nick has helped me with every novel so far, and I appreciate so much his advice and expertise. I'm lucky to have you, Nick!

Thanks to my friend and laser-sharp litigator Joe Hetrick,

Esq., who dropped everything to help me understand the intricacies of damages in mass tort litigation, as well as the economics of a modern law firm practice. Thanks, Joe!

Thanks to Stephanie Kalogredis, Esq., for in-the-clutch trust-and-estates advice. Thanks to Colleen Connor and Sharon Scanlon, two great friends with generous hearts.

Now to my publishing family! A huge thank-you to my amazing editor and dear friend Jennifer Enderlin, who improved this manuscript so much with her expertise and great heart. And big love and thanks to the brilliant, fun gang at St. Martin's Press, starting with the terrific John Sargent, Sally Richardson, Matthew Shear, Matt Baldacci, Jeanne-Marie Hudson, Brian Heller, Jeff Capshew, Nancy Trypuc, Kim Ludlam, John Murphy, John Karle, Dori Weintraub, Stephanie Davis, Paul Hochman, Caitlin Darieff, and all the wonderful sales reps. Big thanks to Rob Grom for an astounding cover design. Also hugs and kisses to Mary Beth Roche, Laura Wilson, Esther Bochner, Brant Janeway, and the great people in audiobooks. I love and appreciate all of you.

Thanks and love to my incredible agent, Molly Friedrich, who has guided me for so long now, and to the amazing Lucy Carson and Nichole LeFebvre.

Thanks and another big hug to my dedicated assistant and friend Laura Leonard. She's invaluable in every way, and has been for over twenty years. Thanks, too, to my friend and assistant Nan Daley, who helped so much with research for this book, as well as for making girl field trips with me! This novel is dedicated to Laura and Nan because it wouldn't have been possible without them.

And to George Davidson, for doing everything else, so that I can be free to write.

Thank you very much to my adorable and brilliant daughter, Francesca, a wonderful writer in her own right, for her love, support, and great humor.

And to my family, for everything.

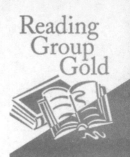

BETRAYED

by Lisa Scottoline

Behind the Novel

- Character Q&A

Keep on Reading

- Ideas for Book Groups
- Reading Group Questions

Special Extra!

- An excerpt from the next Rosato
  & DiNunzio novel, *Corrupted*

Also available as an audiobook
from Macmillan Audio

For more reading group suggestions
visit www.readinggroupgold.com.

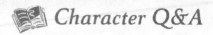

Lisa started her career writing about the beloved characters of Rosato & Associates, now Rosato & DiNunzio. The law firm has been through its share of tough times, difficult cases, and even major changes (can a male lawyer really survive at Rosato?), but they have had equal amounts of laughter, joy, and fun. Throughout the series, you have come to see who Mary, Bennie, Judy, and Anne are as lawyers, citizens, friends, and family members. We thought it would be fun to learn some of the smaller fun facts about the ladies, answered by Lisa, their creator. Many of these are the kind of questions Lisa gets asked all the time in interviews, and a few others, just because.

What is your favorite color?

Mary: Tomato-sauce red

Bennie: True Blue

Judy: Adores all colors.

Anne: "Whatever's trending."

What is your favorite food?

Mary: You need to ask? Pasta.

Bennie: "Opposing counsel."

Judy: "Don't panic, it's organic."

Anne: Air

Who's your favorite Tony?

Mary: Her dad

Bennie: She wishes they would leave her conference room.

Judy: Pigeon Tony

Anne: She is unaware they are three separate people, but they all have crushes on her.

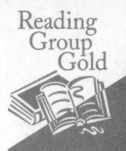

*Which is the better cheesesteak in Philadelphia—
Geno's or Pat's?*

Mary: Pat's

Bennie: Geno's

Judy: (She is a vegetarian, of course.)

Anne: (Doesn't eat red meat.)

Who's your celebrity crush?

Mary: Bradley Cooper

Bennie: Bradley Cooper

Judy: Bradley Cooper

Anne: Bradley Cooper

What's your favorite activity?

Mary: Overcoming insecurity

Bennie: Winning cases

Judy: Painting

Anne: Shopping

What is your must-have item in your purse?

Mary: Mace

Bennie: "My business card."

Judy: "My library card."

Anne: Blotting papers

What is your favorite movie?

Mary: *The Godfather*

Bennie: "I don't have time for movies."

Judy: *Pollock*

Anne: *Notting Hill*

If you were not a lawyer, what would you be?

Mary: A nun

Bennie: A judge

Judy: "I'd work in animal rescue."

Anne: A reconstructive plastic surgeon

Who's your favorite recording artist?

Mary: Taylor Swift

Bennie: The Rolling Stones

Judy: Joni Mitchell

Anne: Beyoncé

What's your **Real Housewives** *tagline?*

Mary: Family is everything, with a side of spaghetti.

Bennie: What are the *Housewives*?

Judy: I don't need a designer label to know who I am.

Anne: Don't hate me because I'm beautiful. Hate me because I won the case.

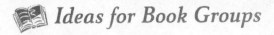

Ideas for Book Groups

I am a huge fan of book clubs because it means people are reading and discussing books. Mix that with wine and carbs, and you can't keep me away. I'm deeply grateful to all who read me, and especially honored when my book is chosen by a book club. I wanted an opportunity to say thank you to those who read me, which gave me the idea of a contest. Every year I hold a book club contest and the winning book club gets a visit from me and a night of fabulous food and good wine. To enter is easy: all you have to do is take a picture of your entire book club with each member holding a copy of my newest hardcover and send it to me by mail or e-mail. No book club is too small or too big. Don't belong to a book club? Start one. Just grab a loved one, a neighbor or friend, and send in your picture of you each holding my newest book. I look forward to coming to your town and wining and dining your group. For more details, just go to **www.scottoline.com**.

Tour time is my favorite time of year because I get to break out my fancy clothes and meet with interesting and fun readers around the country. The rest of the year I am a homebody, writing every day, but thrilled to be able to connect with readers through e-mail. I read all my e-mail, and answer as much as I can. So, drop me a line about books, families, pets, love, or whatever is on your mind at **lisa@scottoline.com**. For my latest book and tour information, special promotions, and updates you can sign up at **www.scottoline.com** for my newsletter.

Lisa Scottoline

*Keep on
Reading*

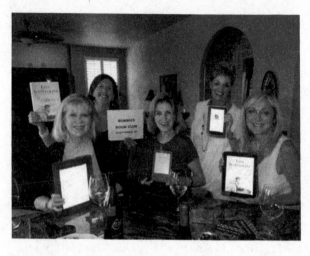

The Bunnies Book Club of Scottsdale, Arizona, submit their photo for Lisa's bookclub contest.

Reading Group Questions

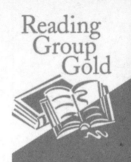

1. Judy and Mary are best friends, but they are very different. For instance, Judy is more able to take risks and roll with the punches than Mary, who likes to plan, process, and is generally more timid. Are you a Judy or Mary? Do you take risks easily or do you avoid them? As you get older, do you take more risks, or less?

2. In *Betrayed*, Judy investigates a death she believes is a murder, and she does this because she cares about justice. Justice is at the heart of so many of Lisa's books because she believes that she has a powerful "justice bone"—a strong urge to see that the right thing happens, and even to make things right, when others do not. Do you have a "justice bone?" Have you ever spoken up, when others would not? What was the result?

3. Judy and her mother vary on their opinions of illegal immigrants, although they both learn a lot about the issue throughout the course of the novel. In writing *Betrayed*, Lisa did extensive research on the topic, and learned a lot herself. Do you identify more with Judy or her mother? What did you learn about illegal immigration that you did not previously know? After reading the book did your opinion change at all? If so, how?

4. Judy and Mary would likely disagree on some of their views of illegal immigrations as well. How do you and your best friend handle situations in which you disagree? Do you avoid topics such as politics, religion, or other hot-button issues, or do you enjoy discussing them with someone you are close with? What is the most significant thing that you and your best friend disagree about?

Keep on Reading

5. Harvesting mushrooms is not a pleasant or an easy job, and one that many would not be willing to do. Would you be willing to do it? What are the limits of what you'd be willing to do for work? What job do you wish you had?

6. Many industries are supported by illegal workers, and doing so has become an "open secret" that is often ignored by the government and law enforcement. Why do you think this holds true? If you were in political office, what changes would you suggest in dealing with this important issue?

7. Having spent so much time with Mary's warm, loving family, Judy comes to the realization that her family felt connected by the activities they did together, whereas Mary's operated on a more emotional level. What kind of connection does your family have? What are your favorite family memories? What is one thing you would change about your family?

8. Lisa often explores, researches, and writes about issues that are relevant to women, and in *Betrayed*, she tackles the extremely important topic of breast cancer. What are some other women's issues that you would like to see Lisa write about? What do you think is the most important issue facing women today? In what ways can women be more supportive of other women?

9. The idea of the traditional family is blurred in *Betrayed*. For a variety of reasons, sometimes we need to create family, and we find it through friendships, communities, or churches. Besides your blood family, who in your life do you consider family?

10. In the novel, Judy feels like she "blew her lead."
    She feels left behind as her best friend makes
    partner, and is getting married. Do you think it
    is possible to be happy for someone else, even
    though you might be jealous at the same time?
    If Mary wasn't getting married, do you think Judy
    would still have felt discontent in her relationship?
    When you feel jealous, does it motivate you to
    work harder for what you want, or does it bring
    you down? In what ways do you think Judy
    and Mary's relationship will change when Mary
    gets married?

*Keep on
Reading*

Turn the page for a sneak peek at
Lisa Scottoline's next novel

CORRUPTED

Available October 2015

Chapter One

Bennie Rosato hadn't taken a murder case in ages, but she'd have to take this one. She'd been working late when the phone rang, with a call she'd been dreading twelve years. It came from a time she didn't want to remember and a place she didn't want to revisit, but she couldn't turn it down. She was a woman of her word.

She'd grabbed her coat, purse, and messenger bag, then hurried out of the office and in no time was sitting in the back of a grimy cab, her thoughts churning. She'd told Jason he should call if he got into trouble and she fully expected he'd get into trouble—or that trouble would get into him. Still she wouldn't have suspected him of murder. Nevertheless, she owed him. She couldn't give his case to an associate. Nobody paid her debts but her.

Traffic stalled and Bennie was too antsy to wait, so when the cab lurched onto Seventh Street, she bailed and decided to walk, despite the ungodly cold, twenty-one degrees in the dead of January and the sky frozen black except for a full moon, round as a bullet hole. She lowered her head, hoisted her bags higher on her shoulder, and powered her way toward the Philadelphia

Police Headquarters, north of the United States Courthouse and the Federal Detention Center, near the tangled ramps to I-95 and the Schuylkill Expressway.

The heels of her boots clacked on the concrete, gritty with salt from the last snow. The sidewalk was empty at midnight, since there were no shops or restaurants around. The only foot traffic was the homeless, rattling cans of coins between the lanes of cars stopped at a red light, heading to the Expressway on-ramp. None of the drivers would lower their windows on a night this cold, or they would use the weather as an excuse. Either way, Bennie didn't judge.

She clutched her quilted coat around her neck, wishing she still had her scarf. Grown women weren't supposed to lose things, but she did, all the time. Her breath made a steamy cloud around her face, and she spotted the incongruously beautiful façade of the local NPR affiliate across the street. It was a sleek modern box that sported a story-high light installation, a glowing screen of powdery pink, pale melon, and robin's-egg blue that washed the grimy city block in pastel watercolors. Not even a fake rainbow could brighten up this section of town.

She passed the bowed cyclone fence that surrounded the police headquarters and took a left turn into its parking lot. There was no pedestrian walkway, and she stopped to let a blue-and-white cruiser exit, spewing a chalky plume of exhaust. She caught a glimpse of a laptop screen glowing inside the car, but it was too dark to see the cops. There was a time she might've recognized them, she was down here so much. But that was then, and this was better.

Bennie crossed behind the cruiser, thinking back to when she'd met Jason. Rosato & Associates had been a boutique law firm, but since then had boomed to a nationally prominent firm, successful enough to promote an associate, thereby becoming Rosato & DiNunzio. Bennie was proud that she'd grown the firm, but lately she was getting a nagging feeling that she'd lost something. Complete control, for one thing, was a thing of the past. Business was booming, but she had no time for her beloved rowing. Plus she hadn't had a date since she and Grady broke up. She thought she was dead below the waist, but for fact that her legs were so dry they itched all winter.

She crossed the vast parking lot, which extended the width of the city block through to Eighth Street. Whitish streaks of salt streaked the asphalt, and the lot seemed more empty than usual. Philly's homicide rate dropped by as much as 20 percent in the winter, murderers being as lazy as everybody else, but that didn't explain the emptiness of the lot. The police were always busier at night, which explained the Homicide Unit's secret sweatshirts which read, Our Day Begins When Yours Ends.

Bennie glanced at the lineup of pool cars used by the detectives, which were parked in designated spaces against the back fence. There were fewer than ever, and the battered Crown Victoria's had been replaced by battered Tauruses. She had read that the force had been reduced, along with other municipal services, funding being a constant struggle in a declining city budget. She kept walking past the parking spaces reserved for the press, but they were vacant, too. In the old days, reporters would have been double-parked, but the newspapers had gone through bankruptcy, cutting back police coverage. Even the scanner had migrated online, so anybody with a laptop could play journalist. Not that Bennie had anything against bloggers. She hated all reporters equally.

She beelined for the building, called the Roundhouse owing to its shape, which was two massive circular sections stuck together like an old-school barbell. The design was certifiably innovative in the '60s, but its precast concrete walls cracked and crumbled, and its windows were three floors of narrow smoked glass, set lengthwise like a prison. Fluorescent lighting from within showed that slatted blinds were broken or missing in almost every window. Bennie was no architecture critic, but something was awry when the not-for-profit NPR had more money to spend on a building than the local constabulary. Maybe the police needed a Suze Orman marathon or Viewers Like You.

PHILADELPHIA POLICE DEPARTMENT, read dark metal letters whose metallic finish had dripped onto the concrete façade, and Bennie looked up at the fourth floor, which held the Homicide Unit. Philadelphia had about three hundred murders a year, and all of the cases were sent here, to the Unit's forty-odd detectives, roughly twelve men to a tour, or shift, deployed in three platoons, A, B, and C. The cases were distributed in a straightforward manner; a detective was stationed at the front desk of the squad room at every tour, and he was called the Up Guy. Whoever was the Up Guy got the case and when he went out on the job, another detective took his place as Up Guy.

HONOR INTEGRITY SERVICE, read a sign with more drippy metal letters, hung on the concrete wall next to a Port-a-John, an overflowing trash can, newspaper boxes, and a mailbox. Bennie opened a single front door of smudged glass and let herself into a hallway paneled with lacquered knotty pine. Mounted on the paneling was a massive wooden shield of the PPD, next to a defunct pay phone, and she walked up to a window of bullet-proof glass. A young uniformed officer came to meet her, wearing a blue shirt, a white Under Armour turtleneck, and the telltale thickness of a Kevlar vest.

"Can I help you, miss?"

Bennie liked him immediately, as she was in her forties and couldn't remember the last time anybody had called her "miss." "I have a client up in Homicide. His name is Jason Leftavick, but I don't know which detective's on the case. First name's Mike, that's all I got."

"Hold on a sec, let me see who caught it." The officer stepped away from the window, consulted an old computer for a moment, then returned. "You want to see Detective Gallagher. He'll meet you upstairs at the Unit. Go to the door on your left. I'll need to see ID, inside."

"Sure, thanks." Bennie waited for the door to buzz, then let herself into the massive round lobby. Its curved wall was covered with the same knotty-pine paneling, and along the perimeter stood tall glass cases that held police uniforms from every decade during the 1900s, like a grade-school display of The Policeman Is Your Friend. Bennie produced her ID, signed the logbook, went through the metal detector, and crossed the empty lobby to the grimy elevator, which she took to the fourth floor.

She took a right and walked along the curved corridor. The wall was covered with the same paneling, and halfway down the hallway stood a set of tall gray lockers and grimy file cabinets. The overhead lights flickered and the floor tile was gray with filth. She passed a bathroom with an open door and a leaking faucet. Running overhead were multicolored wires bundled together, and exposed plumbing wrapped with duct tape. It was as if basic maintenance hadn't been done in years, and Bennie never would've believed that if she hadn't seen it herself.

HOMICIDE, read an old plaque ahead, and the hallway ended in a closed wooden door with a dark window of reinforced glass and a keypad by the knob. She remembered the door used to be propped open all day by a trash can, but a new sign read, SECURITY DOOR, PLEASE ENSURE THAT LOCK HAS ENGAGED UPON ENTRY AND EXIT AT ALL TIMES. She knocked, then waited, facing her own reflection in the window. Her hair was a tangle of long blonde curls twisted into a topknot by a ponytail holder, and she tried to smooth it in place. She wore only light makeup and hadn't bothered to refresh it, so her blue eyes would have to go unlined and her high cheekbones unblushed. She suspected the world-as-we-know-it would not end.

Bennie was fully six feet tall, blessed with a naturally athletic build, a commanding presence that came in handy in a courtroom, but less so on a date. She fell into the Handsome Woman category, though in the window she could see crows' feet deepening around her eyes and laugh lines bracketing her lips, which used to be fuller. She shrugged it off. She didn't earn a living on her looks, so it didn't kill her to lose them, and she had more important things to worry about, like Jason.

The door was opened by a well-built, bald detective with brown eyes, conventionally handsome features, and a ruddy complexion. He looked about her age, but was even taller, maybe six-three, and he flashed a friendly, if professional, smile as he extended a large hand. "You must be Bennie Rosato. I'm Mike Gallagher, good to meet you."

"You too, Detective." Bennie shook his hand, stepping inside. He had on a white shirt with a dark green sweater, khaki slacks, and loafers, and he smelled of a tangy aftershave, a scent memory that took her back. Detectives always dressed well, which she found fitting; a Homicide Unit was no place for casual dress, because murder was the least casual of crimes.

She entered a waiting area only eight feet wide, lined with rubbery black benches. An old-fashioned gumball machine stood between the two benches, but dominating the room were the two large bulletin boards on the walls. WANTED FOR MURDER, CASH REWARD WILL BE PAID FOR INFORMATION LEADING TO ARREST, read a sign above each board, then underneath were thirty-odd photographs of men and women of all races and colors. Each face showed burning eyes and a defiant, yet empty, gaze, though a few were grinning crazily. Bennie didn't know which scared her more.

"Call me Mike, I've heard a lot about you. I know you were a buddy of Azzic's and he spoke well of you. Said you always made him do his job. He moved to Florida, headed for warmer climes. We miss him around here."

"I bet." Bennie felt too antsy for small talk. "So do you think I can see my client?"

"Sure, no problem. Follow me." Detective Gallagher led her past the memorial wall of plaques honoring detectives who had fallen in the line of duty, then into the squad room, which was mostly empty, but utterly run-down. The only remotely modern appliance was a medium-size flat screen television in the back of the room, but otherwise, the Up Guy was on an ancient black phone in front of two old computer monitors, on a battered desk. Ancient gray carrels lined the far wall in front of the windows with the broken slats. The walls were a scuffed light blue, and the drop ceiling a grimy white, with more bundled wiring. The gray tile floor was dirty, and crammed everywhere were random stacks of in-and-out boxes and mismatched file cabinets.

"The squad room's the same, I see." Bennie followed him past the cabinets, which were covered with taped notices about courtroom numbers, Phillies tickets, computer training for the forensics lab, together with bumper stickers for the Phillies and the Eagles, and one that read, YOU BOOKIN'?

"Still a dump, right? They're talking about moving us uptown. God knows when that'll happen." Detective Gallagher stopped in front of the closed door to interview room A. There was a large barrel lock on the outside of the door, and he slid it aside. "Here we go."

"Thanks."

"Take as long as you like, then come find me. My desk is the first one on the right." Detective Gallagher gestured to a connecting room behind him.

"Did you videotape your interview with him?"

"No, the machine is broken. You'll see it dangling over the door in the corner."

"You know, those videotapes are good for us, but they're even better protection for you."

Detective Gallagher snorted. "Tell me about it."

"How about the audio?"

"We gave up on audio recordings a long time ago. They never worked. It sounded like everybody was underwater. The D.A. told us he couldn't use them." Detective Gallagher permitted himself a slight smile, then nodded at the closed door to the interview room. "A word of warning. It's not pretty in there."

"The room? Why am I not surprised?"

"No, your client. And don't blame us, we didn't do it."

"What you mean?" Bennie asked, concerned.

She got her answer after she opened the door.

> "**Scottoline writes riveting thrillers that keep me up all night, with plots that twist and turn.**"
> —HARLAN COBEN

Step into the all-female law firm of Rosato & DiNunzio. . . .

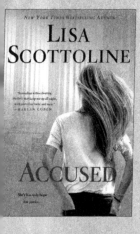 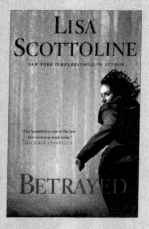 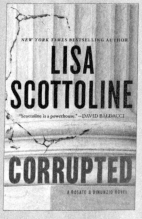

Scottoline is at her best writing the Rosato & Associates stories and this latest is one of her best."

—THE HUFFINGTON POST

"One of the very best writers today."
—MICHAEL CONNELLY

"So many plot twists, the pages seem to turn themselves."
—PEOPLE

St. Martin's Press
St. Martin's Griffin

No one does
EMOTIONAL, POWERFUL, HEARTBREAKING,
or HONEST like *New York Times* bestselling author

LISA SCOTTOLINE

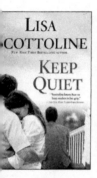
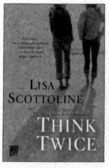
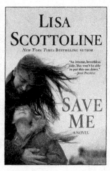
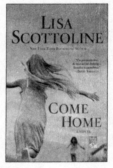

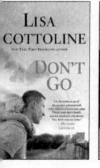
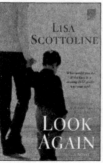
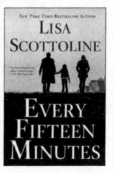

NINE MONTHS

Available
in Hardcover
April 2016

"Lisa and Francesca, mother and daughter, bring you the laughter of their lives."

—Delia Ephron, bestselling author of *Sister Mother Husband Dog*

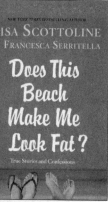

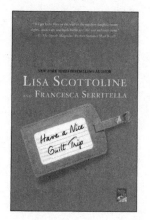

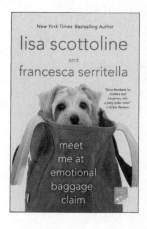

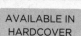

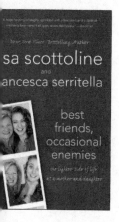

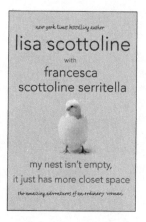

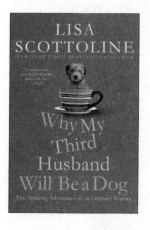

St. Martin's Press

St. Martin's Griffin